Respiratory Disease Series: Diagnostic Tools and Disease Managements

Series Editors

Hiroyuki Nakamura, Ibaraki Medical Center, Tokyo Medical University, Ibaraki, Ibaraki, Japan
Kazutetsu Aoshiba, Ibaraki Medical Center, Tokyo Medical University, Ibaraki, Ibaraki, Japan

This book series cover a variety of topics in respiratory diseases, with each volume providing an overview of the current state of knowledge, recent discoveries and future prospects for each disease. In each chapter the editors pose critical questions, which are often unresolved clinical issues. These are then discussed by the authors, providing insights and suggestions as to which developments need to be addressed. The series offers new information, which will inspire innovative ideas to further develop respiratory medicine.This collection of monographs is aimed at benefiting patients across the globe suffering from respiratory disease.

Edited by established authorities in the field and written by pioneering experts, this book series will be valuable to those researchers and physicians working in respiratory medicine. The series is aimed at a broad readership, and the books will also be a valuable resource for radiologists, emergency medicine physicians, pathologists, pharmacologists and basic research scientists.

Hiroyuki Nagase • Hisatoshi Sugiura
Toshihiro Shirai
Editors

Asthma-COPD Overlap

Updated Concept, Pathophysiology, Diagnosis and Treatment

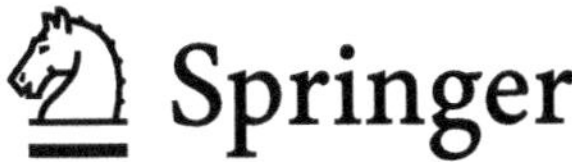

Editors
Hiroyuki Nagase
Division of Respiratory Medicine and Allergology
Teikyo University School of Medicine
Tokyo, Japan

Hisatoshi Sugiura
Department of Respiratory Medicine
Tohoku University Graduate School of Medicine
Sendai, Japan

Toshihiro Shirai
Department of Respiratory Medicine
Shizuoka General Hospital
Shizuoka, Japan

ISSN 2509-5552 ISSN 2509-5560 (electronic)
Respiratory Disease Series: Diagnostic Tools and Disease Managements
ISBN 978-981-96-0219-3 ISBN 978-981-96-0217-9 (eBook)
https://doi.org/10.1007/978-981-96-0217-9

This Springer imprint is published by the registered company Springer Nature Singapore Pte Ltd.
The registered company address is: 152 Beach Road, #21-01/04 Gateway East, Singapore 189721, Singapore

Preface

Asthma and chronic obstructive pulmonary disease (COPD) are two of the most prevalent and challenging respiratory diseases worldwide. For years, clinicians have recognized that some patients exhibit features of both conditions, leading to the identification of a distinct clinical entity known as asthma-COPD overlap (ACO). Despite its significance, ACO has been a topic of intense debate and ongoing research. While the 2020 update of the Global Initiative for Chronic Obstructive Lung Disease (GOLD) recommended focusing on blood eosinophil counts for directing COPD treatment and suggested moving away from the ACO label, there remain compelling reasons to maintain this classification in clinical practice.

First, epidemiological studies have consistently shown that a significant percentage of patients with asthma or COPD exhibit characteristics of both diseases. These patients often require different treatment strategies than those with COPD alone. Moreover, ACO has been linked to unique genetic and epigenetic backgrounds, distinct biomarkers, and specific metabolomic profiles. Importantly, patients with ACO generally experience more severe symptoms, faster lung function decline, and a lower quality of life compared to those with COPD alone, underscoring the need for precise diagnosis and targeted treatment.

Despite the importance of ACO, the lack of a uniform definition and diagnostic criteria has hindered a shared understanding of the condition. Recognizing this, the Japanese Respiratory Society (JRS) published "The JRS Guidelines for the Management of ACO" in December 2017, providing a standardized approach to its identification and management. This guideline was further updated in 2023 to reflect the latest research and clinical insights.

In this book, leading experts in the field offer a comprehensive review of ACO, tracing the evolution of the concept and exploring whether a treatable traits approach can be practically applied. This book covers the epidemiology, pathophysiology, diagnostic criteria, and treatment options for ACO, incorporating the latest data and studies. Controversies surrounding the prognosis of ACO, novel molecular mechanisms such as nitrosative stress, and advanced imaging or physiological techniques like high-resolution computed tomography (HRCT) and forced oscillation are thoroughly examined. Additionally, the book presents the latest animal models of ACO, offering valuable insights into its underlying mechanisms.

Clinical aspects, including the role of biomarkers and the evidence for various treatment options, are discussed in detail. While large-scale studies have often excluded patients with ACO, recent trials involving ICS/LAMA/LABA combination inhalers and biologics offer new hope for effective treatment strategies.

This book aims to be a comprehensive resource on ACO, beneficial not only to residents but also to clinicians, supervisors, and basic researchers. We hope that the insights provided here will enhance understanding and lead to improved patient care.

Tokyo, Japan Hiroyuki Nagase
Sendai, Japan Hisatoshi Sugiura
Shizuoka, Japan Toshihiro Shirai

Contents

Part I
Concept of Asthma COPD Overlap

Chapter 1
Concept of Asthma COPD Overlap: Japanese Guideline and Global Trends—How Was the Concept of Asthma COPD Overlap Developed and Moving Forward?

Mitsuhiro Yamada and Masakazu Ichinose

Abstract Bronchial asthma and chronic obstructive pulmonary disease (COPD) are two of the most frequent respiratory diseases. These two are independent diseases that differ in their pathogenesis and treatment. However, because both diseases often occur in a patient, partly due to the increased incidence of each, and because patients with both diseases may have different medical conditions from those with COPD or asthma alone, the combined condition has been attracting attention from physicians. In light of this situation, the term asthma-COPD overlap (ACO) was introduced by international committees to describe patients with both conditions. However, although many clinical studies on ACO had been published since then, there was no unified definition or diagnostic criteria, which has been a barrier to a true understanding of this condition. Therefore, to provide a uniform definition and diagnostic criteria, the Japanese Respiratory Society published "The JRS Guidelines for the Management of ACO" in December 2017. In this chapter, we will outline the concept of ACO, focusing on the Japanese guidelines, and discuss the future approach to ACO, including developments in other countries, including the international committees.

Keywords ACO · Asthma · COPD · Type 2 airway inflammation · FeNO

M. Yamada
Department of Respiratory Medicine, Tohoku University Graduate School of Medicine, Sendai, Miyagi, Japan

M. Ichinose (✉)
Academic Center of Osaki Citizen Hospital, Osaki, Miyagi, Japan
e-mail: ichinose@h-osaki.jp

H. Nagase et al. (eds.), *Asthma-COPD Overlap*, Respiratory Disease Series: Diagnostic Tools and Disease Managements,
https://doi.org/10.1007/978-981-96-0217-9_1

1 Introduction

Bronchial asthma (hereinafter, asthma) and COPD are two of the most frequent respiratory diseases encountered in clinical settings [1, 2]. These two diseases are independent diseases that differ in their pathogenesis and treatment [3, 4]. In recognizing the difference between asthma and COPD, it is easy to contrast young, non-smoking asthma patients with older COPD patients with a history of heavy smoking. However, in clinical practice, it is true that there are significant numbers of patients who have the characteristics of both asthma and COPD, such as those who are elderly, have a history of heavy smoking, and have variable symptoms characteristic of asthma. Given this situation, the term asthma-COPD overlap (ACO) was introduced by international committees to describe the patients with both conditions [5]. This international document advocates checking symptoms and variability of airflow limitation for COPD and asthma, respectively, and performing the diagnosis of persistent airflow limitation by spirometry for the diagnosis of ACO. On the other hand, the criteria for diagnosis of ACO by round table discussion by Sin et al. [6] are three major criteria: (1) persistent airflow limitation by spirometry, (2) a history of smoking (or air pollution exposure) for more than 10 years, and (3) a history of asthma diagnosis at the age of 40 years or younger (or reversibility of more than 400 mL in FEV_1), and three minor criteria; (1) concomitant atopy or allergic rhinitis, (2) reversibility of >200 mL in FEV_1, and (3) peripheral blood eosinophilia (>300/μl). They recommend that patients who meet all three major criteria and at least one minor criterion be considered for the diagnosis of ACO. This definition by Sin et al. is an ingenious way to find out the characteristics of COPD and asthma and to diagnose ACO, but its shortcoming is that there are few objective indicators. For the criteria to be used widely around the world, it is necessary to make the diagnosis useful in regions with different medical conditions, which is considered unavoidable.

However, for more accurate diagnosis, CT and lung diffusion testing, which are closely related to the destruction of alveolar walls, are useful for the diagnosis of COPD, and measurement of exhaled nitric oxide concentration (FeNO), which correlates well with type 2 airway inflammation, is considered to be a promising diagnostic tool for asthma. Considering the state of medical care in Japan, blood sampling, CT, and FeNO measurement are sufficiently available at general medical institutions, which enable ACO diagnosis with more accurate definitions in Japan. Therefore, because it was thought necessary to present a unified view to facilitate discussions concerning the condition of ACO in Japan, The JRS Guidelines for the Management of ACO was established in December 2017 [7, 8]. In this chapter, the concept of ACO will be outlined along with the concepts of asthma and COPD, which are the underlying diseases. The future approach to ACO will be discussed, including progress in other countries, including international committees.

2 Asthma

In the guidelines by the Japanese Society of Allergology, asthma is characterized by chronic airway inflammation, which clinically manifests as variable airway narrowing (wheezes and dyspnea) and cough [9, 10]. On the other hand, the international guidelines state, "Asthma is a heterogeneous disease, usually characterized by chronic airway inflammation. It is defined by the history of respiratory symptoms such as wheeze, shortness of breath, chest tightness and cough that vary over time and in intensity, together with variable expiratory airflow" [1]. Both guidelines state that asthma results from chronic inflammation of the airways and that variable airway narrowing and clinical symptoms are characteristic of the disease.

Asthma is a heterogeneous inflammatory disease that affects the large and small airways rather than the lung parenchyma [11]. Airway inflammation includes inflammatory cells such as eosinophils, neutrophils, lymphocytes such as type 2 helper cells and type 2 innate lymphoid cells (ILC2), and mast cells, as well as airway component cells such as airway epithelial cells, fibroblasts and airway smooth muscle cells, type 2 cytokines such as interleukin (IL)-4, IL-13 and IL-5, and epithelial-derived cytokines such as IL-33; thymic stromal lymphopoietin (TSLP) and IL-25, are involved [11–13]. Airway narrowing, which is spontaneous or reversible with treatment, is due to airway inflammation and airway hyperresponsiveness. Persistent airway inflammation induces airway injury and subsequent changes in the airway structure (remodeling) that induce irreversible airflow limitation, resulting in severe asthma characterized by irreversible airflow limitation and persistent airway hyperresponsiveness [1, 7, 9].

Asthma includes a cluster of clinical and pathophysiological features due to different pathophysiological processes [11]. For example, atopic asthma, non-atopic asthma, elderly asthma, aspirin-exacerbated respiratory disease (AERD), late-onset asthma, and obesity-associated asthma have been analyzed as representative clusters. This heterogeneity may be explained by the complexity of dysregulation of innate and adaptive inflammatory responses to exogenous allergens and proteases, leading to a spectrum of abnormal tissue remodeling [12]. Type 2 cytokines such as interleukin (IL)-4, IL-13, and IL-5 primarily promote airway eosinophil infiltration, mucus hypersecretion, bronchial hyperreactivity, and mast cell activation. A major subpopulation of asthmatic patients has the molecular features of airway inflammation elicited by type 2 cytokines, so-called type 2 airway inflammation, and responds markedly to inhaled corticosteroids (ICS) [14]. Accumulating evidence from randomized controlled trials, as well as this translational study, highlights the importance of ICS use from the early stages of asthma treatment, as clinical studies have shown that ICS robustly reduce the risk of asthma symptoms, exacerbations, hospitalization, and death [15–17].

Asthma is diagnosed comprehensively by the time course of respiratory symptoms and the results of respiratory function tests [1, 9, 10]. However, as mentioned earlier, asthma includes a wide variety of pathologies (phenotypes), making it difficult to develop clear diagnostic criteria. For this reason, no clear diagnostic criteria have been presented in the Japanese or international guidelines [1, 9, 10]. The Japanese guidelines suggest that diagnosis should be based on the following criteria: (1) recurrent cough (tends to appear at night and early in the morning), (2) fluctuating and reversible airflow limitation, (3) increased airway hyperresponsiveness, (4) the presence of airway inflammation, (5) predisposition to atopy, and (6) exclusion of other diseases [9, 10]. In addition, although algorithms for asthma diagnosis have been proposed in Japanese and international guidelines [1, 10], they have not been established based on evidence. Therefore, although the diagnosis could be evaluated based on drug response if treatment must be prioritized, it is important to reevaluate during the course of the disease.

3 COPD

In the Japanese guidelines, COPD is defined as "a pulmonary disease caused by prolonged inhalation of toxic substances, mainly tobacco smoke, and respiratory function tests show airflow obstruction. Airflow obstruction is caused by a combination of peripheral airway lesions and emphysematous lesions in various proportions. Clinically, the disease presents with slowly progressive dyspnea on exertion and chronic cough and sore throat, but these symptoms may be absent." [18]. On the other hand, the International Committee GOLD definition is "chronic obstructive pulmonary disease (COPD) is a common, preventable, and treatable disease that is characterized by persistent respiratory symptoms and airflow limitation that is due to airway and/or alveolar abnormalities usually caused by significant exposure to noxious particles or gases and influenced by host factors including abnormal lung development. Significant comorbidities may have an impact on morbidity and mortality" [2]. Both definitions describe the etiology and pathogenesis, but the international guidelines first emphasize that COPD is a universal, preventable, and treatable disease.

Tobacco smoke is thought to be the cause of most chronic obstructive pulmonary disease in Japan [19]. Tobacco smoke consists of gaseous and particulate components, each of which can cause inflammation in the airways. The particulate component consists mainly of oil (tar) particles with a diameter of less than 1 μm, which are mainly deposited around the respiratory bronchial region. In smokers, inflammatory cells infiltrate the area without exception [20], which is assumed to be the initial lesion of COPD [21]. In some smokers, such inflammation develops into emphysematous lesions in the periphery by destroying alveoli and airway lesions in the center by expanding inflammation in the airway wall, leading to COPD. The speed of development of these lesions is slow, with a time-lapse of several decades.

However, because nicotine in tobacco is an addictive drug, when smoking begins, the lesions progress without subjective symptoms due to prolonged exposure to tobacco smoke. The progression of emphysematous lesions is irreversible once it occurs. The only known way to prevent or slow the progression of the disease is to not smoke and to stop smoking [22].

The frequency of progression from early lesions to COPD is estimated to be 15–20% among smokers, but in fact, the proportion is even higher in the elderly [2, 18]. Endogenous risk factors for COPD include a genetic background that is sensitive to tobacco smoke [23]. Because no single gene has been identified to explain this, it is expected to involve a complex set of unknown or known candidate genes [24–28]. The presence or absence of this putative genetic susceptibility to tobacco is thought to be a major determinant of whether or not the disease progresses from early lesions to COPD. Smoking susceptibility may also be affected by abnormal lung growth [29].

Unlike asthma, $CD4^+$ T helper 1 (Th1) cells, $CD8^+$ cytotoxic T (Tc) cells, neutrophils, and macrophages primarily affect the small airways and lung parenchyma, causing mucus hypersecretion, alveolar wall destruction (emphysema), and small airway fibrosis in COPD [30, 31]. Both emphysematous lesions and airway lesions in COPD contribute to obstructive disorders. The development of both types of lesions is reflected in a decrease in FEV_1 and FEV_1/FVC on respiratory function tests and manifests itself as slowly progressive dyspnea (shortness of breath). Restricted airflow causes progressive gas trapping in the peripheral lungs during exhalation during exercise, leading to dynamic hyperinflation, which is postulated to be the primary mechanism of exertional dyspnea [32, 33]. Therefore, bronchodilators, such as long-acting muscarinic antagonists (LAMAs) and long-acting beta2 agonists (LABAs), are commonly used as pharmacological therapies for COPD and have been found to reduce pulmonary hyperinflation, dyspnea, and exercise intolerance [34, 35], leading to improved quality of life and reduced frequency of exacerbations [36]. Accumulating evidence shows that LAMAs significantly reduce the frequency of exacerbations and non-serious adverse events and increase the trough forced expiratory volume in FEV_1 compared to LABAs in patients with stable COPD [37].

Decreased physical activity in COPD causes systemic disuse changes, including skeletal muscle, as well as impairing the activities of daily living (ADL) and quality of life (QOL) [38]. In addition, systemic inflammation is generally present, and there are various comorbidities such as cardiovascular disease, hypertension, arteriosclerosis, skeletal muscle dysfunction, osteoporosis, gastrointestinal disorders, depression, and anxiety [39]. The origin of systemic inflammation is unknown. There are two theories about the origin of systemic inflammation: one originates from local inflammation of the lungs [39], and the other originates from inflammation caused by inactivity of the body [40]. However, since physical activity is anti-inflammatory [41], improving and maintaining physical activity is therapeutically important.

4 The Concept of ACO and Its Definition

4.1 The Concept and Definition of ACO in Japanese Guideline

Asthma and COPD are two of the most frequently encountered respiratory diseases [1, 2]. Both have common clinical symptoms such as cough, wheezing, and dyspnea, and both are characterized by chronic airway inflammation and airway remodeling that are deeply involved in their pathogenesis. However, asthma is characterized by eosinophilic airway inflammation, whereas COPD is characterized by neutrophilic airway inflammation, and the anatomical locations of the lesions are different [42]. Furthermore, pathophysiologically, asthma is mainly characterized by type 2 airway inflammation, including type 2 helper T cells (Th2 cells), type 2 innate immune lymphocytes (ILC2), eosinophils, and type 2 cytokines. In contrast, the inflammation induced in COPD is dominated by non-type 2 airway inflammation in which neutrophils, macrophages, cytotoxic T cells, and type 1 helper T cells (Th1 cells) are involved [30, 31]. In recognizing the difference between asthma and COPD, it is easy to contrast young, non-smoking asthma patients with older COPD patients with a history of heavy smoking. However, in clinical practice, it is true that there are significant numbers of patients who have both the characteristics of asthma and COPD, such as those who are elderly, have a history of heavy smoking, and have variable symptoms characteristic of asthma. In view of this situation, the Global Initiative for Asthma (GINA), an international committee to discuss asthma, and GOLD, an international committee to discuss COPD, jointly proposed the Asthma COPD Overlap Syndrome (ACOS) [5].

After this proposal, it was discussed that the term "syndrome" has been used to describe a common condition with no known cause, while "asthma" and "COPD" are diseases with diverse clinical features and pathogenesis caused by various mechanisms. Since it was determined that the term "syndrome" was inappropriate for these reasons, the term "Asthma COPD Overlap (ACO)" was proposed by GINA2017 to replace the term "ACOS."

The pathogenesis of ACO has been widely considered even before GINA and GOLD proposed "ACOS", including overlap syndrome of asthma and COPD [43], mixed asthma-COPD phenotype [44], asthma combined with COPD [45], the coexistence of asthma and COPD [46] and COPD with asthmatic features [47]. When considering the pathogenesis of ACO, it is also important to note that each disease is a risk factor for the development of the other. One of the characteristics of patients with asthma, airway hyperresponsiveness, is a risk factor for the development of COPD. In addition, it has been reported that lung growth is inferior in asthmatics compared to normal subjects, and since lung growth failure is also a risk factor for COPD [29], asthmatics are more prone to COPD than other groups. On the other hand, COPD patients are prone to airway collapse due to a decrease in lung elastic contraction pressure caused by emphysematous changes in the lungs. In other words, a symptom of asthma (paroxysmal airway narrowing) is likely to become apparent in COPD patients, even in cases of very mild asthma with only coughing symptoms that would normally pass unnoticed as asthma.

Although there have been many studies and publications on ACO (or similar conditions) in Japan and elsewhere, the frequency of ACO has been inconsistent, ranging from a few percent to more than 50%, due to the absence of uniform definitions and diagnostic criteria and differences in the population composition studied. In addition, there were no fixed diagnostic criteria. Various clinical indicators such as age, smoking history, allergic history (atopy or allergic rhinitis), symptoms (subjective or objective), diagnosis of asthma (physician's diagnosis or patient's report), FEV_1/FVC after bronchodilator inhalation, airway reversibility test and its reference value, sputum eosinophil count, blood eosinophil count, blood eosinophil ratio, serum IgE level, exhaled nitric oxide concentration (FeNO), and lung diffusing capacity test, had been used with various combinations for such studies.

However, as has been the case in the past, it is not possible to proceed with the discussion of ACO without a unified definition and diagnostic criteria. For example, it is not possible to discuss whether ACO is really an overlap between asthma and COPD, or whether it is a different disease concept from asthma and COPD. Therefore, it was thought necessary to present a unified view to start a discussion on the condition of ACO in Japan. The JRS Guidelines for the Management of ACO" was published in December 2017 [8].

The JRS Guidelines define ACO as "a disease that shows chronic airflow obstruction and has characteristics of both asthma and COPD. The guidelines also provide a conceptual diagram of ACO (Fig. 1.1) and point out that ACO can have a variety of phenotypes, as the underlying asthma and COPD have a variety of phenotypes (Fig. 1.2). Based on the above definition of ACO, the JRS Guidelines present the diagnostic criteria for ACO to check for the presence or absence of features of COPD and asthma in patients over 40 years of age with chronic airflow obstruction with a bronchodilator post-inhalation FEV_1/FVC of less than 70%, and the specific diagnostic procedures (Fig. 1.3). They suggest that the characteristics of asthma may vary with the course of the disease compared to those of COPD, and that it is important to follow up on the presence or absence of asthma characteristics if asthma characteristics cannot be determined when diagnosing ACO. In addition, since symptoms such as cough, sputum, and shortness of breath tend to be underestimated in middle-aged and elderly patients, the guidelines recommend that imaging and functional tests should be performed as much as possible in patients with a history of smoking, which is a risk factor for diseases such as ACO. In addition, tests such as CT, lung diffusing capacity, and FeNO measurement should be performed actively according to the situation in each medical area.

Recently, a prospective, multicenter, observational cohort study has been conducted to investigate patients who meet the JRS ACO diagnostic criteria among COPD patients in clinical practice [7]. The first analysis of this ongoing study of ACO in Japan reported that, at registration, of 708 COPD patients analyzed, 312 (44.1%) were lacking the data for ACO diagnosis to be conducted, suggesting that some of the examinations required for the diagnosis of ACO are not routine in clinical practice. Of the 396 patients with the necessary data for diagnosis, 101 (25.5%) met the JRS diagnostic criteria for ACO and 295 (74.5%) were non-ACO.

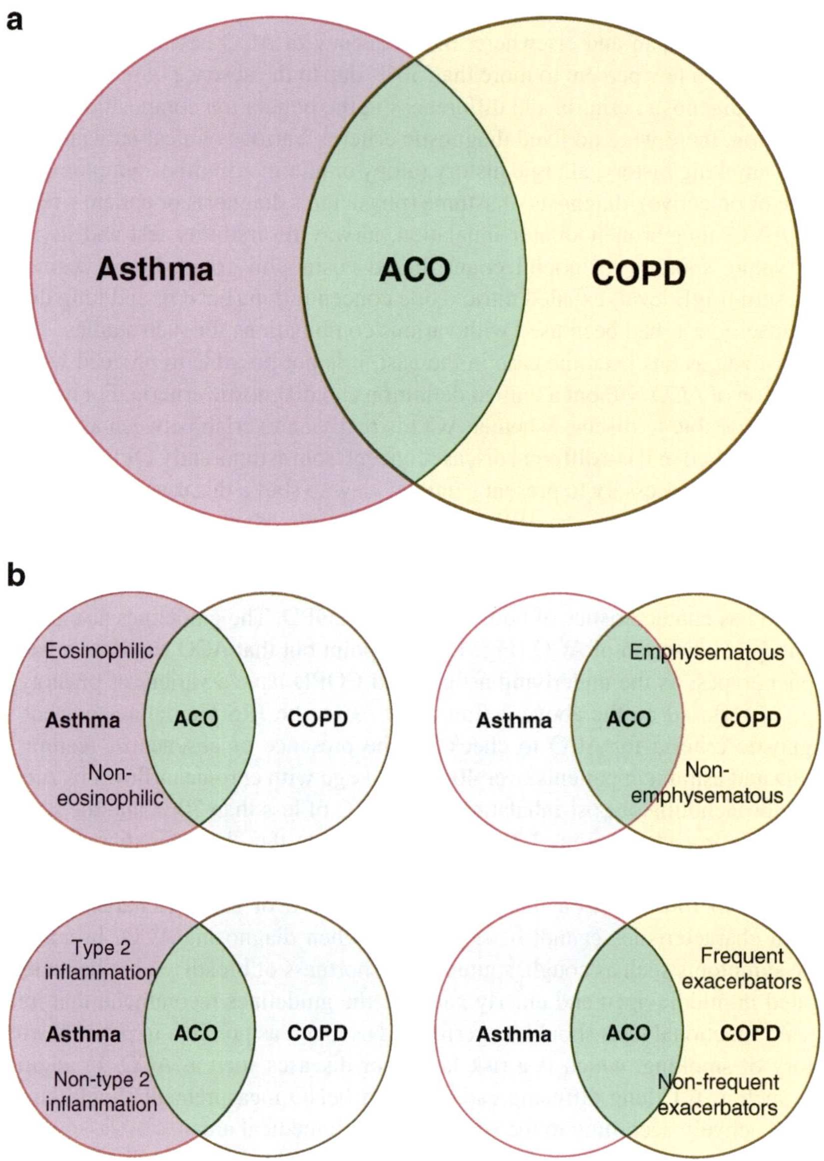

Fig. 1.1 (**a**) Concept of ACO. (**b**) Heterogeneity of ACO due to heterogeneity of asthma and COPD

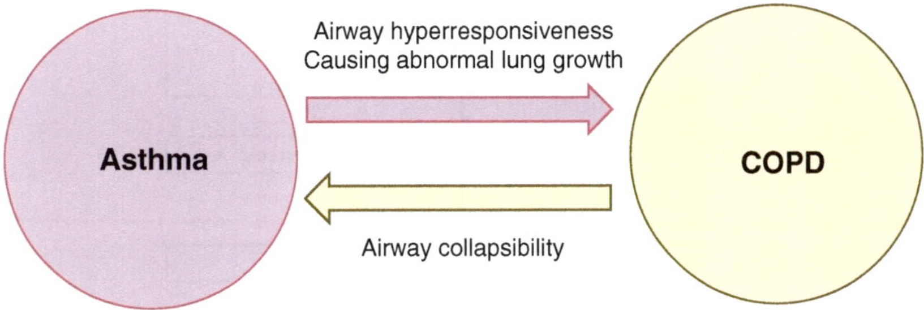

Fig. 1.2 Both of asthma and COPD can become a risk factor for the other disease

4.2 The Global Trend of the Concept for ACO

We also would like to outline the recognition of ACOs in national and international guidelines in chronological order. In 2007, the Canadian COPD guidelines recognized that some patients with COPD may have an asthma component and may require different treatments, especially the early introduction of ICS [48]. Three years later, in 2010, the Japanese COPD guidelines included a chapter on "COPD complicated by asthma," recommending the early introduction of ICS for such patients [49]. These two guidelines did not provide a precise definition of the overlap between COPD and asthma but indicated that some patients may have comorbid features of both diseases, which may affect their treatment. The first national guideline that introduced the term ACO was the Spanish COPD guidelines in 2012, and this document provided the first consensus-based definition of ACO [50].

Critical to the acceptance of ACOs by the medical community was the publication of a joint GINA-GOLD document in 2014, as mentioned earlier. This document provided a list of features that identify COPD or asthma and proposed that an equal number of features of both diseases coexisting in an individual patient should be diagnosed as ACO [5].

However, following the release of the GINA-GOLD joint statement on ACOs in 2014, subsequent updates to the GOLD document did not explicitly include the concept of ACOs in their recommendations for management. Furthermore, the 2020 GOLD update explicitly states that ACOs will no longer be mentioned [51]. This update emphasizes that asthma and COPD are different diseases, although they share some common features and clinical characteristics (e.g., eosinophilia, some degree of reversibility). It further states that asthma and COPD may coexist in individual patients, and if asthma is suspected in a COPD patient, pharmacotherapy should primarily follow the asthma guidelines. Still, pharmacological and non-pharmacological approaches to the COPD portion of the disease may be necessary. However, GOLD recommends using the blood eosinophil count to direct treatment with ICS for COPD.

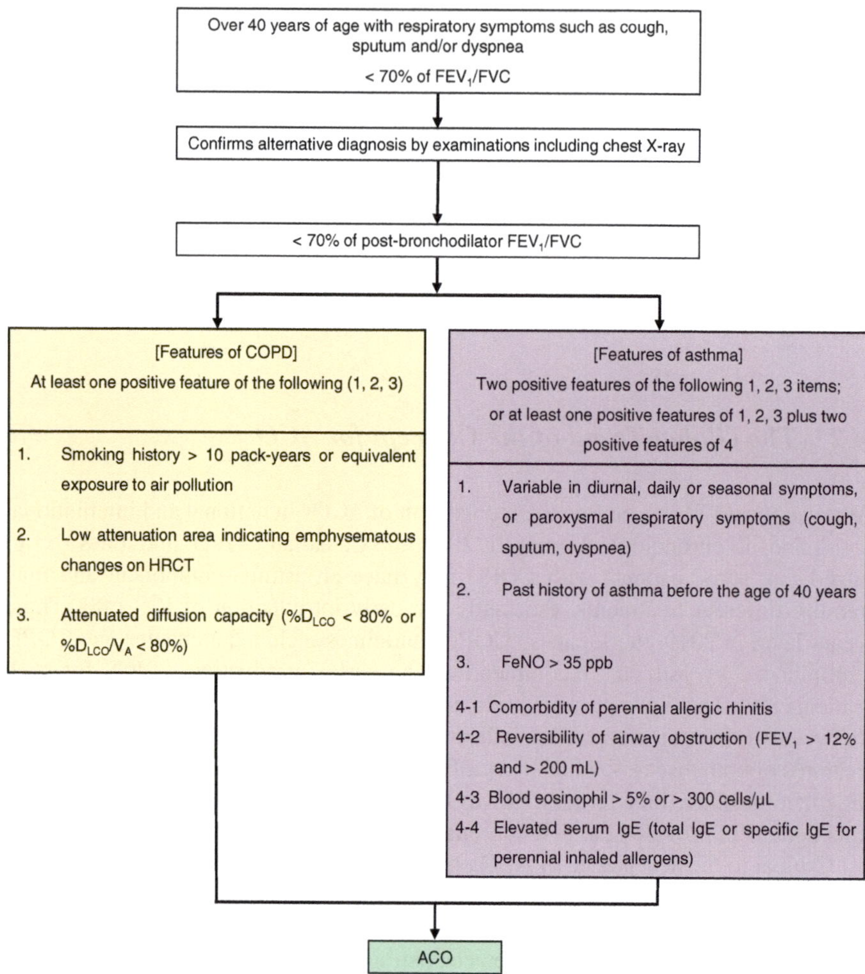

Fig. 1.3 Diagnostic algorithm for ACO in clinical practice. (1) To be diagnosed as ACO, one item of the characteristics of COPD plus two items from 1, 2, and 3 or one item from 1, 2, and 3 and at least two items from criterion 4 of the characteristics of asthma are needed. (2) If the characteristics of COPD alone are present, it is diagnosed as COPD, and if the characteristics of asthma alone are present, it is diagnosed as asthma (with remodeling). (3) If the characteristics of asthma cannot be confirmed when diagnosing ACO, it is important to monitor for the presence of the characteristics of asthma over time. (4) Perennial inhalant antigens include house dust, mites, molds, scales from animals, and feathers, and seasonal inhalant antigens include pollen from trees, plants, and weeds. Note 1. Diseases of differential diagnosis (diffuse panbronchiolitis, congenital sinobronchial syndrome, obstructive panbronchiolitis, bronchiectasis, pulmonary tuberculosis, pneumoconiosis, lymphangioleiomyomatosis, congestive heart failure, interstitial lung disease, and lung cancer) should be ruled out by standard chest x-rays, etc. Note 2. Respiratory symptoms such as cough, sputum, and dyspnea are variable (diurnally, daily, and seasonally) or paroxysmal in asthma and chronic and continuous in COPD. *COPD* chronic obstructive pulmonary disease, *FEV1* forced expiratory volume in one second, *FeNO* fractional exhaled nitric oxide, *FVC* forced vital capacity, *IgE* immunoglobulin E, *DLCO* diffusing capacity of the lung carbon monoxide, *VA* alveolar volume

On the other hand, GINA continues to refer to ACO or "asthma plus COPD" in its latest version of the guidelines as a simple description for patients with the features of both asthma and COPD, emphasizing that these terms do not refer to a single disease entity [1]. Rather, they state that these terms encompass patients with several clinical phenotypes that may be caused by a variety of underlying mechanisms.

Based on an overview of current global trends, it appears that the blood eosinophil count can distinguish eosinophilic COPD phenotypes that may benefit from ICS, while leaving the concept of ACO for patients who simultaneously meet the diagnostic criteria for asthma and COPD, regardless of blood eosinophil count [1–4, 9, 10].

5 Conclusion

In this section, we have outlined the concept and definition of ACO, including international trends. Although there is some lack of agreement on ACO, especially in terms of its pathophysiological significance, we believe that most clinicians and researchers generally agree that appropriate recognition and diagnosis of patients with ACO that do not fit the traditional definition of COPD or asthma is necessary to improve the symptoms and long-term prognosis of ACO patients. It is hoped that basic and clinical research will be continued in the future to further understand the pathogenesis of ACO so that the presence of airflow obstruction and uncontrolled type 2 inflammation in ACO patients can be properly recognized and individualized interventions can improve the prognosis.

References

1. Global Initiative for Asthma (GINA). Global strategy for asthma management and prevention 2021. https://ginasthma.org/wp-content/uploads/2021/05/GINA-Main-Report-2021-V2-WMS.pdf. Accessed 12 Feb 2022.
2. Global Initiative for Chronic Obstructive Lung Disease (GOLD). Global strategy for diagnosis, management and prevention of COPD (2022 Report). https://goldcopd.org/wp-content/uploads/2021/12/GOLD-REPORT-2022-v1.1-22Nov2021_WMV.pdf. Accessed 12 Feb 2022.
3. Fujino N, Sugiura H. ACO (asthma-COPD overlap) is independent from COPD, a case in favor: a systematic review. Diagnostics (Basel). 2021;11(5) https://doi.org/10.3390/diagnostics11050859.
4. Mekov E, Nunez A, Sin DD, Ichinose M, Rhee CK, Maselli DJ, et al. Update on asthma-COPD overlap (ACO): a narrative review. Int J Chron Obstruct Pulmon Dis. 2021;16:1783–99. https://doi.org/10.2147/COPD.S312560.
5. Global Initiative for Asthma (GINA) and Global Initiative for Chronic Obstructive Lung Disease (GOLD). Diagnosis of diseases of chronic airflow limitation: asthma, COPD and Asthma-COPD Overlap Syndrome (ACOS) updated 2015. https://goldcopd.org/wp-content/uploads/2016/04/GOLD_ACOS_2015.pdf. Accessed 12 Feb 2022.

6. Sin DD, Miravitlles M, Mannino DM, Soriano JB, Price D, Celli BR, et al. What is asthma-COPD overlap syndrome? Towards a consensus definition from a round table discussion. Eur Respir J. 2016;48(3):664–73. https://doi.org/10.1183/13993003.00436-2016.
7. Hashimoto S, Sorimachi R, Jinnai T, Ichinose M. Asthma and chronic obstructive pulmonary disease overlap according to the Japanese Respiratory Society diagnostic criteria: the prospective, observational ACO Japan cohort study. Adv Ther. 2021;38(2):1168–84. https://doi.org/10.1007/s12325-020-01573-x.
8. The Japanese Respiratory Society. The JRS guidelines for the management of ACO 2018 (in Japanese). Tokyo: Medical Review; 2017.
9. Nakamura Y, Tamaoki J, Nagase H, Yamaguchi M, Horiguchi T, Hozawa S, et al. Japanese guidelines for adult asthma 2020. Allergol Int. 2020;69(4):519–48. https://doi.org/10.1016/j.alit.2020.08.001.
10. The Japanese Society of allergology. Asthma prevention and management guidelines 2021 (in Japanese). Tokyo: Kyowa Kikaku; 2021.
11. Wenzel SE. Asthma phenotypes: the evolution from clinical to molecular approaches. Nat Med. 2012;18(5):716–25.
12. Lambrecht BN, Hammad H, Fahy JV. The cytokines of asthma. Immunity. 2019;50(4):975–91.
13. Lambrecht BN, Hammad H. The immunology of asthma. Nat Immunol. 2015;16(1):45–56. https://doi.org/10.1038/ni.3049.
14. Woodruff PG, Modrek B, Choy DF, Jia G, Abbas AR, Ellwanger A, et al. T-helper type 2–driven inflammation defines major subphenotypes of asthma. Am J Respir Crit Care Med. 2009;180(5):388–95.
15. Barnes PJ, O'Byrn PM, Rodrigues-Rolsin R. Low dose inhaled budesonide and formoterol in mild persistent asthma. The OPTIMA randomised trial. Am J Respir Crit Care Med. 2001;164:1392–7.
16. Pauwels RA, Pedersen S, Busse WW, Tan WC, Chen Y-Z, Ohlsson SV, et al. Early intervention with budesonide in mild persistent asthma: a randomised, double-blind trial. Lancet. 2003;361(9363):1071–6.
17. Suissa S, Ernst P, Benayoun S, Baltzan M, Cai B. Low-dose inhaled corticosteroids and the prevention of death from asthma. N Engl J Med. 2000;343(5):332–6.
18. The Japanese Respiratory Society. The JRS guidelines for the management of chronic obstructive pulmonary disease 2022 (in Japanese). Tokyo: Medical Review; 2022.
19. Fukuchi Y, Nishimura M, Ichinose M, Adachi M, Nagai A, Kuriyama T, et al. COPD in Japan: the Nippon COPD Epidemiology study. Respirology. 2004;9(4):458–65. https://doi.org/10.1111/j.1440-1843.2004.00637.x.
20. Fraig MM, Shreesha U, Savici D, Katzenstein ALA. Respiratory bronchiolitis: a clinicopathologic study in current smokers, ex-smokers, and never-smokers. Am J Surg Pathol. 2002;26:647–53.
21. Cosio MG, Hale KA, Niewoehner DE, Markert M. Morphologic and morphometric effects of prolonged cigarette smoking on the small airways. Am Rev Respir Dis. 1980;122(2):265–71. https://doi.org/10.1164/arrd.1980.122.2.265.
22. Anthonisen NR, Connett JE, Murray RP. Smoking and lung function of lung health study participants after 11 years. Am J Respir Crit Care Med. 2002;166(5):675–9. https://doi.org/10.1164/rccm.2112096.
23. Ragland MF, Benway CJ, Lutz SM, Bowler RP, Hecker J, Hokanson JE, et al. Genetic advances in COPD: insights from COPDGene. Am J Respir Crit Care Med. 2019; https://doi.org/10.1164/rccm.201808-1455SO.
24. Shrine N, Guyatt AL, Erzurumluoglu AM, Jackson VE, Hobbs BD, Melbourne CA, et al. New genetic signals for lung function highlight pathways and chronic obstructive pulmonary disease associations across multiple ancestries. Nat Genet. 2019;51(3):481–93. https://doi.org/10.1038/s41588-018-0321-7.
25. Sakornsakolpat P, Prokopenko D, Lamontagne M, Reeve NF, Guyatt AL, Jackson VE, et al. Genetic landscape of chronic obstructive pulmonary disease identifies heterogeneous cell-type and phenotype associations. Nat Genet. 2019;51(3):494–505. https://doi.org/10.1038/s41588-018-0342-2.

26. Oelsner EC, Ortega VE, Smith BM, Nguyen JN, Manichaikul AW, Hoffman EA, et al. A genetic risk score associated with chronic obstructive pulmonary disease susceptibility and lung structure on computed tomography. Am J Respir Crit Care Med. 2019;200(6):721–31. https://doi.org/10.1164/rccm.201812-2355OC.
27. Hobbs BD, de Jong K, Lamontagne M, Bosse Y, Shrine N, Artigas MS, et al. Genetic loci associated with chronic obstructive pulmonary disease overlap with loci for lung function and pulmonary fibrosis. Nat Genet. 2017;49(3):426–32. https://doi.org/10.1038/ng.3752.
28. Yamada M, Motoike IN, Kojima K, Fuse N, Hozawa A, Kuriyama S, et al. Genetic loci for lung function in Japanese adults with adjustment for exhaled nitric oxide levels as airway inflammation indicator. Commun Biol. 2021;4(1):1288. https://doi.org/10.1038/s42003-021-02813-8.
29. Lange P, Celli B, Agustí A, Jensen GB, Divo M, Faner R, et al. Lung-function trajectories leading to chronic obstructive pulmonary disease. N Engl J Med. 2015;373(2):111–22. https://doi.org/10.1056/NEJMoa1411532.
30. Barnes PJ. Immunology of asthma and chronic obstructive pulmonary disease. Nat Rev Immunol. 2008;8(3):183–92.
31. Cosio MG, Saetta M, Agusti A. Immunologic aspects of chronic obstructive pulmonary disease. N Engl J Med. 2009;360(23):2445–54.
32. Ofir D, Laveneziana P, Webb KA, Lam Y-M, O'Donnell DE. Mechanisms of dyspnea during cycle exercise in symptomatic patients with GOLD stage I chronic obstructive pulmonary disease. Am J Respir Crit Care Med. 2008;177(6):622–9.
33. Elbehairy AF, Ciavaglia CE, Webb KA, Guenette JA, Jensen D, Mourad SM, et al. Pulmonary gas exchange abnormalities in mild chronic obstructive pulmonary disease. Implications for dyspnea and exercise intolerance. Am J Respir Crit Care Med. 2015;191(12):1384–94.
34. O'Donnell DE, Sciurba F, Celli B, Mahler DA, Webb KA, Kalberg CJ, et al. Effect of fluticasone propionate/salmeterol on lung hyperinflation and exercise endurance in COPD. Chest. 2006;130(3):647–56.
35. O'Donnell DE, Flüge T, Gerken F, Hamilton A, Webb K, Aguilaniu B, et al. Effects of tiotropium on lung hyperinflation, dyspnoea and exercise tolerance in COPD. Eur Respir J. 2004;23(6):832–40.
36. Jones PW, Donohue JF, Nedelman J, Pascoe S, Pinault G, Lassen C. Correlating changes in lung function with patient outcomes in chronic obstructive pulmonary disease: a pooled analysis. Respir Res. 2011;12(1):1–10.
37. Koarai A, Sugiura H, Yamada M, Ichikawa T, Fujino N, Kawayama T, et al. Treatment with LABA versus LAMA for stable COPD: a systematic review and meta-analysis. BMC Pulm Med. 2020;20(1):1–11.
38. Garcia-Rio F, Rojo B, Casitas R, Lores V, Madero R, Romero D, et al. Prognostic value of the objective measurement of daily physical activity in patients with COPD. Chest. 2012;142(2):338–46. https://doi.org/10.1378/chest.11-2014.
39. Barnes PJ, Celli BR. Systemic manifestations and comorbidities of COPD. Eur Respir J. 2009;33(5):1165–85. https://doi.org/10.1183/09031936.00128008.
40. Handschin C, Spiegelman BM. The role of exercise and PGC1α in inflammation and chronic disease. Nature. 2008;454(7203):463–9. https://doi.org/10.1038/nature07206.
41. Pedersen BK. The diseasome of physical inactivity—and the role of myokines in muscle—fat cross talk. J Physiol. 2009;587(Pt 23):5559–68. https://doi.org/10.1113/jphysiol.2009.179515.
42. Jeffery PK. Remodeling and inflammation of bronchi in asthma and chronic obstructive pulmonary disease. Proc Am Thorac Soc. 2004;1(3):176–83. https://doi.org/10.1513/pats.200402-009MS.
43. Kauppi P, Kupiainen H, Lindqvist A, Tammilehto L, Kilpeläinen M, Kinnula VL, et al. Overlap syndrome of asthma and COPD predicts low quality of life. J Asthma. 2011;48(3):279–85. https://doi.org/10.3109/02770903.2011.555576.
44. Miravitlles M, Soler-Cataluña JJ, Calle M, Molina J, Almagro P, Quintano JA, et al. Spanish guideline for COPD (GesEPOC). Update 2014. Arch Bronconeumol. 2014;50 Suppl 1:1–16.

45. Diaz-Guzman E, Khosravi M, Mannino DM. Asthma, chronic obstructive pulmonary disease, and mortality in the U.S. population. COPD. 2011;8(6):400–7. https://doi.org/10.3109/15412555.2011.611200.
46. de Marco R, Pesce G, Marcon A, Accordini S, Antonicelli L, Bugiani M, et al. The coexistence of asthma and chronic obstructive pulmonary disease (COPD): prevalence and risk factors in young, middle-aged and elderly people from the general population. PLoS One. 2013;8(5):e62985. https://doi.org/10.1371/journal.pone.0062985.
47. Hersh CP, Jacobson FL, Gill R, Silverman EK. Computed tomography phenotypes in severe, early-onset chronic obstructive pulmonary disease. COPD. 2007;4(4):331–7. https://doi.org/10.1080/15412550701601274.
48. O'Donnell DE, Aaron S, Bourbeau J, Hernandez P, Marciniuk DD, Balter M, et al. Canadian Thoracic Society recommendations for management of chronic obstructive pulmonary disease—2007 update. Can Respir J. 2007;14 Suppl B(Suppl B):5B–32B. https://doi.org/10.1155/2007/830570.
49. Nagai A. [Guidelines for the diagnosis and management of chronic obstructive pulmonary disease: 3rd edition]. Nihon Rinsho. 2011;69(10):1729–34.
50. Miravitlles M, Soler-Cataluña JJ, Calle M, Molina J, Almagro P, Quintano JA, et al. Spanish COPD Guidelines (GesEPOC): pharmacological treatment of stable COPD. Spanish Society of Pulmonology and Thoracic Surgery. Arch Bronconeumol. 2012;48(7):247–57. https://doi.org/10.1016/j.arbres.2012.04.001.
51. Global Initiative for Chronic Obstructive Lung Disease (GOLD). Global strategy for diagnosis, management and prevention of COPD (2020 Report). https://goldcopd.org/wp-content/uploads/2019/11/GOLD-2020-REPORT-ver1.1wms.pdf. Accessed 12 Feb 2022.

Chapter 2
Concept of Treatable Traits and ACO: Can Treatable Traits Approach Be Applied into Practice?

Hironori Masuko and Nobuyuki Hizawa

Abstract Asthma and chronic obstructive pulmonary disease (COPD) are extremely heterogeneous diseases with respect to symptoms, severity, and response to treatment. The term "asthma–COPD overlap" (ACO) is used to describe a condition that combines the characteristics of both diseases, but it is not a single disease and is equally as diverse. Until the early twenty-first century, the treatment for chronic airway diseases such as asthma and COPD was largely based on an approach termed as one-size-fits-all medicine. However, this approach has been recognized to have limitations in providing appropriate treatment for a variety of conditions that vary from patient to patient. Recently, the importance of understanding the treatable trait has been emphasized for the provision of precision and personalized medicine for treating chronic inflammatory lung disease. The newly proposed concept is known as treatable traits, which implies the traits and characteristics of patients that must be considered to provide optimal treatment. It is a new approach that seeks treatment options in a multidimensional manner based on the clinical traits and characteristics of individual patients without being limited by the conventional diagnosis. This chapter summarizes previous reports on treatable traits in patients with ACO and outlines future perspectives.

Keywords Asthma-COPD overlap · Treatable traits · Phenotype · Endotype

1 Introduction

According to the guidelines of the Japanese Respiratory Society, asthma–chronic obstructive pulmonary disease (COPD) overlap (ACO) is defined as a condition in patients aged >40 years, with a respiratory function test showing an FEV_1/FVC of <70% after inhalation of bronchodilators, and having both features of COPD and

H. Masuko (✉) · N. Hizawa
Department of Pulmonary Medicine, University of Tsukuba, Ibaraki, Japan
e-mail: hmasuko@md.tsukuba.ac.jp

H. Nagase et al. (eds.), *Asthma-COPD Overlap*, Respiratory Disease Series: Diagnostic Tools and Disease Managements,
https://doi.org/10.1007/978-981-96-0217-9_2

asthma [1]. The clinical symptoms common to both asthma and COPD are cough, wheezing, and shortness of breath characterized by chronic airway inflammation and airway remodeling, which are extremely involved in the pathogenesis of the disease [2]. The concept of ACO has been variously termed, such as overlap syndrome of asthma and COPD [3], mixed asthma–COPD phenotype [4], asthma combined with COPD [5], the coexistence of asthma and COPD [6], and COPD with asthmatic features [7].

The Dutch hypothesis, proposed by Dick Orie in 1961, was the first conception of ACO [8]. Asthma and COPD are derived from a common disease known as chronic nonspecific lung disease, and the complex interaction of genetic and environmental factors in their development results in different phenotypes. However, there exists an opposing theory known as the "British Hypothesis," which states that asthma and COPD have separate origins due to their respective genetic characteristics, inflammatory profiles, and treatments [9].

In 2015, a consensus document jointly developed by the Global Initiative for Asthma and Global Initiative for Chronic Obstructive Lung Disease proposed to clinically describe patients who exhibit features of both asthma and COPD, designating them as having ACO [10]. The document specified that an ACO is not a single disease but includes various forms of airway disease. It stated that ACO does not describe the pathophysiology itself, and that there is a concomitant danger in using this umbrella term to refer to patients with ACO with different endotypes and phenotypes as if they were a single disease [11]. Moreover, the document noted that clinical use may require an approach to treatable traits, which will be discussed later.

Although several studies have been conducted on ACO, there is no uniform definition or diagnostic criteria. The frequency of ACO is inconsistent, ranging from a few percent to >50%, depending on the composition of the study population [12]. Regarding the diagnostic criteria, ACO is diagnosed based on a combination of various indicators, including age, smoking history, allergy history (atopy or allergic rhinitis), symptoms, diagnosis of asthma (physician diagnosis and patient report), the FEV_1/FVC after bronchodilator inhalation, airway reversibility tests, sputum eosinophil count, blood eosinophil count/ratio, serum IgE level, exhaled nitric oxide level (FeNO), and diffusion capacity of the lung test. The use of multiple definitions is one of the major limitations in clinical studies on ACO [13, 14]. For instance, clinical studies on asthma and COPD define both diseases relatively strictly to exclude patients who do not meet the "pure type" of both diseases [15]. Although this appears to be the correct approach, it is limited by the available evidence and does not completely describe the spectrum of obstructive airway disease observed in clinical practice.

In a report of cluster analysis using 12 factors known to be associated with exacerbations in 225 Japanese patients with chronic inflammatory lung disease and asthma, COPD, or ACO diagnosed by a respiratory physician, five exacerbation-related clusters were found. Among those, three clusters, namely, eosinophilic type, GERD predominant type, and smokers with impaired lung function type, were found to consist of a mixture of patients with asthma, COPD, and ACO. The presence of exacerbation-related traits beyond conventional disease names was also suggested [16]. The results indicated that the clinical heterogeneity of disease exacerbation may reflect the presence of common exacerbation-prone endotypes across asthma and COPD.

2 Treatable Traits

Until the early twenty-first century, the treatment for chronic airway diseases such as asthma and COPD was largely based on an approach known as one-size-fits-all medicine. This approach was useful for diseases where a single medication could cure the causative agent of the disease, similar to the case of antibiotic use for treating infectious diseases. When this approach is applied to chronic airway diseases, the first step is to label the diagnosis and add (step-up) or discontinue (step-down) drugs under that diagnosis, depending on risk factors, disease severity, and response to treatment. In other words, the dose of inhaled corticosteroids is increased in steps, or long-acting bronchodilators are added. However, this approach has been recognized to have limitations in providing appropriate treatment for a variety of conditions that vary from patient to patient [17, 18], as, for instance, interventions for smokers with "asthma" and patients with "COPD" who have airway reversibility. The newly proposed concept is known as treatable traits, which implies the traits and characteristics of patients that must be considered to provide optimal treatment. Figure 2.1 shows the number of articles with the term "treatable traits" in the title or abstract, which has been rapidly increasing since around 2015, indicating that it is one of the topical issues in chronic airway diseases. This is a new approach that seeks treatment options in a multidimensional manner based on the clinical traits and characteristics of individual patients without being limited by the conventional diagnosis [19, 20]. The primary advantage of this approach is that it can be adapted

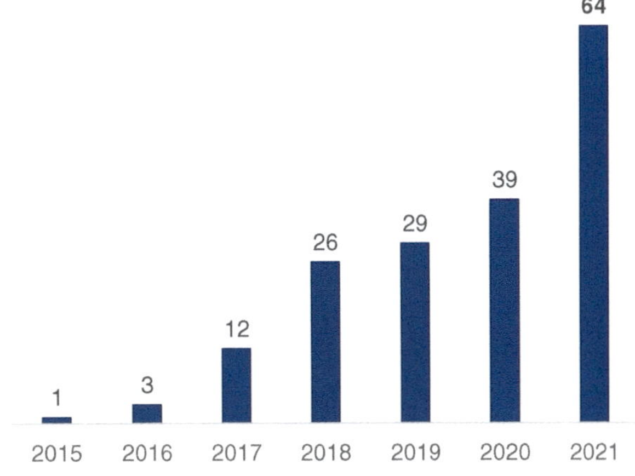

Fig. 2.1 Yearly trend in the number of articles on "treatable traits". "treatable traits" [title/abstract]—Search Results—PubMed (nih.gov)

to conditions for which the diagnosis (asthma or COPD) is not completely established. This situation is often encountered in clinical practice, especially in primary care, making this approach extremely useful.

Treatable traits meet three characteristics. First, the trait is clinically important and associated with a specific disease outcome; second, it is identifiable and measurable, similar to a biomarker; and finally, the trait is treatable. These treatable traits often reflect the clinical phenotype of the disease, or the endotype, which is the molecular biological/genetic mechanism underlying the pathophysiology. Furthermore, these treatable traits are not necessarily limited to intrapulmonary traits alone but include extrapulmonary traits and behavioral and lifestyle risk factors. Therefore, a holistic and multidimensional patient evaluation is necessary to evaluate treatable traits.

Several studies have explored treatable traits in asthma [21, 22]. Pulmonary treatable traits include airflow limitation, eosinophilic airway inflammation, neutrophilic airway inflammation, hypoxemia, and shortness of breath, whereas extrapulmonary treatable traits include atopic predisposition, obesity, depression, anemia, and cardiac disease. In addition, risk factors and behavioral and lifestyle factors such as smoking, sarcopenia, poor inhalation technique, low adherence, and multiple inhalation devices have been documented. There are also some reports on treatable traits in patients with COPD, which include pulmonary factors such as pulmonary hyperinflation, airflow limitation, chronic respiratory failure, repeated exacerbations, and pulmonary hypertension, and extrapulmonary factors such as dyspnea, psychiatric illness, poor exercise tolerance, poor nutrition, obesity, loss of weight, and sleep apnea. Moreover, other risk factors such as smoking and alpha-1-antitrypsin deficiency have been noted [23].

3 Treatable Traits in Patients with ACO

There is still wide debate on whether ACO is simply a combination of the characteristics of both asthma and COPD or whether there exists a distinct pathophysiology [24, 25]. Similarly, there is no clear conclusion on whether the treatable traits of ACO are a combination of the previously mentioned asthma and COPD treatable traits or whether there is a separate and distinct entity. Nevertheless, the concept of treatable traits itself is an approach that was originally proposed to focus more on the pathophysiology of individual patients rather than on the conventional diagnosis of asthma and COPD by disease name. Here, we introduce the reports of treatable traits confirmed in ACO.

The pulmonary-related treatable traits in patients with ACO are listed in Table 2.1, which include airflow limitation, airway smooth muscle contraction, eosinophilic airway inflammation, and pulmonary hyperinflation. Several of these traits have been used as diagnostic criteria for ACO and may reflect the pathogenesis of ACO. Bronchodilator use is recommended for patients with airflow limitations.

Table 2.1 Pulmonary treatable traits in patients with asthma–chronic obstructive pulmonary disease overlap

Treatable traits	Treatment
Pulmonary traits	
Airflow limitation	Bronchodilators
Bacterial colonization	Macrolides, tetracyclines
Bronchiectasis	Macrolides, tetracyclines, nebulized antibiotics/aminoglycosides
Chronic respiratory failure	Oxygen/NIV/lung transplant
Chronic sputum production	Smoking cessation, macrolides, PDE4 inhibitors
Cough reflex hypersensitivity	Gabapentin, P2X3, speech pathology intervention
Emphysema	Lung volume reduction/transplant
Eosinophilic airway inflammation	Corticosteroids/type 2 biologics
Pulmonary hypertension	Oxygen/NIV/lung transplant

NIV Noninvasive ventilation

In patients with ACO with eosinophilic airway inflammation, eosinophils in sputum and eosinophils in peripheral blood and exhaled nitric oxide (FeNO) can be used as biomarkers [26–28].

In 2018, Takayama et al. described that a combined cutoff of FeNO of ≥25 ppb and a blood eosinophil count of ≥250 cells/μL have a 96.1% specificity for differentiating ACO and COPD [29]. Inhaled corticosteroid therapy is recommended for patients with eosinophilic airway inflammation. Emphysema is a treatable trait observed in patients with ACO, but it is not as frequent as in patients with COPD [13, 30]. In 2018, Wang et al. reported that plasma YKL-40, also known as chitinase-3-like-1 protein (CHI3L1), is a promising biomarker to distinguish patients with ACO features from those with COPD [31]. In a study on Japanese subjects, Kanazawa et al. found that YKL-40 lung cis-expression quantitative trait loci are associated with late-onset asthma [32]. It has been difficult to differentiate late-onset asthma from COPD, which can be diagnostic of ACO [33], and YKL-40 may exert some influence on ACO pathogenesis.

Table 2.2 lists extrapulmonary treatable traits found in patients with ACO. ACO and allergic rhinoconjunctivitis [34, 35], atopic dermatitis [36, 37], atopy [38, 39], and other traits are also reasonable and considered diagnostic criteria for ACO in some papers. Other comorbidities known as treatable traits associated with ACO include obesity [3, 40], diabetes [35, 41, 42], lipid abnormalities [42, 43], gastroesophageal reflux disease [44, 45], cerebrovascular disease [46–48], osteoporosis/fracture [49], depression [26, 27, 50], anxiety [26, 27, 48], and malignant tumors [46, 51]; a striking association between ACO and malignancy has been demonstrated for lung cancer as well as other malignancies [46, 51]. Some reports indicate that persistent systemic inflammation is a treatable trait in patients with ACO. In populations with high serum CRP or IL-6, the mortality rate and the frequency of exacerbations is high, suggesting that anti-inflammatory therapy such as statins may be effective in this population [52, 53].

Table 2.2 Extrapulmonary treatable traits in patients with asthma–chronic obstructive pulmonary disease overlap

Treatable traits	Treatment
Extrapulmonary traits	
Anxiety	Anxiolytics
Cachexia	Diet/physical activity
Cardiovascular disease	ACE inhibitors/diuretics/β-blockers
Deconditioning	Rehabilitation
Depression	Cognitive and behavioral therapy
Gastro-esophageal reflux disease	Antacids, lose weight
Obesity	Diet/physical activity/bariatric surgery
Obstructive sleep apnea	Continuous positive airway pressure
Rhinosinusitis	Topical steroids/surgery
Vocal cord dysfunction	Speech pathology therapy

ACE Angiotensin-converting enzyme

Table 2.3 Behavioral/lifestyle risk factors and treatable traits in patients with asthma–chronic obstructive pulmonary disease overlap

Treatable traits	Treatment
Behavioral/lifestyle factors	
Exposure to sensitizing agents	Avoidance/desensitization
Nonadherence to treatment	Reassurance/education/periodic check-up
Polypharmacy	Medication review
Poor family and social support	Family therapy education/self-management support
Poor inhalation technique	Education
Side effects of treatments	Treatment optimization
Smoking	Cessation support

The treatable traits of behavioral and lifestyle factors found in patients with ACO are listed in Table 2.3. Smoking is significantly more frequent in these patients than in patients with only asthma [13, 14, 26, 27]. The evidence is so convincing that several guidelines include smoking exposure as a diagnostic criterion for ACO [1, 54, 55]. This demonstrates the importance of effective smoking cessation strategies in patients with ACO in clinical practice. Another remarkable finding is the poor health-related quality of life observed in patients with ACO, including both respiratory-related quality of life and general health-related quality of life [3, 14, 56]. This evidence is probably related to several comorbidities found in patients with ACO, in addition to the higher frequency and severity of exacerbations. Other behavioral and lifestyle risk factors that can be treated and associated with ACO include low education [57, 58], low family income, and unemployment [46, 59]. It is difficult to state whether these lifestyle habits are a cause or a consequence of disease development. For instance, given the high disease burden of ACO, it is conceivable that the onset of ACO could be a cause of lower productivity and, ultimately, lower household income and unemployment.

4 Randomized Controlled Trials

There is no clear information on the actual therapeutic benefits of applying treatable traits associated with ACO to clinical practice. Moreover, no randomized controlled trials have been conducted on ACO. A useful reference would be the study conducted by McDonald et al. in which treatable traits were used to intervene in severe asthma. This was a multidimensional evaluation of severe persistent asthma in patients aged ≥18 years using pulmonary and extrapulmonary treatable traits and behavioral risk factors [21]. After 16 weeks of treatment, both ACQ and AQLQ scores were significantly improved in the group that received intervention treatment with treatable traits for each patient compared with the usual care group. Although the difficulty of accurately identifying each individual's treatable traits and introducing appropriate treatment for each treatable trait may pose a greater burden on clinicians than ever before, there is a possibility that treatment based on treatable traits could be beneficial. Future randomized controlled trials with similar treatable traits are desirable for not only patients with ACO but also those with COPD.

5 Conclusion

Both asthma and COPD are diverse diseases, and ACO should be considered to include even more complex clinical phenotypes and endotypes. The conventional diagnostic approach and stepping up or down according to the severity and treatment response is burdensome to both patients and the healthcare economy. Precise recognition of the various combinations of treatable traits in patients with ACO may pose some challenges to clinicians, but this is inevitably important for establishing personalized and precision medicine in the future. Although the identification of treatable traits for chronic airway diseases is still insufficient, there is room for debate on the type of treatment most appropriate for each trait. The optimal treatment strategy for each patient is not the one-size-fits-all approach that can be described in guidelines, which may hinder the widespread use of this approach. Nevertheless, future multifaceted studies are required to advance our understanding of ACO pathophysiology and bring the treatable traits approach closer to the ideal.

References

1. The Japanese Respiratory Society. The JRS guidelines for the management of asthma and COPD overlap: ACO; 2018.
2. Hizawa N. Genetic backgrounds of asthma and COPD. Allergol Int. 2009;58:8.
3. Kauppi P, Kupiainen H, Lindqvist A, et al. Overlap syndrome of asthma and COPD predicts low quality of life. J Asthma. 2011;48:279–85.
4. Miravitlles M, Soler-Cataluña JJ, Calle M, et al. Spanish guideline for COPD (GesEPOC). Update 2014. Arch Bronconeumol. 2014;50 Suppl 1:1–16.

5. Diaz-Guzman E, Khosravi M, Mannino DM. Asthma, chronic obstructive pulmonary disease, and mortality in the U.S. population. COPD. 2011;8:400–7.
6. de Marco R, Pesce G, Marcon A, et al. The coexistence of asthma and chronic obstructive pulmonary disease (COPD): prevalence and risk factors in young, middle-aged and elderly people from the general population. PLoS One. 2013;8:e62985.
7. Hersh CP, Jacobson FL, Gill R, Silverman EK. Computed tomography phenotypes in severe, early-onset chronic obstructive pulmonary disease. COPD. 2007;4:331–7.
8. Orie NGM, Sluiter ID, De Vries K, Tammeling GJ, Witkop J. The host factor in bronchitis. In: Orie NGM, Sluiter HJ, editors. Bronchitis. Assen: Royal Vangorcum; 1961. p. 43–59.
9. Venkata AN. Asthma-COPD overlap: review of diagnosis and management. Curr Opin Pulm Med. 2020;26:155–61.
10. Initiatives GaG. Diagnosis of diseases of chronic airfow limitation: asthma, COPD and asthma-COPD overlap syndrome (ACOS) 2015. Available from: https://goldcopd.org/wp-content/uploads/2016/04/GOLD_ACOS_2015.pdf.
11. Fingleton J, Hardy J, Beasley R. Treatable traits of chronic airways disease. Curr Opin Pulm Med. 2018;24:24–31.
12. Tho NV, Park HY, Nakano Y. Asthma-COPD overlap syndrome (ACOS): a diagnostic challenge. Respirology. 2016;21:410–8.
13. Hardin M, Silverman EK, Barr RG, et al. The clinical features of the overlap between COPD and asthma. Respir Res. 2011;12:127.
14. Miravitlles M, Soriano JB, Ancochea J, et al. Characterisation of the overlap COPD-asthma phenotype. Focus on physical activity and health status. Respir Med. 2013;107:1053–60.
15. Gibson PG, Simpson JL. The overlap syndrome of asthma and COPD: what are its features and how important is it? Thorax. 2009;64:728–35.
16. Hyodo K, Masuko H, Oshima H, Shigemasa R, Kitazawa H, Kanazawa J, et al. Common exacerbation-prone phenotypes across asthma and chronic obstructive pulmonary disease (COPD). PLoS One. 2022;17(3):e0264397.
17. Pavord ID, Beasley R, Agusti A, et al. After asthma: redefining airways diseases. Lancet. 2017;391:350–400.
18. Ebmeier S, Thayabaran D, Braithwaite I, Bénamara C, Weatherall M, Beasley R. Trends in international asthma mortality: analysis of data from the WHO Mortality Database from 46 countries (1993–2012). Lancet. 2017;390:935–45.
19. McDonald VM, Hiles SA, Godbout K, Harvey ES, Marks GB, Hew M. Treatable traits can be identified in a severe asthma registry and predict future exacerbations. Respirology. 2019;24:37–47.
20. Gibson PG, McDonald VM, Marks GB. Asthma in the older adult. Lancet. 2010;374:803–13.
21. McDonald VM, Clark VL, Cordova-Rivera L, Wark PAB, Baines KJ, Gibson PG. Targeting treatable traits in severe asthma: a randomised controlled trial. Eur Respir J. 2020;55:1901509.
22. Pavord ID, Beasley R, Agusti A, et al. After asthma: redefining airways diseases. Lancet. 2018;391:350–400.
23. van Dijk M, Gan CT, Koster TD, et al. Treatment of severe stable COPD: the multidimensional approach of treatable traits. ERJ Open Res. 2020;6:00322–2019.
24. Cosío BG, Dacal D, Pérez de Llano L. Asthma-COPD overlap: identification and optimal treatment. Ther Adv Respir Dis. 2018;12:1753466618805662.
25. Barnes PJ. Asthma-COPD overlap. Chest. 2016;149:7–8. https://doi.org/10.1016/j.chest.2015.08.017. Epub 2016 Jan 6. PMID: 26757281.
26. Barrecheguren M, Roman-Rodriguez M, Miravitlles M. Is a previous diagnosis of asthma a reliable criterion for asthma-COPD overlap syndrome in a patient with COPD? Int J Chron Obstruct Pulmon Dis. 2015;10:1745–52.
27. Wurst KE, Rheault TR, Edwards L, Tal-Singer R, Agusti A, Vestbo J. A comparison of COPD patients with and without ACOS in the ECLIPSE study. Eur Respir J. 2016;47:1559–62.
28. Perez de Llano L, Cosio BG, Miravitlles M, Plaza V, Group CS. Accuracy of a new algorithm to identify asthma-COPD overlap (ACO) patients in a cohort of patients with chronic obstructive airway disease. Arch Bronconeumol. 2018;54:198–204.

29. Takayama Y, Ohnishi H, Ogasawara F, Oyama K, Kubota T, Yokoyama A. Clinical utility of fractional exhaled nitric oxide and blood eosinophils counts in the diagnosis of asthma-COPD overlap. Int J Chron Obstruct Pulmon Dis. 2018;13:2525–32.
30. Fu JJ, McDonald VM, Gibson PG, Simpson JL. Systemic inflammation in older adults with asthma-COPD overlap syndrome. Allergy Asthma Immunol Res. 2014;6:316–24.
31. Wang J, Lv H, Luo Z, Mou S, Liu J, Liu C, et al. Plasma YKL-40 and NGAL are useful in distinguishing ACO from asthma and COPD. Respir Res. 2018;19:47.
32. Kanazawa J, Kitazawa H, Masuko H, et al. A cis-eQTL allele regulating reduced expression of CHI3L1 is associated with late-onset adult asthma in Japanese cohorts. BMC Med Genet. 2019;20:58.
33. Abramson MJ, Perret JL, Dharmage SC, McDonald VM, McDonald CF. Distinguishing adult-onset asthma from COPD: a review and a new approach. Int J Chron Obstruct Pulmon Dis. 2014;9:945–62.
34. Kobayashi S, Hanagama M, Yamanda S, Ishida M, Yanai M. Inflammatory biomarkers in asthma-COPD overlap syndrome. Int J Chron Obstruct Pulmon Dis. 2016;11:2117–23.
35. Cosio BG, Perez de Llano L, Lopez Vina A, et al. Th-2 signature in chronic airway diseases: towards the extinction of asthma-COPD overlap syndrome? Eur Respir J. 2017;49:1602397.
36. Park HJ, Byun MK, Kim HJ, et al. Asthma-COPD overlap shows favorable clinical outcomes compared to pure COPD in a Korean COPD cohort. Allergy Asthma Immunol Res. 2017;9:431–7.
37. Wang YC, Jaakkola MS, Lajunen TK, Lai CH, Jaakkola JJK. Asthma-COPD overlap syndrome among subjects with newly diagnosed adult-onset asthma. Allergy. 2018;73:1554–7.
38. Kawamatawong T, Charoenniwassakul S, Rerkpattanapipat T. The asthma and chronic obstructive pulmonary disease overlap syndrome in tertiary care setting Thailand. Asia Pac Allergy. 2017;7:227–33.
39. Ding B, DiBonaventura M, Karlsson N, Ling X. Asthma-chronic obstructive pulmonary disease overlap syndrome in the urban Chinese population: prevalence and disease burden using the 2010, 2012, and 2013 China National Health and Wellness Surveys. Int J Chron Obstruct Pulmon Dis. 2016;11:1139–50.
40. Cosentino J, Zhao H, Hardin M, et al. Analysis of asthma-chronic obstructive pulmonary disease overlap syndrome defined on the basis of bronchodilator response and degree of emphysema. Ann Am Thorac Soc. 2016;13:1483–9.
41. Caillaud D, Chanez P, Escamilla R, Burgel PR, Court-Fortune I, Nesme-Meyer P, et al. Asthma-COPD overlap syndrome (ACOS) vs 'pure' COPD: a distinct phenotype? Allergy. 2017;72:137–45.
42. Ding B, Small M. Treatment trends in patients with asthma-COPD overlap syndrome in a COPD cohort: findings from a real-world survey. Int J Chron Obstruct Pulmon Dis. 2017;12:1753–63.
43. Cosio BG, Soriano JB, Lopez-Campos JL, et al. Distribution and outcomes of a phenotype-based approach to guide COPD management: results from the CHAIN Cohort. PLoS One. 2016;11:e0160770.
44. Koblizek V, Milenkovic B, Barczyk A, et al. Phenotypes of COPD patients with a smoking history in Central and Eastern Europe: the POPE Study. Eur Respir J. 2017;49:1601446.
45. Perez-de-Llano L, Cosio BG, Group CS. Asthma-COPD overlap is not a homogeneous disorder: further supporting data. Respir Res. 2017;18:183.
46. To T, Zhu J, Larsen K, et al. Progression from asthma to chronic obstructive pulmonary disease. is air pollution a risk factor? Am J Respir Crit Care Med. 2016;194:429–38.
47. Wurst KE, St Laurent S, Hinds D, Davis KJ. Disease burden of patients with asthma/COPD overlap in a US claims database: impact of ICD-9 coding-based definitions. COPD. 2017;14:200–9.
48. Shantakumar S, Pwu RF, D'Silva L, et al. Burden of asthma and COPD overlap (ACO) in Taiwan: a nationwide population-based study. BMC Pulm Med. 2018;18:16.
49. Yeh JJ, Wang YC, Kao CH. Asthma-chronic obstructive pulmonary disease overlap syndrome associated with risk of pulmonary embolism. PLoS One. 2016;11:e0162483.

50. Yeh JJ, Lin CL, Hsu WH, Kao CH. The relationship of depression in asthma-chronic obstructive pulmonary disease overlap syndrome. PLoS One. 2017;12:e0188017.
51. Harada T, Yamasaki A, Fukushima T, et al. Causes of death in patients with asthma and asthma-chronic obstructive pulmonary disease overlap syndrome. Int J Chron Obstruct Pulmon Dis. 2015;10:595–602.
52. McDonald VM, Higgins I, Wood LG, Gibson PG. Multidimensional assessment and tailored interventions for COPD: respiratory utopia or common sense? Thorax. 2013;68:691–4.
53. Agusti A, Edwards LD, Rennard SI, et al. Persistent systemic inflammation is associated with poor clinical outcomes in COPD: a novel phenotype. PLoS One. 2012;7:e37483.
54. Plaza V, Alvarez F, Calle M, et al. Consensus on the Asthma-COPD overlap syndrome (ACOS) between the Spanish COPD guidelines (GesEPOC) and the Spanish guidelines on the management of asthma (GEMA). Arch Bronconeumol. 2017;53:443–9.
55. Sin DD, Miravitlles M, Mannino DM, et al. What is asthma-COPD overlap syndrome? Towards a consensus definition from a round table discussion. Eur Respir J. 2016;48:664–73.
56. Llanos JP, Ortega H, Germain G, et al. Health characteristics of patients with asthma, COPD and asthma-COPD overlap in the NHANES database. Int J Chron Obstruct Pulmon Dis. 2018;13:2859–68.
57. Ekerljung L, Mincheva R, Hagstad S, et al. Prevalence, clinical characteristics and morbidity of the Asthma-COPD overlap in a general population sample. J Asthma. 2018;55:461–9.
58. Kumbhare S, Pleasants R, Ohar JA, Strange C. Characteristics and prevalence of asthma/chronic obstructive pulmonary disease overlap in the United States. Ann Am Thorac Soc. 2016;13:803–10.
59. Kim J, Kim YS, Kim K, et al. Socioeconomic impact of asthma, chronic obstructive pulmonary disease and asthma-COPD overlap syndrome. J Thorac Dis. 2017;9:1547–56.

Part II
Epidemiology and Prognosis

Chapter 3
Epidemiology of ACO from Global Data: Does the Prevalence of ACO Vary Among Global Analyses?

Kentaro Machida, Takahiro Matsuyama, Hiromi Matsuyama, Koichi Takagi, and Hiromasa Inoue

Abstract Both asthma and chronic obstructive pulmonary disease (COPD) are well-recognized common pulmonary diseases with different pathophysiologies. Some patients have persistent airflow limitation with coexisting asthma and COPD characteristics, and this condition is called asthma and COPD overlap (ACO). Like asthma and COPD, ACO is considered a heterogenous disease, which makes it difficult to understand the underlying disease mechanism. The prevalence of ACO has varied widely in studies, since there is no universal consensus on definition of and diagnostic criteria for ACO, and its prevalence has been roughly estimated at around 2% in the general population, around 25% in asthma patients, and 30% in COPD patients. The frequency and prognosis of ACO patients were reported to have conflicting results. In general, patients with ACO have more severe symptoms, poor quality of life, rapid lung function decline, lower respiratory function, frequent exacerbations, and hospitalizations compared to patients with asthma or COPD alone; however, the exact disease burden for ACO has not been clarified. It is important to clarify the pathophysiology of ACO and conduct a cohort study and clinical trials using established definitions and diagnostic criteria for pathophysiology, biomarkers and objective measures. This would lead to good clinical practice for ACO patients.

Keywords Asthma–chronic obstructive pulmonary disease overlap (ACO) Asthma · COPD · Prevalence of ACO · Exacerbation

---

K. Machida · T. Matsuyama · H. Matsuyama · K. Takagi · H. Inoue (✉)
Department of Pulmonary Medicine, Graduate School of Medicine and Dental Science, Kagoshima University, Kagoshima, Japan
e-mail: inoue@m2.kufm.kagoshima-u.ac.jp

H. Nagase et al. (eds.), *Asthma-COPD Overlap*, Respiratory Disease Series: Diagnostic Tools and Disease Managements,
https://doi.org/10.1007/978-981-96-0217-9_3

1 Introduction

Asthma and chronic obstructive pulmonary disease (COPD) are two of the most common respiratory diseases worldwide, typically considered to be different diseases caused by different underlying pathophysiological mechanisms [1, 2]. Asthma is recognized as an airway inflammatory disease characterized by airway hyperresponsiveness and reversible airflow obstruction [1]. On the other hand, COPD is a chronic airway inflammatory disease caused by tobacco smoking or a noxious irritant, characterized by progressive and irreversible airflow limitation [2]. The pattern of airway inflammation in asthma and COPD is different: asthma is characterized predominantly by eosinophilic inflammation with $CD4^{+}$ T-lymphocyte and type 2 innate lymphocyte (ILC2) involvement [1], while COPD is characterized predominantly by neutrophilic inflammation with $CD8^{+}$ T-lymphocyte and macrophage involvement [2]. Airway inflammation and clinical features in both diseases are different, and this allows asthma and COPD to be recognized as distinct diseases. However, patients, especially older ones, may sometimes have the clinical features of both diseases [3], and this condition is called asthma–COPD overlap (ACO).

The concept of asthma–COPD overlap syndrome (ACOS) was proposed in 2014 in a joint project of the Global Initiative for Asthma (GINA) and the Global Initiative for Chronic Obstructive Lung Disease (GOLD), where it was defined as persistent airflow limitation with several features usually associated with asthma and several features usually associated with COPD [4]. Use of the modified term "ACO" was recommended by the GINA and GOLD in 2017 because ACO was not considered a single discrete disease entity [5]. However, there is no universal consensus on the definition of and diagnostic criteria for ACO. In addition, the epidemiology of ACO differs depending on the evaluated population. Many epidemiological studies have been reported by various groups using different definitions and diagnostic criteria and evaluating different populations. Therefore, the exact prevalence rate and disease burden of ACO remain unknown. In this review, we will survey the epidemiology of ACO by considering the definitions, diagnostic criteria, and populations in the global data.

2 Definition of and Diagnostic Criteria for ACO

There is no universal consensus on a definition of and diagnostic criteria for ACO. Previous reports have used their own definitions and diagnostic criteria, which makes it difficult to compare the results from different studies. Several studies defined ACO as a fixed airflow obstruction (post-bronchodilator $FEV_1/FVC < 70\%$) with a mixed phenotype with a combination of features of both asthma and COPD [6–13]. A self-reported, physician-diagnosed, or well-documented history and/or current diagnosis of asthma is one of the prominent features of asthma. Variable airflow limitation with reversibility, airway hyperresponsiveness, type 2 inflammation with a high eosinophil count in peripheral blood and/or sputum, serum IgE level, and fractional exhaled of nitric oxide (FeNO) are also concerning asthmatic features [6–15]. The features of COPD include a history of smoking (or equivalent noxious irritants) exposure, and most studies use not fully reversible airflow obstruction as a diagnostic criterion [6, 8, 10–12, 14–19].

The GINA/GOLD joint statement provided a stepwise approach to the diagnosis of ACO with a list of common features of asthma and COPD, and a diagnosis of ACO is suggested if there is a similar number of features of both asthma and COPD [4]. In 2016, a committee of experts recommended using major and minor criteria to identify asthma–COPD overlap and suggested ACO as the existence of all three major criteria: (1) persistent airflow limitation in individuals 40 years of age or older, (2) at least 10 pack-years of tobacco smoking OR equivalent indoor or outdoor air-pollution exposure, and (3) a documented history of asthma before 40 years of age OR a bronchodilator response >400 mL in FEV1, as well as at least one minor criteria: (1) a documented history of atopy or allergic rhinitis, (2) a bronchodilator response of 200 mL in FEV1 and 12% from baseline values on 2 or more visits, or (3) a peripheral blood eosinophil count of 300 cells/μL [20].

The current GINA report states that diagnosis in patients with chronic respiratory symptoms involves a stepwise approach, first recognizing that the patient is likely to have chronic airways disease, then syndromic categorization as characteristic asthma, characteristic COPD, features of both, or other conditions such as bronchiectasis. Lung function testing is essential for confirming persistent airflow limitation, but variable airflow obstruction can be detected with serial peak flow measurements and/or measurements before and after bronchodilator [21]. It is crucial to develop a standardized definition of and diagnostic criteria for ACO.

3 Prevalence of ACO

Previous reports regarding the prevalence of ACO are summarized in Table 3.1. The prevalence of ACO differs depending on the definition and diagnostic criteria, even in the same population [22, 23]. Reports ranged from 0.9% to 4.6% in the general population [6, 7, 10, 13, 17, 24–30], from 23.7% to 27.1% in asthmatic patients [28, 29, 31, 32], and from 4.2% to 50.6% in COPD patients [8, 9, 11, 12, 14–16, 18, 19, 22, 28, 29, 33–35] (Fig. 3.1).

Using the Third National Health and Nutrition Examination Survey (NHANES III) database, Diaz-Guzman et al. reported that the prevalence of ACO, defined as self-reported or physician-diagnosed asthma and COPD, was 2.7% of the general population over the age of 25 in the United States [7]. Using the database of the GEIRD study, de Marco et al. reported that the prevalence of ACO, defined as a physician diagnosis of asthma or COPD (emphysema/chronic bronchitis/COPD), was 1.6%, 2.1%, and 4.5% in the 20–44, 45–64, and 65–84 age groups, respectively, in the general Italian population. In the same study, they reported that the prevalence of ACO among COPD patients was 32.7%, 26.9%, and 25.3% in the 20–44, 45–64, and 65–84 age groups, respectively [13]. In the Latin American population study

Table 3.1 Prevalence of ACO among different population

Author [ref.]	Study design	Subject	Definition of ACO, COPD and asthma	Prevalence of ACO
In general population				
Diaz-Guzman et al. [7]	Cohort	General population, age >25 n = 15,203	ACO: both COPD and ACO COPD: self-reported physician diagnosis of chronic bronchitis or emphysema asthma: self-reported physician diagnosis of asthma	2.7%
de Marco et al. [13]	Cross section	General population, age >20 n = 8360	ACO: both COPD and ACO COPD: self-reported physician diagnosis of chronic bronchitis or emphysema asthma: self-reported physician diagnosis of asthma	1.6% in age 20–40 2.1% in age 45–64 4.5% in age 65–84
de Marco et al. [6]	Cohort	General population, age 20–40 n = 6984	ACO: both current COPD and asthma COPD: post-BD FEV_1/FVC <70% AND (1) symptoms (2) a history of smoking (>10 Pyrs), or occupational exposure Asthma: self-reported asthma AND (1) asthmatic symptoms, medicines in the last year, AHR or transient airflow obstruction (2) self-reported asthma AND AHR	3.1%

Kumbhare et al. [30]	Cross section	General population, age >35 $n = 80{,}498$	ACO: fulfilling all three criteria: (1) self-reported previous history of COPD (2) self-reported previous history of asthma (3) self-reported current asthma	3.2%
Baarnes et al. [26]	Cohort	General population, age 50–64 $n = 57{,}053$	ACO: at least one hospital admission for asthma together with at least one admission for COPD COPD: a history of admissions for COPD Asthma: a history of admissions for asthma	1.2%
Mendy et al. [27]	Cross section	Non-institutionalized civilian age >40 $n = 7570$	ACO: both COPD and asthma COPD: post-BD FEV_1/FVC <70% asthma: self-reported asthma	1.05% 12.59% in COPD 14.60% in asthma
Ekerljung et al. [17]	Cross section	Random sample in general population $n = 1172$ Subjects with suspected asthma $n = 834$ suspected COPD $n = 209$	ACO: post-BD FEV_1/FVC <70% AND At least 1 of 4 criteria (1) a physician-diagnosed asthma with symptoms or asthma medication during the last 12 months (2) post-BD >12% and 200 mL in change FEV_1 (3) self-reported asthma AND a positive methacholine challenge or (4) self-reported asthma AND blood eosinophil count >400/μL	3.4% in the random sample 16.3% in asthma 41.5% in COPD
Hosseini et al. [29]	Meta-analysis	General population (include 27 manuscripts)	ACO: both asthma and COPD	2.0% in the general population 26.5% in asthma 29.6% in COPD

(continued)

Table 3.1 (continued)

Author [ref.]	Study design	Subject	Definition of ACO, COPD and asthma	Prevalence of ACO
Morgan et al. [28]	Cross section	General population, age 35–92 $n = 11{,}923$	ACO: both COPD and asthma COPD; post-BD FEV_1/FVC <LLN asthma; fulfilling 1 of 3 criteria: (1) self-report of wheezing in 1 year (2) self-report of medication use for asthma in 1 year (3) self-report of a physician diagnosis of asthma	3.8%
In COPD patients				
Miravilles et al. [12]	Cross section	COPD patients, age 40–80 $n = 385$	ACO: both COPD and asthma COPD: post-BD FEV_1/FVC <70% Asthma: previously diagnosed with asthma	17.4%
Izquierdo-Alonso et al. [18]	Cross section	COPD patients, age >40 $n = 331$	ACO: post-BD FEV_1/FVC <70% AND DLco/VA ≥80%, absence of pulmonary emphysema in imaging and self-reported physician diagnosis of asthma before age of 40 COPD: post-BD FEV_1/FVC<70%	12.1%
Hardin et al. [11]	Cross section	COPD patients, age 45–80 $n = 3570$	ACO: both COPD and asthma COPD: Post-BD FEV_1/FVC <70%, %FEV_1 <80% Asthma: self-reported physician diagnosis of asthma before age of 40	12.6%
Alshabanat et al. [15]	Meta-analysis	COPD patients (include 17 manuscript)	ACO: post-BD FEV_1/FVC <70% AND physician diagnosed asthma or self-reported physician diagnosis of asthma, post-BD >12% and 200 mL change in FEV_1 from baseline, >20% change in PEF, Airway hyper-responsiveness to methacholine or histamine.	27% in population 28% in hospital-based

Suzuki et al. [19]	Cohort	COPD patients, age > 40 n = 268	ACO: post-BD FEV_1/FVC <70% AND Post-BD >12% and 200 mL in change FEV_1, blood eosinophil count ≧300/μL or presence of specific serum IgE to at least 1 of the 14 inhaled allergens	49.7%
van Boven et al. [8]	Retrospective cohort	Obstructive airway disease, age >18 n = 68,578	ACO: both COPD and asthma COPD: physician diagnosis of COPD Asthma: physician diagnosis of asthma	7.4% in obstructive airway diseases 19.3% in COPD
Cosio et al. [14]	Cohort	COPD patients, age >35 n = 831	ACO: 2 major criteria or 1 major criteria and 2 minor criteria: Major: self-reported previous history of asthma, BDR >15% and 400 mL in change FEV_1 Minor: IgE >100 IU, self-reported history of atopy, BDR >12% and 200 mL change in FEV_1, blood eosinophil >5%	15.0%
Inoue et al. [33]	Cross section	COPD population n = 1008	ACO: stepwise approach in the GINA/GOLD report COPD: FEV_1/FVC <70% in past medical records, age ≥40, current or ex-smoker with a history of ≥ 10 pack-years	4.2–9.2% (depending on the FEV_1 variability cutoff used)
Krishnan et al. [39]	Cohort	Patients currently diagnosed with asthma, COPD, or both in primary care practices. n = 2165	ACO: presence of all four criteria: (1) age ≥40 (2) current or former smoking (3) post-BD FEV_1/FVC <70% (4) post-BD >12% and 200 mL in change FEV_1	20.5% overall (32% diagnosis of both asthma and COPD, 20% diagnosis of COPD only and 14% asthma only)

(continued)

Table 3.1 (continued)

Author [ref.]	Study design	Subject	Definition of ACO, COPD and asthma	Prevalence of ACO
Toledo-Pons et al. [34]	Cohort	COPD patients, age ≥40 $n = 603$	ACO: (1) a concomitant diagnosis of asthma and COPD (smoking asthmatic) (2) COPD with high bronchodilator response (post-BD >15% and 400 mL change in FEV_1) (3) eosinophilic COPD(blood eosinophil count ≧300/μL)	27.35% in fulfilled ≥1 criteria for ACO 13.8% in smoking asthmatics 1.5% in COPD with high bronchodilator response 12.1% in eosinophilic COPD
Barrecheguren et al. [23]	Cohort	COPD patients $n = 522$	ACO: (1) post-BD >12% and 200 mL in change FEV_1 (2) post-BD >15% and 400 mL in change FEV_1 (3) atopy (4) physician diagnosis of asthma (5) reversibility pre-post BD and atopy (6) atopy and a physician diagnosis of asthma (7) reversibility pre-post BD, atopy and physician diagnosis of asthma	50.6%
Kobayashi et al. [41]	Cohort	COPD patients, age ≥40 $n = 387$	ACO: both COPD and asthma COPD: age ≥40 with a smoking history of ≥10 Pyrs Asthma: (1) a history of respiratory symptoms (2) post-BD >12% and 200 mL in change FEV_1	10.6%

Jo et al. [35]	Cohort	COPD patients, age ≥40 $n = 1067$	ACO: fulfilling the following criteria: (1) age >45 with smoking history >10 Pyrs, and post-BD FEV_1/FVC <70% (2) post-BD >15% and 400 mL in change FEV_1 and/or blood eosinophil count ≧300/μL	20.5% 21.4% in non-Hispanic white 17.4% in African American 23.8% in Asian
Hashimoto et al. [36]	Cohort	COPD patients, age ≥40 $n = 396$	Basic characteristics Post-BD FEV_1/FVC <70% in individuals 40 years of age or older Features of COPD (1 item out of 1–3) (1) Smoking history (>10 pack-year) or similar air pollution exposure (2) presence of low attenuation area showing emphysematous lesions on CT (3) Decreased gas exchange (%DLco<80% or %DLco/V_A<80%) Features of asthma (2 items out of 1–3 or at least 1 item out of 1–3 plus 2 items out of 4) (1) Variable or paroxysmal clinical symptoms (2) History of asthma under 40 years (3) Exhaled nitric oxide > 35 ppb (4.1) History of perennial allergic rhinitis (4.2) Bronchodilator response of FEV1 >200 mL and 12% (4.3) Peripheral blood eosinophils >5% or >300 cells/μL (4.4) Elevated IgE level (total or inhaled allergen)	25.5%

(continued)

Table 3.1 (continued)

Author [ref.]	Study design	Subject	Definition of ACO, COPD and asthma	Prevalence of ACO
In asthma patients				
Harada et al. [31]	Retrospective	Asthma patients $n = 650$	ACO: a previous diagnosis of asthma, a smoking history ≥10 Pyrs, post-BD FEV_1/FVC <70%, and symptoms	27.1%
Lee et al. [38]	Cohort	Severe asthma patients $n = 482$	ACO: fulfilling the following criteria: (1) history of smoking (2) fixed airflow limitation (3) post-BD or post-corticosteroid >12% and 200 mL in change FEV_1	23.7%

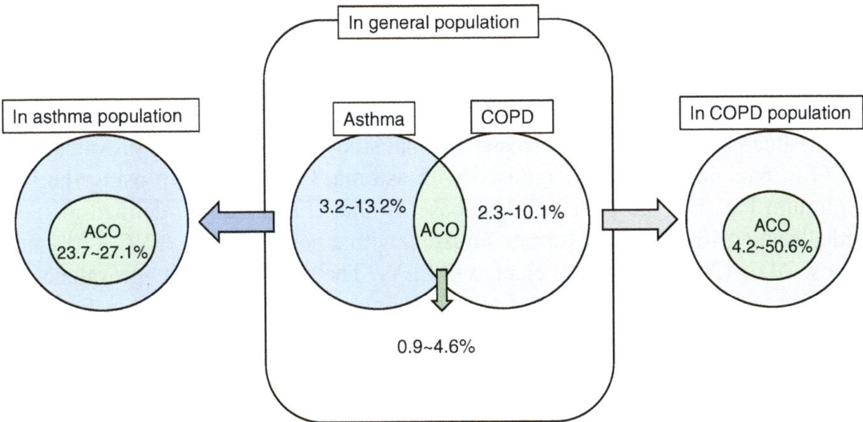

Fig. 3.1 The prevalence rate of ACO among different populations. Prevalence of ACO ranged from 0.9% to 4.6% in the general population, from 23.7% to 27.1% in asthmatic patients, and 4.2% to 50.6% in COPD patients

(PLATINO study), Menezes et al. reported that the prevalence ACO, defined as a combination of features of both asthma and COPD, where the criterion for COPD was a post-bronchodilator (post-BD) FEV_1/FVC ratio <0.70 and the criteria for asthma were a positive answer to the question about wheezing in the last 12 months and post-bronchodilator airflow reversibility, was 1.8% among participants who were over 40 years old [10]. In a cross-sectional cohort study in Japan, Matsumoto et al. reported that the prevalence of ACO, defined as the combination of not fully reversible airflow with variable airflow limitation, post-bronchodilator irreversibility, and no clinical history suggestive of asthma, was 0.9% among the participants who were over 40 years old [24].

In patients with COPD, Alshabanat et al. defined ACO as a combination of post-bronchodilator airflow irreversibility and a diagnosis of asthma, airflow reversibility, peak expiratory flow variability, or airflow hyperresponsiveness. They found that the prevalence of ACO was 27% and 28% in the population- and hospital-based studies, respectively [15]. One study, using the protocol regulating consecutive recruitment, reported that the proportion of patients identified as having ACO based on the stepwise approach in the GINA/GOLD report was 9.2% or 4.2%, depending on the FEV1 variability cutoff used, among the 1008 outpatients medically treated for COPD in a real-life clinical setting [33]. Hashimoto et al. reported the prevalence of ACO, according to the Japanese Respiratory Society (JRS) ACO diagnostic criteria, was 25.5% among patients with COPD [36].

In patients with asthma, Milanese et al. reported that the prevalence of ACO among asthma patients aged 40 years and older was 29% according to the GINA/GOLD ACO definition [32]. Kiljander et al. reported that the prevalence of ACO among asthma patients with a smoking history of at least 10 pack-years was 27.4%, diagnosed by post-bronchodilator irreversible airflow limitation [37]. Lee et al. evaluated the prevalence of ACO among patients with severe asthma using the

Korean severe asthma registry. They reported that the prevalence of ACO in severe asthma patients was 23.7%, diagnosed based on the history of smoking, fixed airflow limitation, and at least 12% and 200 mL increase in FEV1 at post-PD or after corticosteroid treatment [38].

Krishnan et al. conducted a cross-sectional study to determine the prevalence of ACO in patients currently diagnosed with asthma, COPD, or both using the UK Optimum Patient Care Research Database. In that study, ACO is defined as individuals age ≥40, current or former smokers, with a post-BD FEV_1/FVC <70% and a post-BD >12% and 200 mL change in FEV_1. They found an ACO prevalence of 20.5% in patients with a diagnosis of COPD only, 14% in patients with a diagnosis of asthma only, and 32% in patients with a diagnosis of both asthma and COPD [39]. Morgan et al. collected cross-sectional data from four population-based studies and defined COPD as a post-BD FEV_1/FVC ratio below the lower limit of normal; asthma as the history of wheezing or asthma medication use for 12 months or physician's diagnosis based on patient self-reported; and ACO as having both. They reported an ACO prevalence of 3.8%; 43.8% of those with COPD and 21.7% with asthma had ACO among 11,923 participants aged 35 to 92 years [28]. Hosseini et al. conducted a meta-analysis that included 27 studies from population-based and cohort studies to determine the prevalence of ACO and reported an ACO prevalence of 2.0% in the general population, 26.9% in asthma patients, and 29.6% in COPD patients [29].

4 Clinical Manifestations of ACO

4.1 Age and Gender of ACO Patients

Many studies have reported that patients with ACO were older than those with asthma [6, 7, 10, 17, 31, 40]. Comparing ACO and COPD patients, it has been reported both that ACO patients were younger than COPD patients [6–8, 10, 11, 17, 33, 41] and that there was no difference in the mean age of ACO and COPD patients [12, 14, 19, 25].

Regarding gender distributions in ACO patients, some studies report a predominantly male distribution [6, 14, 16, 18, 25], and others show a predominantly female one [7, 8, 10–12, 17, 26]. The main cause of COPD is smoking, which may be affected by gender differences in smoking rates. On the other hand, exposure to biomass fuel is also a cause of COPD, and there is a large population of female patients with COPD in some regions.

In most previous studies, compared to patients with asthma or COPD alone, patients with ACO had a greater burden of symptoms, poor quality of life, rapid lung function decline, lower respiratory function, frequent exacerbations and hospitalizations, and more medical utilization. Patients with ACO reported more wheezing, coughing, and mucus production than patients with asthma or COPD [40]. de Marco et al. showed that ACO patients had higher levels of dyspnea, and the prevalence of patients with an MRC score of 3 or higher was 38.8% in ACO patients, 9.3% in asthma patients, and 20.3% in COPD patients [13]. Lange et al. showed that the annual FEV1 decline of 49.6 ml in ACO patients with late-onset asthma was greater than the annual decline of 39.5 ml in COPD patients in a long-term cohort study [42].

4.2 Exacerbations and Prognosis of ACO

Most studies have reported that the frequency of exacerbations was higher in ACO patients than in asthma [32] or COPD patients [6, 10–12, 23]. However, some other studies have shown that the frequency of exacerbations in ACO patients did not differ from that in COPD patients [14, 18, 19, 41]. In cohort studies, de Marco et al. showed that the frequency of exacerbation in ACO patients was higher than that in COPD patients [6], whereas Cosio et al. found that it was not different between ACO and COPD patients [14].

Long-term prognoses of ACO patients have been reported with conflicting results in several studies, with some showing higher mortality rates in ACO patients than in asthma or COPD patients, while others showed lower mortality rates in ACO patients than in COPD patients. Using the Danish cohort study database, Baarnes et al. reported that the all-cause mortality rate was higher in ACO patients than in those with asthma or COPD alone, particularly in women and younger ACO patients [26]. Diaz-Guzman et al. also showed that ACO patients had a higher risk of death than those with asthma or COPD only [7]. Fu et al. found that the prognosis did not differ among asthma, COPD, and ACO patients in their cohort study [43]. Sorino et al. showed that the 15-year mortality rate of ACO patients aged >65 years enrolled in the SA.R.A. (SAlute Respiratorianell' Anziano, Respiratory Health in the Elderly) study was similar to that of patients with COPD and worse than that of patients with asthma [25]. In their prospective cohort, Cosio et al. reported that patients with COPD who met ACOS criteria had a better one-year survival rate than clinically similar patients with COPD only [14]. In addition, Peltola et al. reported a 10-year survival rate of ACO patients, which was significantly better than that of COPD patients [44]. In the Hokkaido cohort study, Suzuki et al. reported that the 10-year all-cause mortality rate for COPD patients who had two or more asthma-like features was significantly lower than that for patients with one or no asthma-like features [19].

5 Conclusion

ACO patients have features of both asthma and COPD, and ACO includes patients with several clinical phenotypes that are likely caused by a range of different underlying mechanisms. Our answer to the clinical question "Does the prevalence of ACO vary among global analyses?" in this chapter is yes. This variability may be due to differences in ACO definitions, diagnostic criteria, and methodology among the studies. The results of previous studies on the prevalence of ACO varied depending on the definition and diagnostic criteria used and the evaluated populations; however, using similar definitions and diagnostic criteria, the prevalence of ACO evaluated in similar populations showed a similar prevalence rate: the prevalence of ACO was approximately 2% in the general population, 25% in asthma patients, and 30% in COPD patients. The age and gender of ACO patients were also different from those of previous studies. As to the outcome in terms of frequency of exacerbation and prognosis, the majority of previous studies reported that ACO patients had a high symptom burden and a higher frequency of exacerbations and poor prognosis than patients with asthma or COPD alone. Better strategies are needed for diagnosing and classifying ACO, and the search for reliable biomarkers is also important to determine the best treatment for ACO patients.

The GINA and GOLD have now expressed different positions on ACO. The recent publication of GOLD states, "We no longer refer to asthma & COPD overlap (ACO). Instead we emphasize that asthma and COPD are different disorders, although they may share common traits and clinical features (e.g., eosinophilia, some degree of reversibility)." It is not easy to create a universal consensus definition of and diagnostic criteria for ACO; however, it is important to carry out reliable and high-quality clinical research to clarify the exact epidemiology of ACO.

References

1. Lambrecht BN, Hammad H. The immunology of asthma. Nat Immunol. 2015;16(1):45–56. https://doi.org/10.1038/ni.3049.
2. Barnes PJ, Burney PG, Silverman EK, Celli BR, Vestbo J, Wedzicha JA, et al. Chronic obstructive pulmonary disease. Nat Rev Dis Primers. 2015;1:15076. https://doi.org/10.1038/nrdp.2015.76.
3. Gibson PG, Simpson JL. The overlap syndrome of asthma and COPD: what are its features and how important is it? Thorax. 2009;64(8):728–35. https://doi.org/10.1136/thx.2008.108027.
4. Global Initiative for Asthma (GINA). Diagnosis of disease of chronic airflow limitation: asthma, COPD and asthma-COPD overlap syndrome. 2015. https://ginasthma.org/wp-content/uploads/2019/11/GINA-GOLD-ACOS_2015.pdf. Accessed 20 Mar 2022.
5. Global Initiative for Chronic Obstructive Lung Disease (GOLD). Global strategy for the diagnosis, management, and prevention of chronic obstructive pulmonary disease; 2019. https://goldcopd.org/wp-content/uploads/2018/11/GOLD-2019-v1.7-FINAL-14Nov2018-WMS.pdf. Accessed 20 Mar 2022.
6. de Marco R, Marcon A, Rossi A, Antó JM, Cerveri I, Gislason T, et al. Asthma, COPD and overlap syndrome: a longitudinal study in young European adults. Eur Respir J. 2015;46(3):671–9. https://doi.org/10.1183/09031936.00008615.
7. Diaz-Guzman E, Khosravi M, Mannino DM. Asthma, chronic obstructive pulmonary disease, and mortality in the U.S. population. COPD. 2011;8(6):400–7. https://doi.org/10.3109/15412555.2011.611200.
8. van Boven JF, Román-Rodríguez M, Palmer JF, Toledo-Pons N, Cosío BG, Soriano JB. Comorbidome, pattern, and impact of asthma-COPD overlap syndrome in real life. Chest. 2016;149(4):1011–20. https://doi.org/10.1016/j.chest.2015.12.002.

9. Soriano JB, Davis KJ, Coleman B, Visick G, Mannino D, Pride NB. The proportional Venn diagram of obstructive lung disease: two approximations from the United States and the United Kingdom. Chest. 2003;124(2):474–81. https://doi.org/10.1378/chest.124.2.474.
10. Menezes AMB, Montes de Oca M, Pérez-Padilla R, Nadeau G, Wehrmeister FC, Lopez-Varela MV, et al. Increased risk of exacerbation and hospitalization in subjects with an overlap phenotype: COPD-asthma. Chest. 2014;145(2):297–304. https://doi.org/10.1378/chest.13-0622.
11. Hardin M, Cho M, McDonald ML, Beaty T, Ramsdell J, Bhatt S, et al. The clinical and genetic features of COPD-asthma overlap syndrome. Eur Respir J. 2014;44(2):341–50. https://doi.org/10.1183/09031936.00216013.
12. Miravitlles M, Soriano JB, Ancochea J, Muñoz L, Duran-Tauleria E, Sánchez G, et al. Characterisation of the overlap COPD-asthma phenotype. Focus on physical activity and health status. Respir Med. 2013;107(7):1053–60. https://doi.org/10.1016/j.rmed.2013.03.007.
13. de Marco R, Pesce G, Marcon A, Accordini S, Antonicelli L, Bugiani M, et al. The coexistence of asthma and chronic obstructive pulmonary disease (COPD): prevalence and risk factors in young, middle-aged and elderly people from the general population. PLoS One. 2013;8(5):e62985. https://doi.org/10.1371/journal.pone.0062985.
14. Cosio BG, Soriano JB, López-Campos JL, Calle-Rubio M, Soler-Cataluna JJ, de-Torres JP, et al. Defining the asthma-COPD overlap syndrome in a COPD cohort. Chest. 2016;149(1):45–52. https://doi.org/10.1378/chest.15-1055.
15. Alshabanat A, Zafari Z, Albanyan O, Dairi M, FitzGerald JM. Asthma and COPD overlap syndrome (ACOS): a systematic review and meta analysis. PLoS One. 2015;10(9):e0136065. https://doi.org/10.1371/journal.pone.0136065.
16. Pascoe S, Locantore N, Dransfield MT, Barnes NC, Pavord ID. Blood eosinophil counts, exacerbations, and response to the addition of inhaled fluticasone furoate to vilanterol in patients with chronic obstructive pulmonary disease: a secondary analysis of data from two parallel randomised controlled trials. Lancet Respir Med. 2015;3(6):435–42. https://doi.org/10.1016/s2213-2600(15)00106-x.
17. Ekerljung L, Mincheva R, Hagstad S, Bjerg A, Telg G, Stratelis G, et al. Prevalence, clinical characteristics and morbidity of the Asthma-COPD overlap in a general population sample. J Asthma. 2018;55(5):461–9. https://doi.org/10.1080/02770903.2017.1339799.
18. Izquierdo-Alonso JL, Rodriguez-Gonzálezmoro JM, de Lucas-Ramos P, Unzueta I, Ribera X, Antón E, et al. Prevalence and characteristics of three clinical phenotypes of chronic obstructive pulmonary disease (COPD). Respir Med. 2013;107(5):724–31. https://doi.org/10.1016/j.rmed.2013.01.001.
19. Suzuki M, Makita H, Konno S, Shimizu K, Kimura H, Kimura H, et al. Asthma-like features and clinical course of chronic obstructive pulmonary disease. An analysis from the Hokkaido COPD Cohort Study. Am J Respir Crit Care Med. 2016;194(11):1358–65. https://doi.org/10.1164/rccm.201602-0353OC.
20. Sin DD, Miravitlles M, Mannino DM, Soriano JB, Price D, Celli BR, et al. What is asthma-COPD overlap syndrome? Towards a consensus definition from a round table discussion. Eur Respir J. 2016;48(3):664–73. https://doi.org/10.1183/13993003.00436-2016.
21. Global Initiative for Chronic Obstructive Lung Disease (GOLD). Global strategy for the diagnosis, management and prevention of COPD. 2020. https://goldcopd.org/wp-content/uploads/2019/12/GOLD-2020-FINAL-ver1.2-03Dec19_WMV.pdf. Accessed 20 Mar 2022.
22. Jo YS, Lee J, Yoon HI, Kim DK, Yoo CG, Lee CH. Different prevalence and clinical characteristics of asthma-chronic obstructive pulmonary disease overlap syndrome according to accepted criteria. Ann Allergy Asthma Immunol. 2017;118(6):696–703.e1. https://doi.org/10.1016/j.anai.2017.04.010.
23. Barrecheguren M, Pinto L, Mostafavi-Pour-Manshadi SM, Tan WC, Li PZ, Aaron SD, et al. Identification and definition of asthma-COPD overlap: the CanCOLD study. Respirology. 2020;25(8):836–49. https://doi.org/10.1111/resp.13780.

24. Matsumoto K, Seki N, Fukuyama S, Moriwaki A, Kan-o K, Matsunaga Y, et al. Prevalence of asthma with airflow limitation, COPD, and COPD with variable airflow limitation in older subjects in a general Japanese population: the Hisayama Study. Respir Investig. 2015;53(1):22–9. https://doi.org/10.1016/j.resinv.2014.08.002.
25. Sorino C, Pedone C, Scichilone N. Fifteen-year mortality of patients with asthma-COPD overlap syndrome. Eur J Intern Med. 2016;34:72–7. https://doi.org/10.1016/j.ejim.2016.06.020.
26. Baarnes CB, Andersen ZJ, Tjønneland A, Ulrik CS. Incidence and long-term outcome of severe asthma-COPD overlap compared to asthma and COPD alone: a 35-year prospective study of 57,053 middle-aged adults. Int J Chron Obstruct Pulmon Dis. 2017;12:571–9. https://doi.org/10.2147/copd.S123167.
27. Mendy A, Forno E, Niyonsenga T, Carnahan R, Gasana J. Prevalence and features of asthma-COPD overlap in the United States 2007–2012. Clin Respir J. 2018;12(8):2369–77. https://doi.org/10.1111/crj.12917.
28. Morgan BW, Grigsby MR, Siddharthan T, Chowdhury M, Rubinstein A, Gutierrez L, et al. Epidemiology and risk factors of asthma-chronic obstructive pulmonary disease overlap in low- and middle-income countries. J Allergy Clin Immunol. 2019;143(4):1598–606. https://doi.org/10.1016/j.jaci.2018.06.052.
29. Hosseini M, Almasi-Hashiani A, Sepidarkish M, Maroufizadeh S. Global prevalence of asthma-COPD overlap (ACO) in the general population: a systematic review and meta-analysis. Respir Res. 2019;20(1):229. https://doi.org/10.1186/s12931-019-1198-4.
30. Kumbhare S, Pleasants R, Ohar JA, Strange C. Characteristics and prevalence of asthma/Chronic obstructive pulmonary disease overlap in the United States. Ann Am Thorac Soc. 2016;13(6):803–10. https://doi.org/10.1513/AnnalsATS.201508-554OC.
31. Harada T, Yamasaki A, Fukushima T, Hashimoto K, Takata M, Kodani M, et al. Causes of death in patients with asthma and asthma-chronic obstructive pulmonary disease overlap syndrome. Int J Chron Obstruct Pulmon Dis. 2015;10:595–602. https://doi.org/10.2147/copd.S77491.
32. Milanese M, Di Marco F, Corsico AG, Rolla G, Sposato B, Chieco-Bianchi F, et al. Asthma control in elderly asthmatics. An Italian observational study. Respir Med. 2014;108(8):1091–9. https://doi.org/10.1016/j.rmed.2014.05.016.
33. Inoue H, Nagase T, Morita S, Yoshida A, Jinnai T, Ichinose M. Prevalence and characteristics of asthma-COPD overlap syndrome identified by a stepwise approach. Int J Chron Obstruct Pulmon Dis. 2017;12:1803–10. https://doi.org/10.2147/copd.S133859.
34. Toledo-Pons N, van Boven JFM, Román-Rodríguez M, Pérez N, Valera Felices JL, Soriano JB, et al. ACO: time to move from the description of different phenotypes to the treatable traits. PLoS One. 2019;14(1):e0210915. https://doi.org/10.1371/journal.pone.0210915.
35. Jo YS, Hwang YI, Yoo KH, Lee MG, Jung KS, Shin KC, et al. Racial differences in prevalence and clinical characteristics of asthma-chronic obstructive pulmonary disease overlap. Front Med (Lausanne). 2021;8:780438. https://doi.org/10.3389/fmed.2021.780438.
36. Hashimoto S, Sorimachi R, Jinnai T, Ichinose M. Asthma and chronic obstructive pulmonary disease overlap according to the Japanese respiratory society diagnostic criteria: the prospective, observational ACO Japan cohort study. Adv Ther. 2021;38(2):1168–84. https://doi.org/10.1007/s12325-020-01573-x.
37. Kiljander T, Helin T, Venho K, Jaakkola A, Lehtimäki L. Prevalence of asthma-COPD overlap syndrome among primary care asthmatics with a smoking history: a cross-sectional study. NPJ Prim Care Respir Med. 2015;25:15047. https://doi.org/10.1038/npjpcrm.2015.47.
38. Lee H, Kim SH, Kim BK, Lee Y, Lee HY, Ban GY, et al. Characteristics of specialist-diagnosed asthma-COPD overlap in severe asthma: observations from the Korean Severe Asthma Registry (KoSAR). Allergy. 2021;76(1):223–32. https://doi.org/10.1111/all.14483.
39. Krishnan JA, Nibber A, Chisholm A, Price D, Bateman ED, Bjermer L, et al. Prevalence and characteristics of asthma-chronic obstructive pulmonary disease overlap in routine primary care practices. Ann Am Thorac Soc. 2019;16(9):1143–50. https://doi.org/10.1513/AnnalsATS.201809-607OC.

40. Senthilselvan A, Beach J. Characteristics of asthma and COPD overlap syndrome (ACOS) in the Canadian population. J Asthma. 2019;56(11):1129–37. https://doi.org/10.1080/02770903.2018.1531997.
41. Kobayashi S, Hanagama M, Ishida M, Ono M, Sato H, Yamanda S, et al. Clinical characteristics and outcomes of patients with asthma-COPD overlap in Japanese patients with COPD. Int J Chron Obstruct Pulmon Dis. 2020;15:2923–9. https://doi.org/10.2147/copd.S276314.
42. Lange P, Çolak Y, Ingebrigtsen TS, Vestbo J, Marott JL. Long-term prognosis of asthma, chronic obstructive pulmonary disease, and asthma-chronic obstructive pulmonary disease overlap in the Copenhagen City Heart study: a prospective population-based analysis. Lancet Respir Med. 2016;4(6):454–62. https://doi.org/10.1016/s2213-2600(16)00098-9.
43. Fu JJ, Gibson PG, Simpson JL, McDonald VM. Longitudinal changes in clinical outcomes in older patients with asthma, COPD and asthma-COPD overlap syndrome. Respiration. 2014;87(1):63–74. https://doi.org/10.1159/000352053.
44. Peltola L, Pätsi H, Harju T. COPD comorbidities predict high mortality—asthma-COPD-overlap has better prognosis. COPD. 2020;17(4):366–72. https://doi.org/10.1080/15412555.2020.1783647.

Chapter 4
Epidemiology of ACO Defined by the JRS Guidelines: What Is the Prevalence of ACO in Japan?

Kuniaki Hirai and Hiroyuki Nagase

Abstract The Japanese Respiratory Society (JRS) published the first guideline in Japan for asthma–chronic obstructive pulmonary disease (COPD) overlap (ACO) in 2018. Distinguishing between COPD, asthma, and ACO is clinically important because of the different treatment strategies based on the diagnosis. The JRS ACO guidelines, which include several inflammatory indices, are detailed; however, the prevalence of ACO based on the JRS guidelines remained not fully analyzed.

Six studies can be used to investigate prevalence based on the JRS guidelines. In summary, 19.3–44.7% of patients with COPD were diagnosed with ACO. Additionally, asthma diagnosis before the age of 40 years has resulted in ACO diagnosis in patients with COPD (84.0–100%). Only two studies have investigated the prevalence of ACO among patients with asthma, reporting 31.3% and 55.5%, respectively, and requiring further study.

The prevalence of ACO varied depending on the study population, but all reports indicated a certain proportion of patients with ACO diagnosed according to the JRS guidelines. Physicians should actively identify ACO in patients with both COPD and asthma who can be optimally treated with additional inhaled corticosteroids and long-acting muscarinic antagonists.

Keywords Asthma–COPD overlap · Epidemiology · Japanese Respiratory Society guidelines · Prevalence

K. Hirai
Department of Medicine, Division of Respiratory Medicine and Allergology, Showa University School of Medicine, Tokyo, Japan

H. Nagase (✉)
Division of Respiratory Medicine and Allergology, Department of Medicine, Teikyo University School of Medicine, Tokyo, Japan
e-mail: nagaseh@med.teikyo-u.ac.jp

H. Nagase et al. (eds.), *Asthma-COPD Overlap*, Respiratory Disease Series: Diagnostic Tools and Disease Managements,
https://doi.org/10.1007/978-981-96-0217-9_4

1 Introduction

The Japanese Respiratory Society (JRS) published the first guideline in Japan for diagnosing asthma–chronic obstructive pulmonary disease (COPD) overlap (ACO), which combines the pathophysiology of asthma and COPD, in 2018 [1]. The diagnostic criteria for ACO in JRS contain more items to be evaluated than other diagnostic criteria adopted in clinical studies (Table 4.1). Several ACO diagnostic criteria recommend achieving the asthma component in a single item, such as an asthma history or a positive blood eosinophils criteria, whereas JRS requires the satisfaction of multiple items (see Chap. 1). Therefore, the prevalence of ACO according to the JRS guidelines is expected to differ from that of other diagnostic criteria. However, no report summarized the prevalence of ACO using the JRS diagnostic criteria.

Distinguishing between COPD and ACO is clinically important. The Japanese COPD guideline does not recommend the initial use of inhaled corticosteroids (ICS) for patients with COPD but proposes using ICS for patients with ACO;

Table 4.1 Diagnostic criteria for ACO in clinical studies

	Study design	Prevalence of ACO	Definition of ACO, asthma, and COPD
Pascoe et al. [17]	COPD Age: >40 years	66%	ACO: Blood eosinophil count of >2% and COPD
Cosio et al. [18]	COPD Cohort Age: >35 years	15.0%	ACO: COPD+ 2 or 1 major and 2 minor criteriaMajor: Self-reported history of asthma Reversibility: FEV1 change of >15% and 400 mL Minor: IgE of >100 IU Self-reported history of atopy 2 separated reversibility of >12% and 200 mL Blood eosinophil count of >5%
van Boven et al. [19]	Obstructive Airway diseases (OAD) Age: >18 years	7.4% in OAD 19.3% in COPD	ACO: Combination of asthma and COPD Asthma: physician diagnosis on the medical record COPD: physician diagnosis on the medical record
Menezes et al. [20]	General population Age >40 years	1.8%	ACO: post-BD FEV1/FVC of <70% and Reversibility (12% and 200-mL change in FEV1)
Hardin et al. [21]	COPD Age: 45–80 years	12.6%	ACO: Combination of self-reported physician diagnosis of asthma before the age of 40 years and COPD
Suzuki et al. [22]	COPD Cohort Age: >40 years	49.7%	ACO: post-BD FEV1/FVC <70% and COPD and Reversibility: 12% and 200-mL change in FEV1 Blood eosinophil count of 300 cells/μL, or the presence of at least one specific serum IgE

therefore, the treatment strategies for COPD and ACO greatly vary [2]. ICS has reduced the risk of acute exacerbations in some patients with COPD; however, ICS increases the risk of various comorbidities such as pneumonia and osteoporosis [3–6]. Acute exacerbations are less frequent in Japanese patients with COPD than in other countries [7]. Additionally, aging [7] and low body mass index [8, 9], which are risk factors for pneumonia due to ICS, are more prevalent in Japanese patients. Therefore, the balance between the advantages and disadvantages of ICS should be carefully considered, especially in Japan [10]. The differential diagnosis between asthma and ACO is crucial because the ACO guidelines of JRS recommend the use of ICS + long-acting beta agonist + long-acting muscarinic antagonist (LAMA) [1], and ACO diagnosis will increase the chances of prescribing LAMA in patients with asthma.

JRS's ACO guidelines are very detailed, and fully assessing the diagnosis of ACO in all patients with COPD and asthma in real-world settings may be difficult. Therefore, investigating the prevalence of ACO by JRS guidelines will help clinicians decide on evaluating ACO if the prevalence is high. Six available studies estimate the epidemiology of ACO using the JRS guidelines, and this chapter summarizes the prevalence of ACO in patients with COPD or asthma by reviewing the literature.

2 Prevalence and Characteristics of ACO Among Patients with COPD

2.1 *Reported Prevalence of ACO Among Patients with COPD Based on JRS Guidelines*

Diagnosing ACO among patients with COPD is important because ICS should be administered to all patients with ACO but not to patients with pure COPD [2]. This chapter focuses on the prevalence of ACO among patients with COPD based on the JRS guidelines.

Nagase et al. reported the prevalence of ACO and its characteristics in patients with COPD, focusing on serum immunoglobulin E (IgE) (Table 4.2) [11]. Of the 76 patients with COPD, 44.7% were diagnosed with ACO. Patients with ACO were more likely to be positive for House dust and *D. pteronyssinus*-specific IgE antibodies, and more of those with higher IgE classes may be diagnosed with ACO. The probability of being ACO is >60% if both specific IgE antibodies are classified as 1 or 2, and the probability of being ACO is ≥80% in class 3 or higher. An active survey for ACO diagnosis should be performed when specific antibodies for House dust or *D. pteronyssinus*, commonly measured in routine practice, are positive in patients with COPD.

Table 4.2 Participants' background in studies evaluating the prevalence of ACO

Study	Participants	N	Prevalence of ACO	ICS user (%)	Blood eosinophil Count (%)	Total IgE (IU/mL)	FeNO (ppb)
Nagase [11]	COPD	76	44.7%	19.7%	231 ± 167 (3.6 ± 2.5)	310.4 ± 487.7	26.4 ± 16.1
Hashimoto et al. [12]	COPD	396	25.5%	45.5%	241.1 ± 277.9 (3.8 ± 3.8)	415.1 ± 837.9	27.4 ± 23.5
Yamamura et al. [13]	Airflow limitation	170	30.6%	No data	237.8 ± 257.6 (No data)	298 (7–8632)	31.7 ± 26.4
Hirai et al. [14]	COPD	197	19.3%	0.0%	198.1 ± 153.1 (3.2 ± 2.1)	282.3 ± 546.1	28.7 ± 21.6
Tanaka [15]	Asthma	211	31.3%	94.8%	369.6 ± 343.9 (5.9 ± 5.1)	889.2 ± 1997.5	54.8 ± 44.8
Ishikawa et al. [16]	Severe asthma	20	55.0%	100.0%	497.8 ± 147.5 (6.6 ± 1.2)	1731.5 ± 1245.2	No data

Hashimoto et al. is currently conducting a prospective cohort study of ACO in 708 patients with COPD [12]. This observational study revealed that data at enrollment indicated that 396 of 708 patients with COPD were evaluated for ACO, of which 101 (25.5%) were diagnosed with ACO (Table 4.2). Of the 396 patients evaluated for ACO, 76.5% of patients with ACO were treated by ICS and 36.3% of patients with no ACO received ICS. This result revealed that 23.5% of patients with ACO were not prescribed ICS and 36.3% of non-ACO COPD patients were prescribed ICS, which may potentially limit the efficacy. This study reveals that assessing ACO can provide a more appropriate treatment for patients with COPD.

Yamamura et al. retrospectively analyzed 1348 patients who visited the outpatient department of respiratory medicine [13]. Among the 170 patients with persistent airflow limitation, 111 were evaluated according to JRS's ACO guidelines, and 34 (30.6%) were diagnosed with ACO (Table 4.2). This study revealed a different prevalence of ACO from the actual prevalence because the study population included patients with asthma with persistent airflow limitation.

Hirai et al. investigated the prevalence of ACO in patients with COPD who were not prescribed ICS (Table 4.2) [14]. Of the 197 patients with COPD, 38 were diagnosed with ACO, indicating that ICS was necessary in approximately 20% of the patients whose respiratory physicians had assumed that ICS was unnecessary.

We attributed the differences in the prevalence of ACO in the above studies to variations in participant characteristics. In particular, Nagase reported a higher proportion of ACO among patients with COPD than Hirai [11, 14]. Additionally, Nagase reported higher peripheral blood eosinophils and total IgE than Hirai, indicating that more patients with features of type 2 inflammation were included in Nagase's study (Table 4.2). In contrast, Hirai excluded ICS-treated COPD, which may have resulted in the exclusion of patients with COPD with type 2 inflammation.

Summarizing the above four studies, 19.3–44.7% of patients with COPD were diagnosed with ACO according to the JRS criteria. An active survey for ACO in patients with COPD is highly recommended based on the considerably high prevalence of ACO among patients with COPD.

2.2 *Impact of History of Asthma Before the Age of 40 Years on Diagnosing ACO Among Patients with COPD*

One of the diagnostic criteria for JRS's ACO guidelines is a history of asthma before the age of 40 years. It is an extremely easy evaluation item that can be confirmed only by interview and is frequently used in other ACO diagnostic criteria (Table 4.1).

Interestingly, Hashimoto [12] reported that 23 of the 24 patients (95.8%) who were diagnosed with asthma before the age of 40 were classified as ACO. Additionally, Hirai [14] reported that 14 out of 15 patients with COPD (93.3%) who were pointed out to have asthma before the age of 40 years had ACO. Moreover, Yamamura reported that 18 of 18 patients with COPD who had asthma before age 40 had ACO (100%) [13]. Nagase revealed that 21 of 25 patients diagnosed with asthma before the age of 40 years had ACO (84.0%). Thus, according to the JRS diagnostic criteria for ACO, a history of asthma diagnosis before the age of 40 years was very likely to be ACO in patients with COPD (84.0–100%). An active survey for ACO should be performed if a patient with COPD has a history of asthma before the age of 40 years, or an ICS prescription should be considered if scrutiny for ACO cannot be performed. Conversely, Hashimoto et al. investigated the influence of a history of asthma diagnosis "after" the age of 40 years on ACO diagnosis. Of the 151 patients with a history of asthma diagnosis after age 40 years, 44 had ACO (28.8%), indicating a lower probability of ACO than that of a history of asthma diagnosis before age 40 years.

2.3 Impact of FeNO and Variable Respiratory Symptoms on Diagnosing ACO Among Patients with COPD

FeNO of >35 ppb and the presence of variable or paroxysmal respiratory symptoms are the major criteria for the characteristics of asthma in the ACO guidelines of JRS, in addition to asthma diagnosis before the age of 40 years. The proportion of patients with ACO with FeNO of >35 ppb was 13 of 33 (39.4%), 16 of 86 (18.6%), 27 of 41 (65.9%), and 22 of 24 (91.7%) reported by report Nagase, Hashimoto, Hirai, and Yamamura, respectively, indicating the variable impact of FeNO on the diagnosis.

Among patients with COPD with the presence of variable or paroxysmal respiratory symptoms, Hashimoto, Hirai, and Yamamura revealed that 42 of 126 patients (33.3%), 18 of 30 patients (60.0%), and 23 of 27 patients (85.2%) had ACO, indicating the variable impact of the presence of variable or paroxysmal respiratory symptoms on the diagnosis, revealing a higher impact of history of asthma diagnosis before age 40 years as compared to FeNO or variable symptoms.

2.4 Comparison of the Clinical Characteristics of ACO and COPD Based on JRS Diagnostic Criteria

No statistically significant difference was observed, but Nagase, Yamamura, and Hirai reported that patients with ACO had lower %FEV1 than those with COPD. Hashimoto revealed slightly higher %FEV1 in patients with ACO than those with COPD. Hirai indicated that patients with ACO had a worse COPD Assessment Test (CAT) score than those with COPD (15.5 vs. 11.0; $P = 0.02$) and a worse mMRC score (1.6 vs. 1.2; $P < 0.01$). Conversely, Hashimoto reported no significant difference in scores of CAT (10.7 vs. 10.1) and mMRC (1.0 vs. 1.1) between patients with ACO and COPD. The reason for the differences in subjective symptoms among patients with ACO, despite the use of identical diagnostic criteria, may be the usage rate of ICS in patients with ACO. Hirai revealed that all patients with ACO did not use ICS, whereas Hashimoto indicated that 76.5% of patients with ACO used ICS. Patients with ACO without ICS may be more symptomatic than those with COPD, and subjective symptoms may not differ between patients with ACO and COPD with ICS.

3 Prevalence of ACO Among Patients with Asthma

Only two studies have investigated the prevalence of ACO according to the JRS guidelines in patients with asthma. Tanaka retrospectively revealed that 66 of 211 patients with asthma (31.3%) were diagnosed with ACO (Table 4.2) [15]. However, the actual prevalence of ACO in patients with asthma may be higher because not all patients have undergone the chest CT scan or DLco testing. Ishikawa et al. revealed that 11 of 20 (55.5%) patients with severe asthma treated by mepolizumab over the age of 65 years had ACO (Table 4.2) [16]), revealing the potentially high prevalence of ACO among elderly patients with severe asthma and the need for a survey of ACO in such patients to determine the optimal prescription of LAMA. However, the prevalence of ACO in asthma has remained insufficiently investigated so far, and further research results are warranted.

4 Conclusion

Prevalence rates varied based on the study, but all reports indicated a certain proportion of patients with ACO based on the JRS criteria. The treatment strategy differs depending on ACO diagnosis among patients with COPD or asthma; thus, active survey for ACO is strongly recommended for patients with obstructive lung diseases.

References

1. Japanese Respiratory Society. [The JRS guidelines for the management of ACO 2018]. Tokyo: Medical Review; 2018 (in Japanese).
2. Japanese Respiratory Society. [The JRS guidelines for the management of chronic obstructive pulmonary disease 2018]. Tokyo: Medical Review; 2018 (in Japanese).
3. Suissa S, Dell'Aniello S, Ernst P. Comparative effects of LAMA-LABA-ICS vs LAMA-LABA for COPD: cohort study in real-world clinical practice. Chest. 2020;157(4):846–55.
4. Suissa S, Dell'Aniello S, Ernst P. Comparative effectiveness and safety of LABA-LAMA vs LABA-ICS treatment of COPD in real-world clinical practice. Chest. 2019;155(6):1158–65.

5. Janson C, Lisspers K, Ställberg B, Johansson G, Gutzwiller FS, Mezzi K, Mindeholm L, Bjerregaard BK, Jorgensen L, Larsson K. Osteoporosis and fracture risk associated with inhaled corticosteroid use among Swedish COPD patients: the ARCTIC study. Eur Respir J. 2021;57(2):2000515.
6. Chiu KL, Lee CC, Chen CY. Evaluating the association of osteoporosis with in-haled corticosteroid use in chronic obstructive pulmonary disease in Taiwan. Sci Rep. 2021;11(1):724.
7. Ishii T, Nishimura M, Akimoto A, James MH, Jones P. Understanding low COPD exacerbation rates in Japan: a review and comparison with other countries. Int J Chron Obstruct Pulmon Dis. 2018;13:3459–71.
8. Crim C, Dransfield MT, Bourbeau J, Jones PW, Hanania NA, Mahler DA, Vestbo J, Wachtel A, Martinez FJ, Barnhart F, Lettis S, Calverley PM. Pneumonia risk with in-haled fluticasone furoate and vilanterol compared with vilanterol alone in patients with COPD. Ann Am Thorac Soc. 2015;12(1):27–34.
9. Crim C, Calverley PM, Anderson JA, Celli B, Ferguson GT, Jenkins C, Jones PW, Willits LR, Yates JC, Vestbo J. Pneumonia risk in COPD patients receiving inhaled corticosteroids alone or in combination: TORCH study results. Eur Respir J. 2009;34(3):641–7.
10. Agusti A, Fabbri LM, Singh D, Vestbo J, Celli B, Franssen FME, Rabe KF, Papi A. Inhaled corticosteroids in COPD: friend or foe? Eur Respir J. 2018;52(6):1801219.
11. Toyota H, Sugimoto N, Kobayashi K, Suzuki Y, Takeshita Y, Ito A, Ujino M, Tomyo F, Sakasegawa H, Koizumi Y, Kuramochi M, Yamaguchi M, Nagase H. Comprehensive analysis of allergen-specific IgE in COPD: mite-specific IgE specifically related to the diagnosis of asthma-COPD overlap. Allergy Asthma Clin Immunol. 2021;17(1):13.
12. Hashimoto S, Sorimachi R, Jinnai T, Ichinose M. Asthma and chronic obstructive pulmonary disease overlap according to the Japanese respiratory society diagnostic criteria: the prospective, observational ACO Japan cohort study. Adv Ther. 2021;38(2):1168–84.
13. Yamamura K, Hara J, Kobayashi T, Ohkura N, Abo M, Akasaki K, Nomura S, Yuasa M, Saeki K, Terada N, Matsuoka H, Tambo Y, Nishikawa S, Sone T, Kimura H, Kasahara K. The prevalence and clinical features of asthma-COPD overlap (ACO) definitively diagnosed according to the Japanese Respiratory Society Guidelines for the Management of ACO 2018. J Med Invest. 2019;66(1.2):157–64.
14. Hirai K, Tanaka A, Homma T, Kawahara T, Oda N, Mikuni H, Uchida Y, Uno T, Miyata Y, Inoue H, Ohta S, Yamaguchi F, Suzuki S, Sagara H. Prevalence and clinical features of asthma-COPD overlap in patients with COPD not using inhaled corticosteroids. Allergol Int. 2021;70(1):134–5.
15. Sato H, Tanaka A, Hirai K, Ebato T, Inoue H, Homma T, Ohta S, Suzuki S, Sagara H. A comparative study of asthma with airflow limitation and asthma-COPD overlap using the forced oscillation technique. Showa Univ J Med Sci. 2021;3(32):25–33.
16. Isoyama S, Ishikawa N, Hamai K, Matsumura M, Kobayashi H, Nomura A, Ueno S, Tanimoto T, Maeda H, Iwamoto H, Hattori N. Efficacy of mepolizumab in elderly patients with severe asthma and overlapping COPD in real-world settings: a retrospective observational study. Respir Investig. 2021;59(4):478–86.
17. Pascoe S, Locantore N, Dransfield MT, Barnes NC, Pavord ID. Blood eosinophil counts, exacerbations, and response to the addition of inhaled fluticasone furoate to vilanterol in patients with chronic obstructive pulmonary disease: a secondary analysis of data from two parallel randomised controlled trials. Lancet Respir Med. 2015;3(6):435–42.
18. Cosio BG, Soriano JB, López-Campos JL, Calle-Rubio M, Soler-Cataluna JJ, de-Torres JP, Marín JM, Martínez-Gonzalez C, de Lucas P, Mir I, Peces-Barba G, Feu-Collado N, Solanes I, Alfageme I, Casanova C, CHAIN Study. Defining the asthma-COPD overlap syndrome in a COPD cohort. Chest. 2016;149(1):45–52.
19. van Boven JF, Román-Rodríguez M, Palmer JF, Toledo-Pons N, Cosío BG, So-riano JB. Comorbidome, pattern, and impact of asthma-COPD overlap syndrome in real life. Chest. 2016;149(4):1011–20.

20. Menezes AMB, Montes de Oca M, Pérez-Padilla R, Nadeau G, Wehrmeister FC, Lopez-Varela MV, Muiño A, JRB J, Valdivia G, Tálamo C, PLATINO Team. In-creased risk of exacerbation and hospitalization in subjects with an overlap phenotype: COPD-asthma. Chest. 2014;145(2):297–304.
21. Hardin M, Cho M, McDonald ML, Beaty T, Ramsdell J, Bhatt S, van Beek EJ, Make BJ, Crapo JD, Silverman EK, Hersh CP. The clinical and genetic features of COPD-asthma overlap syndrome. Eur Respir J. 2014;44(2):341–50.
22. Suzuki M, Makita H, Konno S, Shimizu K, Kimura H, Kimura H, Nishimura M, Hokkaido COPD Cohort Study Investigators. Asthma-like features and clinical course of chronic obstructive pulmonary disease. An analysis from the Hokkaido COPD cohort study. Am J Respir Crit Care Med. 2016;194(11):1358–65.

Chapter 5
Prognosis and Characteristics of ACO: What Are the Specific Characteristics of ACO?

Seiichi Kobayashi

Abstract Asthma–chronic obstructive pulmonary disease (COPD) overlap (ACO) is not a single disease entity but rather includes several different clinical phenotypes reflecting different underlying mechanisms. ACO is a clinical description of patients with persistent airflow limitation and clinical features consistent with both asthma and COPD. Patients with ACO are younger than those with COPD but older than those with asthma. Patients with ACO have a shorter smoking history and a higher body mass index than patients with COPD. Patients with ACO have been recognized to have a greater burden of symptoms, poorer quality of life, more frequent exacerbations, and higher mortality than those with asthma or COPD alone. However, the findings of several recent studies have been controversial. Inflammatory biomarkers, including fractional exhaled nitric oxide, blood eosinophil count, and total immunoglobulin E levels, are significantly higher in patients with ACO than in those with COPD alone. The difference in maintenance therapy, such as inhaled corticosteroids, could result in disagreement of outcomes in ACO. ACO may not be associated with poor clinical features or outcomes in patients with COPD if appropriate and adequate treatment is administered.

Keywords Asthma · Asthma–COPD overlap (ACO) · COPD · Exacerbations · Mortality

S. Kobayashi (✉)
Department of Respiratory Medicine, Japanese Red Cross Ishinomaki Hospital, Ishinomaki, Japan
e-mail: skoba-thk@umin.ac.jp

H. Nagase et al. (eds.), *Asthma-COPD Overlap*, Respiratory Disease Series: Diagnostic Tools and Disease Managements,
https://doi.org/10.1007/978-981-96-0217-9_5

1 Introduction

Asthma and chronic obstructive pulmonary disease (COPD) show different patterns of clinical features and have been regarded as two distinct entities [1, 2], but some patients present with features of both asthma and COPD [3]. The term asthma–COPD overlap (ACO) was introduced to describe these patients.

Since the Global Initiative for Asthma (GINA) and the Global Initiative for Chronic Obstructive Lung Disease (GOLD) issued a joint document describing asthma–COPD overlap syndrome (ACOS) in 2014, the clinical characteristics and outcomes of this overlap have attracted interest. The word "syndrome" was removed from ACOS to become "ACO" because it is not a single disease entity but rather includes several different clinical phenotypes reflecting different underlying mechanisms. ACO is now considered a clinical description for patients with persistent airflow limitation and clinical features consistent with both asthma and COPD [1]. Therefore, controversial issues exist regarding its concept and clinical manifestations.

Patients with ACO have been recognized to have a greater burden of symptoms, poorer quality of life (QOL), more frequent exacerbations, higher mortality, and greater use of healthcare resources than those with asthma or COPD alone. However, the findings of several recent studies have been controversial.

In this review, the clinical manifestations and outcomes of ACO are described, focusing on specific characteristics and prognoses compared with those of asthma or COPD.

2 Clinical Manifestations of ACO

2.1 Patient Characteristics

A systematic review and meta-analysis showed that patients with ACO were significantly younger than patients with COPD and older than those with asthma [4]. Patients with ACO had a shorter smoking history and a higher body mass index than those with COPD. No significant difference was found in sex and smoking status (active, ex, or never smoker) between patients with ACO and those with COPD. Patients with ACO tended to use more medications, including inhaled corticosteroids (ICS).

2.2 Symptoms and Health-Related QOL

Patients with ACO have more dyspnea than those with only asthma [5, 6] or COPD [5, 7–10]. Patients with ACO have more wheezing than patients with COPD alone [5, 7–9]. More cases of cough and phlegm have also been reported compared with

COPD [5, 7]. Health-related QOL is lower in patients with ACO than in patients with asthma [11] or COPD alone [7–10, 12].

A case-control study was conducted by de Marco et al. in the frame of the Gene Environment Interaction in Respiratory Diseases Project [5]. Among 8360 general Italian population aged 20–84 years, the prevalence of ACO was 1.6%, 2.1%, and 4.5% in the 20–44, 45–64, and 65–84 age groups, respectively. A higher prevalence of dyspnea, which was evaluated using the Medical Research Council (MRC) dyspnea scale (score ≥3), was observed in the ACO group (38.8%) compared with the COPD (20.8%) and asthma groups (9.3%). Patients in the ACO group were more likely to have cough or phlegm (overlap, 61.7%; COPD, 54%; asthma, 23.1%) and wheezing (overlap, 78.7%; COPD, 42.7%; asthma, 43.4%).

Milanese et al. conducted the Elderly Subjects with Asthma study, a multicenter observational study performed in 16 Italian pulmonology and allergy clinics [6]. A total of 350 elderly patients with asthma aged >64 years were enrolled over 6 months, and 101 patients were classified as having ACO. The ACO group showed a higher modified MRC (mMRC) dyspnea score than the asthma group ($P = 0.010$).

Menezes et al. [7] analyzed data from the Latin American Project for the Investigation of Obstructive Lung Disease study, a multicenter population-based survey conducted in five Latin American cities. Of the 5044 subjects, 767 were classified as having COPD ($n = 594$), asthma ($n = 84$), or ACO ($n = 89$). The prevalence of cough and phlegm was higher in the ACO group (50.6% and 42.7%, respectively) than in the asthma group (41.7% and 39.3%, respectively) or COPD group (27.4% and 25.4%, respectively) ($P < 0.001$). The ACO group showed more dyspnea than the COPD group (65.2% vs. 47.4%, $P < 0.010$). Wheezing was equally observed by all patients with asthma and overlap syndrome (both 100%), whereas it was significantly lower in patients with COPD (29.3%, $P < 0.001$). After adjusting for confounders, ACO was associated with a worse self-reported general health status than COPD.

Miravitlles et al. conducted an epidemiological, cross-sectional, population-based study at 11 centers throughout Spain, which included 3885 adults aged 40–80 years [8]. A total of 385 patients were classified as having COPD, and 67 of them were classified as having asthma overlap. Miravitlles et al. found that the overlap group had a higher prevalence of dyspnea than the COPD group ($P < 0.001$). Patients with overlapping phenotypes were also more likely to report wheezing compared with the COPD group (92.5% vs. 58.2%, $P < 0.001$). By contrast, the proportion of patients reporting cough and sputum production did not differ between those with asthma and COPD overlap and those with COPD. This overlap phenotype significantly worsened health-related QOL as evaluated using the St. George's Respiratory Questionnaire (SGRQ).

The evaluation of COPD longitudinally to identify predictive surrogate endpoints study, which was a 3-year non-interventional longitudinal prospective cohort study, was conducted at 46 centers in 12 countries [9]. Among the 1976 patients with COPD, 493 (25%) had ACO. Patients with ACO showed more dyspnea

(60% vs. 51%, $P < 0.01$) and wheezing (89% vs. 72%, $P < 0.01$), whereas the presence of cough (52% vs. 52%) and phlegm (64% vs. 63%) was not significant. After adjusting for age, sex, baseline forced expiratory volume in 1 s (FEV_1), and prior exacerbation history, the SGRQ total score was higher, indicating lower QOL in patients with ACO.

Barrecheguren et al. analyzed data from the Canadian Cohort Obstructive Lung Disease [10]. This was a prospective, multicenter study that recruited 1561 patients with COPD, smokers with normal post-bronchodilator spirometry, and healthy controls. Patients with ACO presented more dyspnea with an MRC score ≥3 compared with patients without ACO (13.8% vs. 5.3%, $P < 0.05$). For all ACO definitions, the mean score of the COPD assessment test (CAT), which is an eight-item questionnaire with possible scores ranging from 0 to 40, with higher scores indicating worse QOL, was higher. Moreover, symptomatic patients with CAT scores ≥10 were also significantly higher. Similarly, individuals with ACO had significantly worse SGRQ scores. Worse physical QOL was evaluated using the 36-Item Short Form Survey.

By contrast, the findings of several studies in Japan differ from the results of the aforementioned studies.

Inoue et al. conducted a multicenter, cross-sectional, observational study that enrolled outpatients receiving medical treatment for COPD in Japan [13]. Of the 1008 patients with stable COPD, 167 (16.6%) had syndromic features of ACO. Patients identified as having ACO were of significantly younger age, had a shorter duration of COPD, lower number of pack-years, better lung function, and milder dyspnea symptoms than patients with COPD alone.

Kobayashi et al. conducted a prospective cohort study analyzing data from community-dwelling outpatients with COPD enrolled in the Ishinomaki COPD Network [14]. Patients with features of asthma who had a history of respiratory symptoms that varied over time and intensity, together with documented variable expiratory airflow limitation, were identified and then defined as having ACO. Among the 387 patients with COPD, 41 (10.6%) were identified as having ACO. Patients with ACO tended to be younger, have a higher body mass index, have a shorter smoking history, and use more respiratory medications, particularly ICS. The lung function, mMRC score, and CAT score did not differ between the groups.

Hirai et al. recently conducted a multicenter, cross-sectional study of COPD and investigated the clinical features of patients with ACO treated without ICS [15]. A total of 197 patients with COPD were included in this study, and 38 (19.3%) met the ACO diagnostic criteria, according to the Japanese guidelines. No statistical differences were found in age, sex, smoking habit, pack-years, respiratory function, and respiratory medication between patients with ACO and those with COPD only. However, statistically significant differences were noted in the CAT and mMRC scores between the ACO and COPD-only groups. The results of this study indicated that ICS-naïve patients have more respiratory symptoms.

2.3 Physiology

Pulmonary function testing is performed to diagnose and evaluate airflow limitation in obstructive pulmonary diseases, including asthma and COPD. FEV_1 measured using spirometry showed disease severity. Several studies have demonstrated lower FEV_1 in patients with ACO than in patients with asthma [6, 7, 16]. By contrast, some studies reported lower [7, 8, 10, 16, 17], whereas others reported similar values [9, 12] in patients with ACO compared with those with COPD alone.

The diffusing capacity of the lungs for carbon monoxide (DLCO) measures the ability of the lungs to transfer gas from inhaled air into the alveoli. DLCO is decreased in patients with emphysema but tends to be normal or high in patients with asthma. DLCO was similar between patients with ACO and those with COPD [18] but was significantly reduced compared with patients with asthma [19].

Lange et al. reported a decline in lung function by analyzing data from the Copenhagen City Heart Study [20]. The multivariable-adjusted decline in FEV_1 in ACO with early-onset asthma was 27.3 mL/year, which did not differ significantly from the decline of 20.9 mL/year in healthy never-smokers. FEV_1 decline in individuals with ACO with late-onset asthma was 49.6 mL/year, which was higher than the decline in ACO with early-onset asthma ($P = 0.0001$), the decline of 39.5 mL/year in COPD ($P = 0.003$), and the decline in healthy never-smokers ($P < 0.0001$).

Exercise tolerance and daily physical activity progressively decreased as COPD progressed. The 6-minute walk test is commonly used to assess changes in exercise capacity following pulmonary rehabilitation in patients with COPD. Exercise tolerance evaluated using the 6-minute walk test was not significant for ACO and COPD [8, 17].

2.4 Biomarkers

Previous studies have attempted to identify the ACO phenotype by using various criteria. Thus, awareness of the importance of recognizing ACO using biomarkers has increased.

Inflammatory biomarkers, such as fractional exhaled nitric oxide (FENO), blood eosinophils, and allergen-specific immunoglobulin E (IgE), are sometimes used to distinguish between asthma and COPD [1]. Typically, asthma is characterized predominantly by inflammation involving eosinophils, whereas inflammation involving neutrophils is dominant in COPD. FENO and blood eosinophil count, which increase in patients with asthma, have been considered biomarkers of local and systemic eosinophilic inflammation. Total serum IgE and antigen-specific IgE levels were also elevated in patients with allergic asthma.

Previous studies observed increased FENO levels in a subset of patients with COPD [21, 22], and increased blood and sputum eosinophil counts in patients with COPD were associated with asthmatic symptoms [23].

Kobayashi and colleagues identified patients with ACO presenting features of asthma, including both variable respiratory symptoms and variable expiratory airflow limitation, in a COPD outpatient cohort [24]. They also demonstrated that inflammatory biomarkers, including FENO, blood eosinophil count, and IgE, increased in ACO patients. The mean FENO level was significantly higher in patients with ACO than in those without ACO (38.5 ppb vs. 20.3 ppb, $P < 0.001$). The blood eosinophil count and percentage were significantly increased in patients with ACO (295/mm^3 vs. 212/mm^3, $P = 0.032$; 4.7% vs. 3.2%, $P = 0.003$, respectively). The total IgE level was also significantly higher, and antigen-specific IgE was observed more frequently in patients with ACO. These results were confirmed in subsequent studies [25–27]. FENO and blood eosinophils have been proposed as potential biomarkers of ACO.

2.5 *Radiology*

Chest radiography may show hyperinflation in patients with airflow limitation; therefore, it generally does not help differentiate among asthma, COPD, and ACO.

Chest computed tomography (CT) revealed low-attenuation areas denoting either air trapping or emphysematous change, bronchial wall thickening, and features of pulmonary hypertension in COPD. In stable asthma, chest CT findings are often normal, but air trapping and increased bronchial wall thickness may be observed. The imaging features of ACO measured using quantitative CT analysis were less emphysema and more airway disease than COPD alone [12].

2.6 *Comorbidities*

The most frequently reported comorbidities of asthma include rhinitis, sinusitis, gastroesophageal reflux disease (GERD), obesity, and food allergy [1]. In patients with COPD, cardiovascular disease, osteoporosis, depression/anxiety, GERD, and lung cancer are commonly reported [2].

An epidemiological study using data from the Behavioral Risk Factor Surveillance System survey that included 90,851 participants showed that subjects with ACO had at least one comorbidity (90%) more often than those with COPD (84%), asthma (71%), or controls (58%) [28]. The ACO group had higher rates of cardiovascular diseases, cerebrovascular diseases, arthritis, diabetes, and obesity. Similarly, in a retrospective study of patients with a physician-confirmed diagnosis of asthma and COPD, patients with ACO had higher rates of allergic rhinitis, GERD, anxiety, and osteoporosis [29]. These studies have demonstrated that increased rates of comorbidities have also been linked to increased healthcare and medication use.

Several studies have examined the Charlson comorbidity index (CCI). CCI is a widely used scoring system for comorbidities that predict mortality risk. Miravittles et al. reported that the CCI was significantly higher in patients with ACO than in those with COPD (overlap, 1.44; COPD, 0.89; $P = 0.001$) [8]. However, each comorbid condition was considered individually, and the difference was significant only for diabetes. Fu et al. found no significant difference in CCI at baseline between the three groups (asthma, 3.5; COPD, 4; overlap, 4; $P = 0.82$) and identified a significant increase in total CCI for all groups at follow-up [17]. In a Japanese cohort study, CCI was not significantly different between ACO and COPD alone [14].

3 Clinical Outcomes of ACO

3.1 Exacerbations

In most cross-sectional studies, the frequency of exacerbations in patients with ACO is higher than that in patients with asthma [6] and COPD [7, 8, 12]. However, Izquierdo-Alonso et al. reported that the exacerbation rate in patients with ACO was not different from that in patients with COPD [30].

A large epidemiological study in the USA showed more hospitalizations and emergency department visits for patients with ACO than for patients with COPD [31]. Similarly, two large epidemiological studies in Latin America and Spain showed a significantly higher frequency of exacerbations in patients with ACO than in patients with COPD [7, 8]. The results of the Copenhagen City Heart Study demonstrated a significantly higher risk of severe exacerbations in patients with ACO, particularly in those with late-onset asthma than in those with asthma or COPD alone [20].

In cohort studies, the frequency of exacerbations in patients with ACO was higher than that in patients with COPD [9, 10], whereas Cosio et al. reported no difference between patients with ACO and those with COPD [32].

In Japan, the frequency of exacerbations in patients with ACO has been reported in only a few studies. Among the cross-sectional and cohort studies, the rate of exacerbations in patients with ACO was not different from that in patients with COPD. In a multicenter, cross-sectional study of 1008 patients with COPD, the rate of exacerbations in the previous year at baseline was not significantly different between patients with ACO and those with COPD alone [13]. A prospective, 3-year-follow-up cohort study demonstrated no difference in the annual rate of all exacerbations and severe exacerbations requiring hospital admission between patients with ACO and those with COPD alone (0.20 vs. 0.14, 0.12 vs. 0.10, events per person, respectively) [14]. The frequency of exacerbations among patients classified as having asthma, COPD, and ACO is summarized in Table 5.1.

Table 5.1 Frequency of exacerbation (per year) among patients classified ACO, asthma alone, and COPD alone

Study	Evaluation	Number of participants	ACO	Asthma	COPD	*P*-value
Menezes et al. (2014) [7]	Previous history	Asthma, $n = 84$ COPD, $n = 594$ ACO, $n = 89$	1.5 ± 6.4	0.3 ± 0.9	0.3 ± 2.2	0.002
Miravitlles et al. (2013) [8]	Previous history	COPD, $n = 385$ ACO, $n = 67$	1.8		0.5	<0.001
Wurst et al. (2016) [9]	Previous history	COPD, $n = 1483$ ACO, $n = 493$	1.6		1.1	<0.01
Hardin et al. (2014) [12]	Previous history	COPD, $n = 3120$ ACO, $n = 450$	1.2 ± 1.6		0.7 ± 1.2	<0.001
Inoue et al. (2017) [13]	Previous history	COPD, $n = 915$ ACO, $n = 93$	0.570		0.491	0.502
Kobayashi et al. (2020) [14]	3-year follow up	COPD, $n = 321$ ACO, $n = 38$	0.20 ± 0.37		0.14 ± 0.31	0.338

Notes: Data are shown as mean ± SD. Abbreviations: *ACO* Asthma–COPD overlap

3.2 *Mortality*

In epidemiological studies, Kumbhare et al. [33] investigated mortality among 4434 patients with obstructive lung disease, based on self-reported diagnoses of asthma, COPD, and ACO, compared with the US general population. Mortality rates from cardiovascular disease and malignancy were similar across the disease categories. However, patients with ACO had a disproportionately higher number of deaths from chronic respiratory disease than the other groups, although this was not statistically significant compared with COPD after adjusting for age, sex, and smoking status.

Similar results were obtained by Baarnes et al. [31] in a 35-year prospective study that enrolled over 57,000 adults aged 50–64 years. All-cause mortality was significantly higher among participants with ACO than among those with asthma or COPD alone, particularly among women and younger participants. In a prospective population-based study in Denmark with 8382 participants, patients with ACO associated with late-onset asthma had the worst survival with a reduced life expectancy of 12.8 years compared with healthy never-smokers, which was significantly worse than the 10.1 years of reduced survival of patients with COPD and 3.3 years of patients with asthma. Patients with ACO associated with early-onset asthma had a similar survival compared with those with COPD (9.3 years reduction in survival) [20].

By contrast, the results of several cohort studies are inconsistent with those obtained in the succeeding studies. A multicenter, prospective study of 831 patients with obstructive lung disease showed a 1-year survival rate of 94.7% for ACO compared with 87.3% for COPD ($P < 0.05$) [32]. Another prospective study of 1976 patients with COPD demonstrated that mortality rates during the 3-year follow-up were similar in patients with COPD with (10%) and without (9%) ACO [9]. A retrospective observational study of 891 patients with COPD showed that patients with ACO had the best long-term prognosis compared to the three other COPD phenotypes, including non-exacerbators, exacerbators with chronic bronchitis, and emphysema exacerbations [34]. However, no significant differences in mortality were found after adjusting for potential confounders, suggesting that these observations were primarily driven by between-group differences in COPD severity and comorbidities.

In Japan, only a few studies have reported on the prognosis of patients with ACO. The results of the Hokkaido cohort study demonstrated a significantly reduced 10-year mortality in patients with COPD who had at least two of the so-called asthma-like features (positive bronchodilator test, increased blood eosinophils, and/or atopy) compared with patients with COPD with 0 or 1 of these features [35]. Kobayashi et al. analyzed prospectively collected data from the Ishinomaki COPD Network registry and demonstrated that 3-year mortality was significantly higher in patients with COPD alone than in those with ACO (12.9% vs. 0%; $P = 0.037$) [14]. The estimated survival rate at 3 years was significantly worse in patients with COPD alone than in those with ACO (hazard ratio, 0.87; 95% confidence interval, 0.83–0.90). Yamauchi et al. conducted a retrospective study using a national inpatient database in Japan [36]. Of the 30,405 eligible patients, in-hospital mortality in patients with ACO, asthma alone, and COPD alone was 2.3%, 1.2%, and 9.7%, respectively. Patients with COPD had significantly higher mortality than patients with ACO (odds ratio, 1.96; 95% confidence interval, 1.38–2.79); patients with asthma alone showed lower mortality (0.70; 0.50–0.97).

4 Discussion

The reported characteristics and outcomes of ACO remain controversial. Possible reasons for this are the age and sex differences of the study populations. Another reason is the regional differences in the healthcare system. A possible major reason is the different diagnostic criteria used by different investigators.

Although the standard of care has not been established in ACO, the results of several studies suggest that differences in maintenance therapy could result in disagreement in outcomes in ACO. Bronchodilators, such as long-acting muscarinic antagonists and long-acting β_2-agonists, are commonly used maintenance medications in COPD that improve symptoms, lung function, and health status and reduce exacerbation rates [2], and ICS are the most effective controllers used in asthma treatment [1]. Treatment with ICS increases the risk of pneumonia in patients with COPD; thus, ICS should be used in patients who can be expected to respond to corticosteroid therapy. A better response to ICS was demonstrated in selected COPD patients who had a history of exacerbations and higher concentrations of blood eosinophils [37–39]. The GOLD report no longer refers to ACO but recommends the use of blood eosinophil counts at ≥300 cells/μL to direct additional therapy with ICS [2]. Blood eosinophils were significantly increased in patients with ACO [24, 27]. Thus, ICS treatment may be considered for patients with ACO. Currently, ICS-containing therapy is recommended for patients with features of asthma and COPD to reduce the risk of severe exacerbation and death [1]. Recently, Hirai et al. demonstrated that ACO without ICS use has a significant effect on the frequency of acute exacerbations [15]. ACO may not be associated with poor outcomes in patients receiving appropriate and adequate treatment.

5 Conclusion

Patients with ACO have been recognized to have a greater burden of symptoms, poorer QOL, more frequent exacerbations, and higher mortality than those with asthma or COPD alone. However, the findings of several recent studies are controversial, suggesting that ACO may not be associated with poor outcomes in patients receiving appropriate and adequate treatment.

References

1. Global Initiative for Asthma. Global strategy for asthma management and prevention (2021 update). http://www.ginasthma.org/. Accessed 11 Mar 2022.
2. Global Initiative for Chronic Obstructive Lung Disease. Global strategy for the diagnosis, management and prevention of COPD (2022 report). http://www.goldcopd.org/. Accessed 11 Mar 2022.
3. Gibson PG, Simpson JS. The overlap syndrome of asthma and COPD: what are its features and how important is it? Thorax. 2009;64:728–35. https://doi.org/10.1136/thx.2008.108027.
4. Alshabanat A, Zafari Z, Albanyan O, Dairi M, FitzGerald JM. Asthma and COPD overlap syndrome (ACOS): a systematic review and meta analysis. PLoS One. 2015;10:e0136065. https://doi.org/10.1371/journal.pone.0136065.
5. de Marco R, Pesce G, Marcon A, Accordini S, Antonicelli L, Bugiani M, et al. The coexistence of asthma and chronic obstructive pulmonary disease (COPD): prevalence and risk factors in young, middle-aged and elderly people from the general population. PLoS One. 2013;8(5):e62985. https://doi.org/10.1371/journal.pone.0062985.
6. Milanese M, Di Marco F, Corsico AG, Milanese M, Di Marco F, Corsico AG, et al. Asthma control in elderly asthmatics. An Italian observational study. Respir Med. 2014;108:1091–9. https://doi.org/10.1016/j.rmed.2014.05.016.
7. Menezes AMB, Montes de Oca M, Pérez-Padilla R, Nadeau G, Wehrmeister FC, Lopez-Varela MV, et al. Increased risk of exacerbation and hospitalization in subjects with an overlap phenotype: COPD-asthma. Chest. 2014;145(2):297–304. https://doi.org/10.1378/chest.13-0622.
8. Miravitlles M, Soriano JB, Ancochea J, Muñoz L, Duran-Tauleria E, Sánchez G, et al. Characterisation of the overlap COPD-asthma phenotype. Focus on physical activity and health status. Respir Med. 2013;107(7):1053–60. https://doi.org/10.1016/j.rmed.2013.03.007.
9. Wurst KE, Rheault TR, Edwards L, Tal-Singer R, Agusti A, Vestbo J. A comparison of COPD patients with and without ACOS in the ECLIPSE study. Eur Respir J. 2016;47:1559–62.

10. Barrecheguren M, Pinto L, Mostafavi-Pour-Manshadi SM, Tan WC, Li PZ, Aaron SD, et al. Identification and definition of asthma-COPD overlap: the CanCOLD study. Respirology. 2020;25:836–49. https://doi.org/10.1111/resp.13780.
11. Kauppi P, Kupiainen H, Lindqvist A, Tammilehto L, Kilpeläinen M, Kinnula VL, et al. Overlap syndrome of asthma and COPD predicts low quality of life. J Asthma. 2011;48:279–85. https://doi.org/10.3109/02770903.2011.555576.
12. Hardin M, Cho M, McDonald ML, Beaty T, Ramsdell J, Bhatt S, et al. The clinical and genetic features of COPD-asthma overlap syndrome. Eur Respir J. 2014;44:341–50. https://doi.org/10.1183/09031936.00216013.
13. Inoue H, Nagase T, Morita S, Yoshida A, Jinnai T, Ichinose M. Prevalence and characteristics of asthma-COPD overlap syndrome identified by a stepwise approach. Int J Chron Obstruct Pulmon Dis. 2017;12:1803–10. https://doi.org/10.2147/COPD.S133859.
14. Kobayashi S, Hanagama M, Ishida M, Ono M, Sato H, Yamanda S, et al. Clinical characteristics and outcomes of patients with asthma-COPD overlap in Japanese patients with COPD. Int J Chron Obstruct Pulmon Dis. 2020;15:2923–9. https://doi.org/10.2147/COPD.S276314.
15. Hirai K, Tanaka A, Homma T, Kawahara T, Oda N, Mikuni H, et al. Prevalence and clinical features of asthma-COPD overlap in patients with COPD not using inhaled corticosteroids. Allergol Int. 2021;70:134–5. https://doi.org/10.1016/j.alit.2020.07.009.
16. Chung JW, Kong KA, Lee JH, Lee SJ, Ryu YJ, Chang JH. Characteristics and self-rated health of overlap syndrome. Int J Chron Obstruct Pulmon Dis. 2014;9:795–804. https://doi.org/10.2147/COPD.S61093.
17. Fu JJ, Gibson PG, Simpson JL, McDonald VM. Longitudinal changes in clinical outcomes in older patients with asthma, COPD and asthma-COPD overlap syndrome. Respiration. 2014;87:63–74. https://doi.org/10.1159/000352053.
18. Kitaguchi Y, Yasuo M, Hanaoka M. Comparison of pulmonary function in patients with COPD, asthma–COPD overlap syndrome, and asthma with airflow limitation. Int J Chron Obstruct Pulmon Dis. 2016;11:991–7. https://doi.org/10.2147/COPD.S105988.
19. Tommola M, Ilmarinen P, Tuomisto LE, Lehtimäki L, Haanpää J, Niemelä O, et al. Differences between asthma–COPD overlap syndrome and adult-onset asthma. Eur Respir J. 2017;49:1602383. https://doi.org/10.1183/13993003.02383-2016.
20. Lange P, Çolak Y, Ingebrigtsen TS, Vestbo J, Marott JL. Long-term prognosis of asthma, chronic obstructive pulmonary disease, and asthma-chronic obstructive pulmonary disease overlap in the Copenhagen City Heart study: a prospective population-based analysis. Lancet Respir Med. 2016;4:454–62. https://doi.org/10.1016/S2213-2600(16)00098-9.
21. Donohue JF, Herje N, Crater G, Rickard K. Characterization of airway inflammation in patients with COPD using fractional exhaled nitric oxide levels: a pilot study. Int J Chron Obstruct Pulmon Dis. 2014;9:745–51. https://doi.org/10.2147/COPD.S44552.
22. Tamada T, Sugiura H, Takahashi T, Matsunaga K, Kimura K, Katsumata U, et al. Biomarker-based detection of asthma-COPD overlap syndrome in COPD populations. Int J Chron Obstruct Pulmon Dis. 2015;10:2169–76. https://doi.org/10.2147/COPD.S88274.
23. Kitaguchi Y, Komatsu Y, Fujimoto K, Hanaoka M, Kubo K. Sputum eosinophilia can predict responsiveness to inhaled corticosteroid treatment in patients with overlap syndrome of COPD and asthma. Int J Chron Obstruct Pulmon Dis. 2012;7:283–9. https://doi.org/10.2147/COPD.S30651.
24. Kobayashi S, Hanagama M, Yamanda S, Ishida M, Yanai M. Inflammatory biomarkers in asthma-COPD overlap syndrome. Int J Chron Obstruct Pulmon Dis. 2016;11:2117–23. https://doi.org/10.2147/COPD.S113647.
25. Goto T, Camargo CA Jr, Hasegawa K. Fractional exhaled nitric oxide levels in asthma–COPD overlap syndrome: analysis of the National Health and Nutrition Examination Survey, 2007–2012. Int J Chron Obstruct Pulmon Dis. 2016;11:2149–55. https://doi.org/10.2147/COPD.S110879.

26. Chen FJ, Huang XY, Liu YL, Lin GP, Xie CM. Importance of fractional exhaled nitric oxide in the differentiation of asthma-COPD overlap syndrome, asthma, and COPD. Int J Chron Obstruct Pulmon Dis. 2016;11:2385–90. https://doi.org/10.2147/COPD.S115378.
27. Takayama Y, Ohnishi H, Ogasawara F, Oyama K, Kubota T, Yokoyama A. Clinical utility of fractional exhaled nitric oxide and blood eosinophils counts in the diagnosis of asthma-COPD overlap. Int J Chron Obstruct Pulmon Dis. 2018;13:2525–32. https://doi.org/10.2147/COPD.S167600.
28. Kumbhare S, Pleasants R, Ohar JA, Strange C. Characteristics and prevalence of asthma/chronic obstructive pulmonary disease overlap in the United States. Ann Am Thorac Soc. 2016;13:803–10. https://doi.org/10.1513/AnnalsATS.201508-554OC.
29. van Boven JF, Román-Rodríguez M, Palmer JF, Toledo-Pons N, Cosío BG, Soriano JB. Comorbidome, pattern, and impact of asthma-COPD overlap syndrome in real life. Chest. 2016;149:1011–20. https://doi.org/10.1016/j.chest.2015.12.002.
30. Izquierdo-Alonso JL, Rodriguez-Gonzálezmoro JM, de Lucas-Ramos P, Unzueta I, Ribera X, Antón E, et al. Prevalence and characteristics of three clinical phenotypes of chronic obstructive pulmonary disease (COPD). Respir Med. 2013;107:724–31. https://doi.org/10.1016/j.rmed.2013.01.001.
31. Baarnes CB, Andersen ZJ, Tjønneland A, Ulrik CS. Incidence and long-term outcome of severe asthma-COPD overlap compared to asthma and COPD alone: a 35-year prospective study of 57,053 middle-aged adults. Int J Chron Obstruct Pulmon Dis. 2017;12:571–9. https://doi.org/10.2147/COPD.S123167.
32. Cosio BG, Soriano JB, López-Campos JL, Calle-Rubio M, Soler-Cataluna JJ, de-Torres JP, et al. Defining the asthma-COPD overlap syndrome in a COPD cohort. Chest. 2016;149:45–52. https://doi.org/10.1378/chest.15-1055.
33. Kumbhare S, Strange C. Mortality in asthma-chronic obstructive pulmonary disease overlap in the United States. South Med J. 2018;111:293–8. https://doi.org/10.14423/SMJ.0000000000000807.
34. Golpe R, Suárez-Valor M, Martín-Robles I, Sanjuán-López P, Cano-Jiménez E, Castro-Añón O, et al. Mortality in COPD patients according to clinical phenotypes. Int J Chron Obstruct Pulmon Dis. 2018;13:1433–9. https://doi.org/10.2147/COPD.S159834.
35. Suzuki M, Makita H, Konno S, Shimizu K, Kimura H, Kimura H, et al. Asthma-like features and clinical course of chronic obstructive pulmonary disease. An analysis from the Hokkaido COPD Cohort Study. Am J Respir Crit Care Med. 2016;194:1358–65. https://doi.org/10.1164/rccm.201602-0353OC.
36. Yamauchi Y, Yasunaga H, Matsui H, Hasegawa W, Jo T, Takami K, et al. Comparison of in-hospital mortality in patients with COPD, asthma and asthma-COPD overlap exacerbations. Respirology. 2015;20:940–6. https://doi.org/10.1111/resp.12556.
37. Lipson DA, Barnhart F, Brealey N, Brooks J, Criner GJ, Day NC, et al. Once-daily single-inhaler triple versus dual therapy in patients with COPD. N Engl J Med. 2018;378:1671–80. https://doi.org/10.1056/NEJMoa1713901.
38. Rabe KF, Martinez FJ, Ferguson GT, Wang C, Singh D, Wedzicha JA, et al. Triple inhaled therapy at two glucocorticoid doses in moderate-to-very-severe COPD. N Engl J Med. 2020;383:35–48. https://doi.org/10.1056/NEJMoa1916046.
39. Harries TH, Rowland V, Corrigan CJ, Marshall IJ, McDonnell L, Prasad V, et al. Blood eosinophil count, a marker of inhaled corticosteroid effectiveness in preventing COPD exacerbations in post-hoc RCT and observational studies: systematic review and meta-analysis. Respir Res. 2020;2:3. https://doi.org/10.1186/s12931-019-1268-7.

Chapter 6
Prognosis of COPD with Asthma-Like Features and ACO: Is the Prognosis of COPD and ACO Different?

Masaru Suzuki

Abstract Some patients with COPD have asthma-like features, such as significant bronchodilator reversibility, blood eosinophilia, and/or atopy, but they may not be clinically diagnosed with asthma. According to some proposed diagnostic criteria for ACO, a physician's confirmed diagnosis of asthma or typical respiratory symptoms of asthma is not necessarily required for a diagnosis of ACO. As such, patients with COPD could be labeled as having ACO simply because of the presence of asthma-like features. This chapter summarizes the evidence for the prognosis of COPD with asthma-like features and ACO. The impact of asthma-like features or ACO on lung function declines, exacerbations, and mortality varied between studies. The interpretation of results from each study requires caution. Various factors should be considered when interpreting results, including the ACO diagnostic criteria, disease severity, sample size, and follow-up period. Such variations can affect ACO prognosis. The condition shows heterogeneous phenotypes, even among patients classified as having ACO.

Keywords COPD · Asthma · ACO · Overlap · Prognosis · Lung function decline · Exacerbation · Mortality

1 Introduction

Since the concept of ACO was introduced, varying diagnostic criteria have been proposed by several different groups. Importantly, some patients with COPD have asthma-like features, such as significant bronchodilator reversibility, blood eosinophilia, and/or atopy, but they may not be clinically diagnosed with asthma.

M. Suzuki (✉)
Department of Respiratory Medicine, Faculty of Medicine, Hokkaido University, Sapporo, Japan
e-mail: suzumasa@med.hokudai.ac.jp

H. Nagase et al. (eds.), *Asthma-COPD Overlap*, Respiratory Disease Series: Diagnostic Tools and Disease Managements,
https://doi.org/10.1007/978-981-96-0217-9_6

The Hokkaido COPD cohort study, conducted in Japan, reported that 50% of patients with COPD were not clinically diagnosed with asthma but presented with at least one asthma-like feature (21% bronchodilator reversibility, 19% blood eosinophilia, and 25% atopy) [1]. According to some proposed diagnostic criteria for ACO, a physician's confirmed diagnosis of asthma or typical respiratory symptoms of asthma is not necessarily required for a diagnosis of ACO [2–5]. As such, patients with COPD could be labeled as having ACO simply because of the presence of asthma-like features. This chapter summarizes the evidence for the prognosis of COPD with asthma-like features and ACO by considering lung function, exacerbations, and mortality. Evidence suggests conflicting results, which may be due to inconsistencies in the definition of ACO.

2 Presence of Asthma-Like Features or ACO and Lung Function Decline

A COPD diagnosis is based on the presence of airflow limitation that is not fully reversible. Lung function, measured by the decline in the forced expiratory volume in 1 second (FEV_1), is one of the most important outcome determinants in patients with COPD. Earlier studies, such as the Inhaled Steroids in Obstructive Lung Disease in Europe (ISOLDE) study [6] and the Lung Health Study [7], investigated the association between bronchodilator reversibility and the decline in FEV_1 in patients with COPD. The ISOLDE study was a 3-year randomized controlled trial to test the effect of inhaled fluticasone propionate 500 μg twice daily on the rate of decline in FEV_1 in patients with non-asthmatic COPD [8]. There was no relationship between the absolute or percentage predicted changes in FEV_1 after bronchodilator use and the subsequent rate of decline in FEV_1 [6]. The Lung Health Study reported that baseline bronchodilator responses did not correlate with a subsequent decline in FEV_1 during the 11-year follow-up period [7]. The Hokkaido COPD cohort study [1] and the Korean Obstructive Lung Disease (KOLD) study conducted in South Korea [9] also showed that the sole presence of bronchodilator reversibility did not affect the decline in FEV_1. In contrast, the Evaluation of COPD Longitudinally to Identify Predictive Surrogate Endpoints (ECLIPSE) study showed that the presence of bronchodilator reversibility was associated with a slower annual decline in FEV_1, with the effect on the annual change in FEV_1 was −17 mL/year [10]. Since 72% of the subjects in the ECLIPSE study used inhaled corticosteroids (ICS), this favorable effect of bronchodilator reversibility on lung function decline may be related to the therapeutic effect of ICS.

The Hokkaido COPD cohort study reported that the presence of blood eosinophilia at baseline (≥300 cells/μL) in patients with non-asthmatic COPD was associated with a slower annual decline in FEV_1 over 5 years than in patients without any asthma-like features (bronchodilator reversibility, blood eosinophilia, and atopy) (−22 mL/year vs. −34 mL/year) [1]. Furthermore, the study showed a significant association between the number of asthma-like features and a slower decline in FEV_1 [1]. The Korean COPD Subgroup Study (KOCCOS) conducted in South Korea also reported that patients with eosinophilic COPD had a slower decline in FEV_1 over 3 years compared to patients with non-eosinophilic COPD (−12.2 mL/year vs. −19.4 mL/year) [11]. In contrast, the KOLD study showed no difference in the annual decline in FEV_1 among COPD patients with persistently high blood eosinophils (≥300 cells/μL), persistently low blood eosinophils (<300 cells/μL), and variable blood eosinophils [12]. Although ICS treatment can reduce the rate of decline in FEV_1 in patients with eosinophilic COPD [13], there were no differences in ICS use between patients with eosinophilic and non-eosinophilic COPD in these three studies [1, 11, 12]. Therefore, the presence of blood eosinophilia does not appear to contribute to the rapid decline in lung function in patients with COPD.

Several reports have shown a rapid decline in lung function in ACO. The Canadian Cohort Obstructive Lung Disease (CanCOLD) study, conducted in Canada, investigated the clinical outcomes of patients with ACO using multiple definitions. The results indicated a trend for a higher annual decline in FEV_1 in patients with any ACO criteria than in those who did not have ACO (−49.6 mL/year vs. −38.1 mL/year). In particular, patients with ACO (as defined by bronchodilator reversibility >400 mL and 15%) had the highest annual decline in FEV_1 (−81.1 mL/year) [14]. The Copenhagen City Heart study, a longitudinal population-based study over 18–22 years, reported that ACO patients with late-onset asthma (after 40 years of age) had a higher annual decline in FEV_1 (−49.6 mL/year) than ACO patients with early-onset asthma (−27.3 mL/year), patients with COPD (−39.5 mL/year), and patients with asthma alone (−25.6 mL/year) [15]. In contrast, Fu et al., in their 4-year prospective study of older (age >55 years) patients with obstructive airway diseases, reported that there was no significant difference in FEV_1 decline among patients with COPD, asthma, and ACO [16]. In contrast, the European Community Respiratory Health Survey (ECRHS) study showed that young adults (aged 20–40 years) with ACO had a slower annual decline in FEV_1 than those with COPD (−25.9 mL/year vs. −37.3 mL/year) [17]. The KOLD study also showed a slower annual decline in FEV_1 in patients with ACO than those with COPD (−13.9 mL/year vs. −29.3 mL/year) [9]. Altogether, the available evidence demonstrates that there are conflicting results regarding the effects of ACO on lung function.

3 Presence of Asthma-Like Features or ACO and Exacerbations

The ISOLDE study showed that the presence of bronchodilator reversibility was not associated with exacerbation frequency [6]. Likewise, the Hokkaido COPD cohort study showed that the sole presence of bronchodilator reversibility to a β2-agonist (salbutamol) at baseline was not related to exacerbation-free survival [1]. In contrast, the same study reported that COPD patients who were consistently reversible to anticholinergic agent (oxitropium), but not to salbutamol, were significantly associated with the early development of the first exacerbation event [18]. This result suggests that some of them present a consistently increased airway cholinergic tone, as reflected by high bronchodilator reversibility to oxitropium, and may be susceptible to exacerbation. Alternatively, this may also suggest that repeated exacerbations increased the airway cholinergic tone, resulting in high bronchodilator reversibility to anticholinergic agents. Marín et al. reported that the rate of hospitalization for patients with COPD was significantly lower, while the time to the first hospitalization was prolonged in patients with positive bronchodilator reversibility (39.3 months vs. 32.4 months) [19]. Kim et al. investigated the impact of bronchodilator reversibility according to various criteria on the risk of severe COPD exacerbations in four prospective COPD cohorts conducted in South Korea. They reported that positive bronchodilator reversibility according to the GOLD criteria (>200 mL and 12%) was significantly associated with a decreased risk of severe COPD exacerbations (adjusted odds ratio 0.38) [20]. In this study, there was a significant interaction between ICS/long-acting β2-agonists (LABA) treatment and the effect of bronchodilator reversibility on severe COPD exacerbations, suggesting that positive bronchodilator reversibility could predict a response to ICS/LABA treatment [20].

In patients with COPD, blood eosinophilia has been reported to be associated with an increased exacerbation risk. For example, the Copenhagen General Population Study reported that COPD patients with blood eosinophil levels >343 cells/μL had a higher incidence of severe exacerbations (incidence risk ratio 1.76) and moderate exacerbations (incidence risk ratio 1.15) during a median of 3.3 years of follow-up [21]. The KOCCOS study also reported that patients with eosinophilic COPD had more frequent exacerbations than those with non-eosinophilic COPD (adjusted odds ratio 1.49) [11]. A post-hoc analysis of data from two randomized controlled trials of vilanterol or vilanterol plus fluticasone furoate showed that the exacerbation rates increased progressively with increasing eosinophil counts in patients treated with vilanterol alone [22]. Moreover, this study and other reports [23, 24] showed that ICS treatment was more effective in preventing exacerbations in patients with COPD with higher blood eosinophil counts. In contrast, several cohort studies reported no association between blood eosinophil counts and the development of exacerbations [1, 12, 25], which might be affected by ICS treatment. The Hokkaido COPD cohort study showed no association between the presence of multiple asthma-like features and exacerbation-free survival [1]. Taken together, blood eosinophilia does not have at least a beneficial effect on the development of exacerbations in patients with COPD.

In the Genetic Epidemiology of COPD (COPDGene) study, patients with COPD who reported a history of physician-diagnosed asthma before the age of 40 years had a higher percentage of frequent exacerbations (42.7% vs. 18%) and severe exacerbations (32.8% vs. 17.6%) in the year prior to enrolment compared to patients with COPD only [26]. The Latin American Project for the Investigation of Obstructive Lung Disease (PLATINO) study also reported that patients with ACO, defined by the presence of wheezing in the previous year and bronchodilator reversibility, experienced more exacerbations in the past year than patients with

COPD (15.7% vs. 5.2%, adjusted prevalence ratio 2.11) [27]. The ECRHS, a population-based study, showed a higher prevalence of hospital admission in patients with ACO than in those with COPD alone (15.8% vs. 8.1%) [17]. The Copenhagen City Heart study, another well-known population-based study, reported that patients with ACO and late-onset asthma (after the age of 40 years) experienced the most hospital admissions due to exacerbations. They also showed that patients with ACO and early-onset asthma also had a higher risk of admissions than patients with COPD, when adjusted for covariates [15]. Several other studies have shown that patients with ACO have more frequent exacerbations than patients with COPD [14, 28, 29]. Although other studies have shown no difference in exacerbation frequency between patients with ACO and COPD [5, 30–32], ACO is likely to negatively impact exacerbations in general. Importantly, there is heterogeneity in the biological response to COPD exacerbations [33], and the exacerbations associated with ACO may be predominantly eosinophilic.

4 Presence of Asthma-Like Features or ACO and Mortality

Hansen et al. reported that bronchodilator reversibility was associated with better survival after controlling for baseline FEV_1 during a median of 11.2 years of follow-up, but this association became non-significant after controlling for the best FEV_1 [34]. Marín et al. showed that all-cause mortality was significantly reduced in those with COPD and bronchodilator reversibility during approximately 5.8 years of follow-up (10.5% vs. 17%) [19]. The Understanding Potential Long-term Improvements in Function with Tiotropium (UPLIFT) trial, a 4-year placebo-controlled clinical trial evaluating the effects of tiotropium, also demonstrated that all-cause mortality tended to be lower in patients with COPD with bronchodilator reversibility, regardless of the responsiveness definition used [35]. In contrast, the KOLD study reported that patients with COPD and persistently high blood eosinophil counts had a better survival rate than those with persistently low blood eosinophil counts during a median of 6.0 years of follow-up (adjusted mortality rate ratio 0.29) [12]. The Hokkaido COPD cohort study showed that COPD patients with multiple asthma-like features had significantly better 10-year all-cause mortality than those with one or no asthma-like features (Fig. 6.1) [1]. In this study, the presence of multiple asthma-like features was associated with the baseline characteristics of younger age, higher body mass index, better diffusion capacity, and less emphysema than those with one or no asthma-like features. This suggests that the presence of multiple asthma-like features may be associated with a unique phenotype of COPD with milder clinical presentation and better outcomes. In addition, patients with multiple asthma-like features had better survival when ICS was prescribed than those with one or no asthma-like features treated with ICS, which implies a better response to ICS treatment in patients with multiple asthma-like features [1]. Therefore, the presence of asthma-like features does not necessarily contribute to worse mortality in patients with COPD.

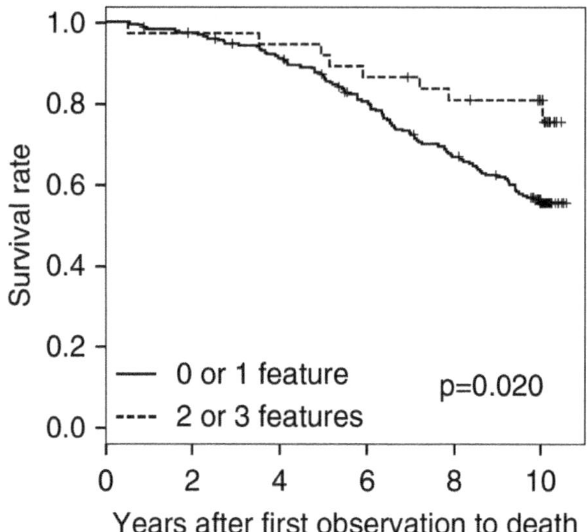

Fig. 6.1 Kaplan–Meier curves for all-cause mortality according to the number of asthma-like features from the Hokkaido COPD cohort study. (Adapted with permission of the American Thoracic Society. Copyright © 2022 American Thoracic Society. All rights reserved. Cite: Suzuki et al. [1]. The American Journal of Respiratory and Critical Care Medicine is an official journal of the American Thoracic Society. Readers are encouraged to read the entire article for the correct context at https://www.atsjournals.org/doi/abs/10.1164/rccm.201602-0353OC. The authors, editors, and The American Thoracic Society are not responsible for errors or omissions in adaptations)

Conflicting results regarding mortality in patients with ACO have been reported. The ECLIPSE and other studies reported no difference in mortality rates between patients with ACO and COPD [16, 36, 37]. In NHANES III, a population-based study in which diagnosis was defined by self-reported questions, coexisting COPD and asthma had the highest risk for mortality (hazard ratio 1.45), followed by current COPD (hazard ratio 1.28) and current asthma (hazard ratio 1.04) in survival models adjusting for factors including baseline lung function [38]. Another report using data from the NHANES III showed that deaths resulting from chronic lower respiratory disease were higher in patients with ACO (21.4%) than in those with COPD (12.6%) and asthma (9.5%) [39]. Data from the Lung Health Study showed that patients with ACO, defined as COPD with airway hyperreactivity in a methacholine provocation test, had a higher increased risk of respiratory mortality (hazard ratio 2.38) [40]. The Danish Diet, Cancer, and Health (DCH) study, another large population-based study, also reported that the mortality rate was higher in patients with ACO (defined as at least one admission for asthma and one for COPD) (25.9 per 1000 person-years) than in those with COPD (23.1 per 1000 person-years) and asthma alone (7.9 per 1000 person-years) [41].

Several studies have reported better survival in patients with ACO. The CHAIN study in Spain showed better 1-year mortality in patients with ACO than in those with COPD [5]. Notably, in the CHAIN study, only 22% of the subjects in the ACO group had a previous history of asthma because the diagnostic criteria for ACO included several asthma-like features (i.e., bronchodilator reversibility, blood eosinophilia, high blood total IgE levels, or history of atopy) and did not require a physician's confirmed diagnosis of asthma [5]. This indicates that many patients with COPD who were labeled as ACO in the CHAIN study had asthma-like features alone. Similarly, in the Hokkaido COPD cohort study, patients with COPD and multiple asthma-like features had better survival [1]. Bai et al. reported that patients with COPD had a higher mortality risk than those with ACO, during a median follow-up period of 3.8 years (hazard ratio 3.93), despite more frequent exacerbations in the past 12 months in patients with ACO [29]. A study using data from the Diagnosis Procedure Combination database, a nationwide inpatient database in Japan, demonstrated that all-cause in-hospital mortality was lower in the ACO group (2.3%) than in the COPD group (9.7%) [42]. Peltola et al. also reported that the survival of patients with ACO was significantly better than that of patients with COPD after COPD exacerbation requiring hospitalization (4.7 years vs. 1.7 years) [43]. In this report, there were no differences in the underlying causes of death between the ACO and COPD groups [43]. Lastly, the Copenhagen City Heart Study demonstrated that ACO patients with late-onset asthma (after the age of 40 years) had the worst all-cause and respiratory mortality, while the mortality of ACO patients with early-onset asthma was better than that of patients with COPD (Fig. 6.2) [15]. This result suggests that the prognosis of patients with ACO is affected by the definition and diagnosis of ACO.

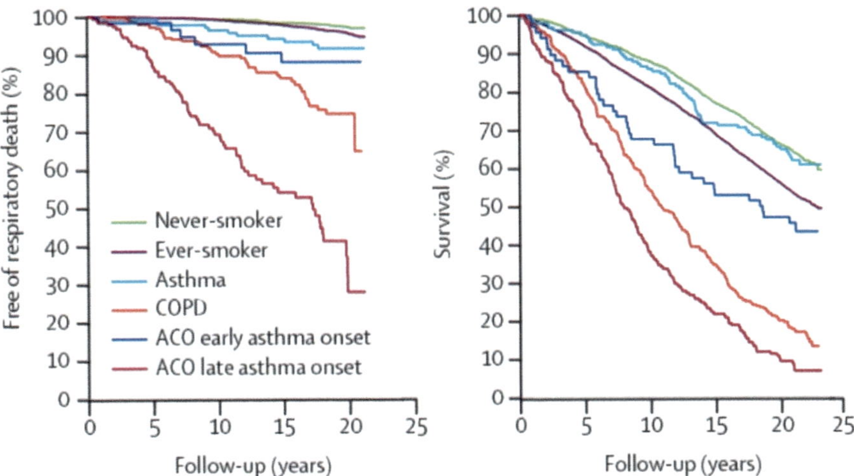

Fig. 6.2 Kaplan–Meier curves for respiratory mortality (left) and all-cause mortality (right) from the Copenhagen City Heart Study. (Reprinted from Lange et al. [15], with permission from Elsevier)

5 Conclusion

The impact of asthma-like features or ACO on lung function, exacerbations, and mortality varied between studies. Interpretation of the results from each study requires caution. When interpreting the results, variations in the diagnostic criteria for ACO, disease severity, sample size, and follow-up period must be considered. Such variations affect the prognosis of ACO and remind us that heterogeneous phenotypes exist, even among patients classified as having ACO. To accurately understand the pathogenesis of ACO and to predict treatment response and prognosis, it is important to describe ACO beyond the disease label of "asthma" and "COPD."

References

1. Suzuki M, Makita H, Konno S, Shimizu K, Kimura H, et al. Asthma-like features and clinical course of chronic obstructive pulmonary disease. An analysis from the Hokkaido COPD cohort study. Am J Respir Crit Care Med. 2016;194(11):1358–65.
2. Marsh SE, Travers J, Weatherall M, Williams MV, Aldington S, Shirtcliffe PM, et al. Proportional classifications of COPD phenotypes. Thorax. 2008;63(9):761–7.
3. Soler-Cataluña JJ, Cosío B, Izquierdo JL, López-Campos JL, Marín JM, Agüero R, et al. Consensus document on the overlap phenotype COPD-asthma in COPD. Arch Bronconeumol. 2012;48(9):331–7.
4. Golpe R, Pérez de Llano L. Are the diagnostic criteria for asthma-COPD overlap syndrome appropriate in biomass smoke-induced chronic obstructive pulmonary disease? Arch Bronconeumol. 2016;52(2):110.
5. Cosio BG, Soriano JB, López-Campos JL, Calle-Rubio M, Soler-Cataluna JJ, de-Torres JP, et al. Defining the Asthma-COPD overlap syndrome in a COPD cohort. Chest. 2016;149(1):45–52.
6. Calverley PM, Burge PS, Spencer S, Anderson JA, Jones PW. Bronchodilator reversibility testing in chronic obstructive pulmonary disease. Thorax. 2003;58(8):659–64.
7. Anthonisen NR, Lindgren PG, Tashkin DP, Kanner RE, Scanlon PD, Connett JE, et al. Bronchodilator response in the lung health study over 11 years. Eur Respir J. 2005;26(1):45–51.
8. Burge PS, Calverley PM, Jones PW, Spencer S, Anderson JA, Maslen TK. Randomised, double blind, placebo controlled study of fluticasone propionate in patients with moderate to severe chronic obstructive pulmonary disease: the ISOLDE trial. BMJ. 2000;320(7245):1297–303.
9. Park HY, Lee SY, Kang D, Cho J, Lee H, Lim SY, et al. Favorable longitudinal change of lung function in patients with asthma-COPD overlap from a COPD cohort. Respir Res. 2018;19(1):36.
10. Vestbo J, Edwards LD, Scanlon PD, Yates JC, Agusti A, Bakke P, et al. Changes in forced expiratory volume in 1 second over time in COPD. N Engl J Med. 2011;365(13):1184–92.
11. Jo YS, Moon JY, Park YB, Kim YH, Um SJ, Kin WJ, et al. Longitudinal changes in forced expiratory volume in 1 s in patients with eosinophilic chronic obstructive pulmonary disease. BMC Pulm Med. 2022;22(1):91.
12. Shin SH, Park HY, Kang D, Cho J, Kwon SO, Park JH, et al. Serial blood eosinophils and clinical outcome in patients with chronic obstructive pulmonary disease. Respir Res. 2018;19(1):134.
13. Barnes NC, Sharma R, Lettis S, Calverley PM. Blood eosinophils as a marker of response to inhaled corticosteroids in COPD. Eur Respir J. 2016;47(5):1374–82.
14. Barrecheguren M, Pinto L, Mostafavi-Pour-Manshadi SM, Tan WC, Li PZ, Aaron SD, et al. Identification and definition of asthma-COPD overlap: the CanCOLD study. Respirology. 2020;25(8):836–49.

15. Lange P, Çolak Y, Ingebrigtsen TS, Vestbo J, Marott JL. Long-term prognosis of asthma, chronic obstructive pulmonary disease, and asthma-chronic obstructive pulmonary disease overlap in the Copenhagen City Heart study: a prospective population-based analysis. Lancet Respir Med. 2016;4(6):454–62.
16. Fu JJ, Gibson PG, Simpson JL, McDonald VM. Longitudinal changes in clinical outcomes in older patients with asthma, COPD and asthma-COPD overlap syndrome. Respiration. 2014;87(1):63–74.
17. de Marco R, Marcon A, Rossi A, Antó JM, Cerveri I, Gislason T, et al. Asthma, COPD and overlap syndrome: a longitudinal study in young European adults. Eur Respir J. 2015;46(3):671–9.
18. Konno S, Makira H, Suzuki M, Shimizu K, Kimura H, Kimura H, et al. Acute bronchodilator responses to β2-agonist and anticholinergic agent in COPD: their different associations with exacerbation. Respir Med. 2017;127:14–20.
19. Marín JM, Ciudad M, Moya V, Carrizo S, Bello S, Piras B, et al. Airflow reversibility and long-term outcomes in patients with COPD without comorbidities. Respir Med. 2014;108(8):1180–8.
20. Kim J, Kim WJ, Lee CH, Lee SH, Lee MG, Shin KC, et al. Which bronchodilator reversibility criteria can predict severe acute exacerbation in chronic obstructive pulmonary disease patients? Respir Res. 2017;18(1):107.
21. Vedel-Krogh S, Nielsen SF, Lange P, Vestbo J, Nordestgaard BG. Blood eosinophils and exacerbations in chronic obstructive pulmonary disease. The Copenhagen General Population Study. Am J Respir Crit Care Med. 2016;193(9):965–74.
22. Pascoe S, Locantore N, Dransfield MT, Barnes NC, Pavord ID. Blood eosinophil counts, exacerbations, and response to the addition of inhaled fluticasone furoate to vilanterol in patients with chronic obstructive pulmonary disease: a secondary analysis of data from two parallel randomised controlled trials. Lancet Respir Med. 2015;3(6):435–42.
23. Bafadhel M, Peterson S, De Blas MA, Calverley PM, Rennard SI, Richter K, et al. Predictors of exacerbation risk and response to budesonide in patients with chronic obstructive pulmonary disease: a post-hoc analysis of three randomised trials. Lancet Respir Med. 2018;6(2):117–26.
24. Pascoe S, Barnes N, Brusselle G, Compton C, Criner GJ, Dransfield MT, et al. Blood eosinophils and treatment response with triple and dual combination therapy in chronic obstructive pulmonary disease: analysis of the IMPACT trial. Lancet Respir Med. 2019;7(9):745–56.
25. Hastie AT, Martinez FJ, Curtis JL, Doerschuk CM, Hansel NN, Christenson S, et al. Association of sputum and blood eosinophil concentrations with clinical measures of COPD severity: an analysis of the SPIROMICS cohort. Lancet Respir Med. 2017;5(12):956–67.
26. Hardin M, Silverman EK, Barr RG, Hansel NN, Schroeder JD, Make BJ, et al. The clinical features of the overlap between COPD and asthma. Respir Res. 2011;12(1):127.
27. Menezes AMB, Montes de Oca M, Pérez-Padilla R, Nadeau G, Wehrmeister FC, Lopez-Varela MV, et al. Increased risk of exacerbation and hospitalization in subjects with an overlap phenotype: COPD-asthma. Chest. 2014;145(2):297–304.
28. Miravitlles M, Soriano JB, Ancochea J, Muñoz L, Duran-Tauleria E, Sánchez G, et al. Characterisation of the overlap COPD-asthma phenotype. Focus on physical activity and health status. Respir Med. 2013;107(7):1053–60.
29. Bai JW, Mao B, Yang WL, Liang S, Lu HW, Xu JF. Asthma-COPD overlap syndrome showed more exacerbations however lower mortality than COPD. QJM. 2017;110(7):431–6.
30. Izquierdo-Alonso JL, Rodriguez-Gonzálezmoro JM, de Lucas-Ramos P, Unzueta I, Ribera X, Antón E, et al. Prevalence and characteristics of three clinical phenotypes of chronic obstructive pulmonary disease (COPD). Respir Med. 2013;107(5):724–31.
31. Kobayashi S, Hanagama M, Yamanda S, Ishida M, Yanai M. Inflammatory biomarkers in asthma-COPD overlap syndrome. Int J Chron Obstruct Pulmon Dis. 2016;11:2117–23.
32. Inoue H, Nagase T, Morita S, Yoshida A, Jinnai T, Ichinose M. Prevalence and characteristics of asthma-COPD overlap syndrome identified by a stepwise approach. Int J Chron Obstruct Pulmon Dis. 2017;12:1803–10.
33. Bafadhel M, McKenna S, Terry S, Mistry V, Reid C, Haldar P, et al. Acute exacerbations of chronic obstructive pulmonary disease: identification of biologic clusters and their biomarkers. Am J Respir Crit Care Med. 2011;184(6):662–71.

34. Hansen EF, Phanareth K, Laursen LC, Kok-Jensen A, Dirksen A. Reversible and irreversible airflow obstruction as predictor of overall mortality in asthma and chronic obstructive pulmonary disease. Am J Respir Crit Care Med. 1999;159(4 Pt 1):1267–71.
35. Hanania NA, Sharafkhaneh A, Celli B, Decramer M, Lystig T, Kesten S, et al. Acute bronchodilator responsiveness and health outcomes in COPD patients in the UPLIFT trial. Respir Res. 2011;12(1):6.
36. Wurst KE, Rheault TR, Edwards L, Tal-Singer R, Agusti A, Vestbo J. A comparison of COPD patients with and without ACOS in the ECLIPSE study. Eur Respir J. 2016;47(5):1559–62.
37. Sorino C, Pedone C, Scichilone N. Fifteen-year mortality of patients with asthma-COPD overlap syndrome. Eur J Intern Med. 2016;34:72–7.
38. Diaz-Guzman E, Khosravi M, Mannino DM. Asthma, chronic obstructive pulmonary disease, and mortality in the U.S. population. COPD. 2011;8(6):400–7.
39. Kumbhare S, Strange C. Mortality in asthma-chronic obstructive pulmonary disease overlap in the United States. South Med J. 2018;111(5):293–8.
40. Tkacova R, Dai DLY, Vonk JM, Leung JM, Hiemstra PS, van den Berge M, et al. Airway hyperresponsiveness in chronic obstructive pulmonary disease: a marker of asthma-chronic obstructive pulmonary disease overlap syndrome? J Allergy Clin Immunol. 2016;138(6):1571–9.
41. Baarnes CB, Andersen ZJ, Tjønneland A, Ulrik CS. Incidence and long-term outcome of severe asthma-COPD overlap compared to asthma and COPD alone: a 35-year prospective study of 57,053 middle-aged adults. Int J Chron Obstruct Pulmon Dis. 2017;12:571–9.
42. Yamauchi Y, Yasunaga H, Matsui H, Hasegawa W, Jo T, Takami K, et al. Comparison of in-hospital mortality in patients with COPD, asthma and asthma-COPD overlap exacerbations. Respirology. 2015;20(6):940–6.
43. Peltola L, Pätsi H, Harju T. COPD comorbidities predict high mortality—Asthma-COPD-overlap has better prognosis. COPD. 2020;17(4):366–72.

Chapter 7
Causes of Death in Patients with Asthma-Chronic Obstructive Pulmonary Disease Overlap: Is There Any Difference Compared to Asthma?

Akira Yamasaki, Tomoya Harada, and Katsuyuki Tomita

Abstract Patients with asthma-chronic obstructive pulmonary disease (COPD) overlap (ACO) show both asthma and COPD features. The mortality rate of ACO is reportedly lower or higher than that of asthma or COPD alone, probably because of differences in diagnostic labeling, cohort size, severity, and mortality rate definition among studies. The cause-specific mortality rate per 1000 person-years is 2.29 to 25.9 for ACO and 1.39 to 11.7 for asthma. The most common causes of mortality are cancer and cardiovascular diseases, and the causes of death in individuals with asthma and ACO are comparable. However, ACO is associated with more comorbidities compared with asthma, and some of these comorbidities affect mortality and cause of death.

The impact of coronavirus disease 2019 (COVID-19), which is caused by the severe acute respiratory syndrome coronavirus 2 (SARS-CoV-2), on asthma and ACO-related mortality is critical. COPD, but not asthma, has been linked to SARS-CoV-2 infection and its severity, and patients with ACO are more likely to develop severe COVID-19 infection compared with patients with asthma.

Thus, comorbidities, including malignant diseases, influence the prognoses of ACO and asthma. Several infectious diseases, including COVID-19, also affect ACO-related mortality. Controlling comorbidities and contagious diseases can improve ACO prognosis.

Keywords ACO · Asthma · COPD · COVID-19 · Comorbidity

A. Yamasaki (✉) · T. Harada
Division of Respiratory Medicine and Rheumatology, Department of Multidisciplinary Internal Medicine, Faculty of Medicine, Tottori University, Yonago, Japan
e-mail: yamasaki@tottori-u.ac.jp

K. Tomita
Department of Respiratory Medicine, National Hospital Organization Yonago Medical Center, Yonago, Japan

H. Nagase et al. (eds.), *Asthma-COPD Overlap*, Respiratory Disease Series: Diagnostic Tools and Disease Managements,
https://doi.org/10.1007/978-981-96-0217-9_7

1 Introduction

Asthma-chronic obstructive pulmonary syndrome (COPD) overlap (ACO) is a disorder that has both asthma and COPD symptoms. When compared with asthma or COPD alone, the prognosis of ACO is debatable, with some studies reporting a favorable prognosis and others reporting the opposite. One explanation for this difference is the method of calculating the mortality rate. Furthermore, while asthma or COPD can be considered as the cause of death, the same cannot be said of ACO because, as mentioned before, it is a condition. Therefore, examining the cause of death in patients with ACO and the difference in the cause of death between patients with ACO and those with only asthma or only COPD can yield interesting results. Furthermore, the impact of coronavirus disease 2019 (COVID-19), which is caused by the severe acute respiratory syndrome-coronavirus-2 (SARS-CoV-2), on ACO-related mortality, asthma, and ACO is a major concern. The causes of death in individuals with asthma, COPD, and ACO are discussed in this article. Moreover, this study discusses the association of COVID-19 with asthma and ACO.

2 Number of Deaths Among Patients with Asthma, COPD, or ACO

Asthma is a prevalent respiratory condition that affects people all over the world. In 2019, asthma affected an estimated 262 million individuals worldwide, with 461,000 deaths [1]. The proportion of elderly patients reported to have died of asthma is high in the United States, United Kingdom, and Japan [2–4]. Elderly patients with asthma exhibit two phenotypes: late-onset asthma and long-standing asthma [5]. Smoking and obesity are associated with late-onset asthma, whereas atopy and family history are associated with long-standing asthma. The mortality rate for senior asthma patients is five times higher than for young individuals [5]. Moreover, Nakazawa et al. reported that 20% of patients who died of asthma had pulmonary emphysematous changes [6]. Therefore, a certain proportion of elderly individuals who die of asthma may have COPD features.

COPD is the world's third biggest cause of death, accounting for 3.23 million deaths in 2019. Currently, it is the eighth largest cause of death among men globally, as reported in 2019. In 2020, 16,127 individuals died of COPD in Japan, with a mortality rate of 13.1%, and the percentage of deaths from COPD compared with that from any other cause was 1.2% in 2020. It is noteworthy that COPD, as a single respiratory disease is one of the leading causes of death worldwide, including Japan.

The number of deaths from ACO has not been reported globally or in Japan because ACO is a heterogeneous condition and is not the name of a particular disease. If a patient with ACO dies of an asthma attack, the cause of death is speculated to be asthma, and if a patient with ACO dies of COPD exacerbation, the cause of death is speculated to be COPD. Asthma, COPD, and ACO have prevalence rates of

6.2% (5.0–7.4%), 4.9% (4.3–5.5%), and 2.0% (1.4–2.6%) in the general population, respectively [7]. According to a recent meta-analysis, ACO was found to be prevalent in 29.6% of the patients with COPD and 26.5% of the patients with asthma [7]. Therefore, a certain number of patients with ACO die of asthma or COPD.

3 Mortality Rate of Patients with ACO

Mortality rate can be indicated in three ways: cause-specific mortality rate (CMR), case fatality rate (CFR), and standardized mortality ratio (SMR). Generally, CMR describes the mortality rate of a particular disease. It is defined as the number of deaths from an illness that occurs within the total population at any given time. The CMR is distinct from the CFR in that the latter quantifies the severity of a disease by expressing the total number of deaths as a percentage of all reported cases at a given time. As age and sex are confounding factors, standardized or adjusted rates allow for differences in age and sex distributions in the populations under study. The SMR, a comparable statistic for evaluating disease burden and lethal disease intensity, is widely used by registrar generals for summarizing time trends and regional differences. It is computed by dividing the observed mortality rates in each population, for example, the number of deaths in a group of ACO patients, by the expected mortality rates in the same group predicted by age- and sex-specific mortality rates for a standard population. The SMR is the ratio of fatalities observed in a population during a particular period to deaths expected if the research population had the same age-specific mortality rates as the reference population. If the rate is larger than 1%, the population under study is deemed to have an excess mortality rate.

3.1 CMR for ACO

Some studies have used CMRs based on community-based follow-up data for patients suffering from asthma, COPD, and ACO [8–10]. Table 7.1 shows the CMR comparisons found in various studies. Baarnes et al. described CMRs for asthma, COPD, and ACO based on patient age. The ACO group was confirmed to have the highest CMR (25.9/1000 person-years), followed by the COPD and asthma groups (23.1 and 7.9 per 1000 person-years, respectively) (regarding CMR, ACO>COPD>asthma) [8]. For patients with ACO until the age of 65 years, men had a higher CMR than women, whereas the opposite was observed for patients aged ≥65 years. Kendzerska et al. demonstrated that the CMR of ACO was similar to that of COPD and subsequently that of asthma (regarding CMR, ACO≈COPD>ACO). According to this study, individuals with ACO were notably older than those with asthma [9]. Diaz-Guzman et al. reported that COPD showed the highest CMR compared with asthma or ACO (COPD>ACO>asthma) [10]. These discrepancies may

Table 7.1 Review of cause-specific mortality rates for asthma-chronic obstructive pulmonary disease (COPD) overlap (ACO)

Author (year)	Research type	Target	Mortality rate (per 1000 person-years)
Baarnes et al. [8] (2017)	Prospective cohort	• Study site: Denmark • 57,053 adults • Follow-up period: Long term (35 years) • Diagnosis of ACO: Physician-based, using ICD codes on discharge	ACO ($n = 662$) Total: 25.9 Female sex: 25.5 55–65 years: 12.9 >75 years: 57.2 COPD ($n = 3375$) Total: 23.1 Female sex: 19.6 55–65 years: 7.2 >75 years: 75.5 Asthma ($n = 1183$) Total: 7.9 Female sex: 6.9 55–65 years: 4.6
Kendzerska et al. [9] (2015)	Retrospective cohort	• Study site: Ontario, Canada • 2012, 7,589,414 adults • Diagnosis of ACO: Physician-diagnosed	ACO Total: 2.29 COPD Total: 2.25 Asthma Total: 1.39
Diaz-Guzman et al. [10] (2011)	Prospective cohort	• Study site: USA • 15,203 individuals • Follow-up period: Long term (up to 18 years) • Diagnosis of ACO: Physician-based	ACO ($n = 357$) Total: 28.3 COPD ($n = 815$) Total: 36.1 Asthma ($n = 709$) Total: 11.7

be due to differences in the prevalence rates of diseases. Although it is not clearly defined, there are more relevant published articles on the mortality rates of ACO compared with those of other asthma-related comorbidities.

3.2 *CFR for ACO*

Several studies have reported CFRs for asthma, COPD, and ACO (Table 7.2) [11–15]. However, these studies have shown that CFRs for ACO widely range from 0% to 20% for similar proportions of patients diagnosed with the aforementioned conditions; this is not surprising, given the extensive variations in the approaches employed in different studies. In some studies, initial patient selection was based on all identified cases in a nationwide database of cases, whereas in some studies, thoroughly diagnosed but highly selective patients were chosen from a tertiary referral inpatient setting. Follow-up intervals ranged from 5 to 33 years, and crude mortality numbers inevitably increase with more extended follow-up periods; that is, as a

Table 7.2 Review of case fatality rates (CFRs) for asthma-chronic obstructive pulmonary disease (COPD) overlap (ACO)

Author (year)	Research type	Target	CFR (%)
Kobayashi et al. [11] (2020)	Prospective	• Assessment: CFR • Study setting: Ishinomaki in Japan • Follow-up period: Short term (3 years) • Diagnosis of ACO: Physiological lung function criteria	ACO ($n = 38$) Total: 0% COPD ($n = 321$) Total: 12.9%
Sorino et al. [12] (2016)	Retrospective	• Study setting: Italy • 24 centers • Diagnosis of ACO: Physiological lung function criteria • Follow-up period: Long term (15 years)	ACO ($n = 118$) Total: 7.2% COPD ($n = 205$) Total: 9.1% Asthma ($n = 159$) Total: 4.7%
Harada et al. [13] (2015)	Retrospective	• Study setting: Yonago in Japan • 650 patients followed up from Jan 2000 to Mar 2012 • Diagnosis of ACO: GINA criteria	ACO ($n = 176$) Total: 18.8% Asthma ($n = 474$) Total: 11.4%
Yamauchi et al. [14] (2015)	Retrospective	• Study setting: Japan • All-cause in-hospital mortality • Diagnosis of ACO: Physician-based, using ICD codes on discharge	ACO ($n = 6279$) Total: 2.3% COPD ($n = 4261$) Total: 9.7% Asthma ($n = 19{,}865$) Total: 1.2%
Fu et al. [15] (2014)	Prospective cohort	• Study setting: Newcastle in Australia • 650 patients followed up from July 2006 to Dec 2011 • Diagnosis of ACO: Physiological lung function criteria	ACO ($n = 55$) Total: 20.0% COPD ($n = 36$) Total: 13.9% Asthma ($n = 8$) Total: 0%

cohort ages, there will be more cases of death. Numerous biological, social, political, and environmental elements can alter a population's CFRs [11–15].

Soriano et al. reported that the CFR for ACO was lower than that for COPD alone in a 15-year follow-up study [12]. Yamauchi et al. used a nationwide database in Japan to show that COPD had a higher in-hospital CFR (9.7%) compared with ACO (2.3%) or asthma alone (1.2%) [14]. This reasonably significant difference in CFR might indicate a link between comorbidities in asthma and COPD or could suggest that patients with COPD alone had a higher risk of death throughout the research due to their advanced age compared with those with asthma or ACO [14]. Obstructive respiratory diseases, including asthma, COPD, and ACO, may be characterized by their CFRs, and the causes of death, in descending order, are projected to be asthma, COPD, and ACO. In one study, patients with COPD had worse outcomes than those with asthma and ACO because their body mass index, airflow obstruction level, dyspnea level, and exercise index were lower [15]. Several studies have discovered that people with ACO have a lower overall quality of life and are more likely to be hospitalized for exacerbations than people with asthma or COPD alone [9, 14].

3.3 SMR for ACO

SMR for ACO was reanalyzed using data published by Kendzerska et al. [9] and additional general population and mortality data in Ontario during the same period (Fig. 7.1). The authors found that SMR for ACO was higher among patients aged ≥65 years, with no difference in sex during the reanalysis. According to previous studies, patients with ACO are more likely to be younger women, have a higher body mass index, and have a more significant load of comorbidities compared with patients with asthma or COPD alone [16, 17]. The re-calculated SMR also demonstrated that age was an independent factor affecting ACO-related mortality.

4 Causes of Death in Patients with Asthma, COPD, and ACO

The actual causes of mortality among patients with asthma, COPD, and ACO are unknown. Table 7.3 summarizes the three major causes of mortality in patients with the aforementioned conditions. The order of causes of death probably differs because of differences in the study period and number of participants among various studies. However, malignant diseases (especially lung cancer), cardiovascular disorders, and respiratory diseases are essentially the leading causes of death in patients with asthma and those with ACO.

One study evaluated patients with asthma using ICD-10 from 2001 to 2007 in the United Kingdom. When asthma was recorded as the underlying cause, the leading cause of death was pneumonia, followed by chronic ischemic heart disease (IHD) and COPD, in this order. In contrast, when asthma was a contributing cause of death, the leading cause was chronic IHD, followed by acute myocardial infarction and COPD, in this order [4]. In another study, 13 cardiovascular diseases (29.3%), solid tumors (20.7%), and infections (14.6%) were the most common causes of death in patients with asthma in Spanish secondary and tertiary hospitals. In the same study, solid tumors (26.6%), acute respiratory insufficiency (25.5%), and infections were the causes of death in patients with COPD (16.3%) [18]. A study from the United States examined 4434 patients with asthma, COPD, or ACO and found that cardiovascular diseases and malignancies were the leading causes of

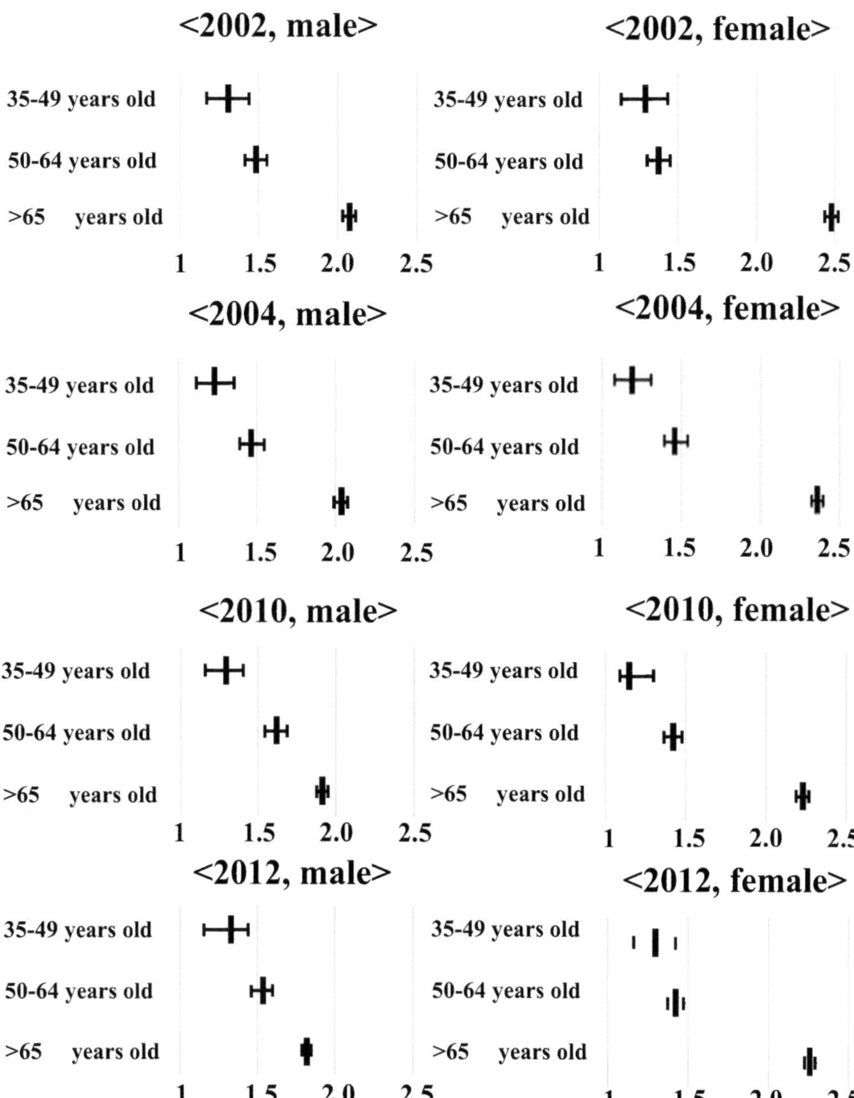

Fig. 7.1 Standardized mortality rate for asthma-chronic obstructive pulmonary syndrome overlap reanalyzed using data published by Kendzerska et al. [9] and additional data for the general population and mortality in the same period in Ontario

death in all groups [19]. A report from Australia showed that the leading causes of death in patients with asthma were influenza and pneumonia, while COPD and coronary heart disease were the second and third most common causes of death, respectively.

Table 7.3 The three major leading causes of death in patients with asthma, chronic obstructive pulmonary disease (COPD), and asthma-COPD overlap (ACO)

Country	Asthma	COPD	ACO	Reference
United Kingdom	Asthma as an underlying cause 1. Pneumonia 2. Chronic ischemic heart disease 3. COPD Asthma as a contributing cause 1. Chronic ischemic heart disease 2. Acute myocardial infarction 3. COPD	–	–	[4]
Spain	1. Cardiovascular disease 2. Solid malignancies 3. Infections	1. Solid malignancies 2. Acute respiratory failure 3. Cardiovascular disease	–	[18]
United States	1. Cardiovascular disease 2. Malignant neoplasm 3. Chronic lower respiratory diseases	1 Cardiovascular disease 2. Malignant neoplasm 3. Chronic lower respiratory diseases	1 Cardiovascular disease 2. Malignant neoplasm 3. Chronic lower respiratory diseases	[19]
Australia	1. Influenza and pneumonia 2. COPD 3. Coronary heart disease	1. Influenza and pneumonia 2. Coronary heart diseases 3. Heart failure and complications and ill-defined heart diseases	–	[20]
Finland	–	1. Respiratory causes 2. Cardiovascular diseases 3. Neoplasms	1. Respiratory causes 2. Cardiovascular diseases 3. Neoplasms	[17]
Japan	1. Malignant disease 2. Solid malignancies 3. Sudden death/unknown	–	1. Malignant diseases 2. Pneumonia 3. Cardiovascular disease	[13]

In contrast, in patients with COPD, the leading causes of death were influenza and pneumonia, followed by coronary heart disease and heart failure with complications and ill-defined heart diseases [20]. Pelota et al. reported that the underlying causes of mortality did not differ between the ACO and COPD groups [17]. In Finland, respiratory causes were the most common, while cardiovascular diseases and neoplasms were the second and third leading causes of death, respectively, in patients with asthma as well as those with COPD. From 2000 to 2012, Harada et al. investigated the causes of mortality in patients with asthma and those with ACO [13]; in patients with ACO, the leading cause of death was malignant diseases, followed by pneumonia and cardiovascular diseases, in this order. In patients with asthma, the leading cause of death was malignant diseases, while the second and third leading causes of death were pneumonia and sudden death/unknown, respectively [13]. The authors found that malignant disorders were a more significant cause of death than benign diseases, with lung cancer and gastrointestinal cancer being the most common causes of death in asthma-only ($n = 474$) and ACO ($n = 176$) patients. Young et al. reported that COPD was an independent risk factor for lung cancer development, irrespective of smoking exposure [21] and that patients in the ACO group were older and smoked more pack-year cigarettes than did those in the asthma group; this explained why the ACO group had a greater lung cancer prevalence. Charokopos et al. found that the risk of lung cancer in patients with ACO is similar to that in patients with COPD [22]. They also found the following lung cancer incidence rates per 1000 person-years: ACO, 3.2; COPD, 11.7; smokers with asthma, 1.8; smokers with normal spirometry values, 4.1 [22]. Thus, COPD, whether coupled with asthma or not, is a risk factor for lung cancer development. The use of inhaled corticosteroids (ICS) is not associated with a lower risk of lung cancer [23]. A 10-year cohort study (the Hokkaido cohort study) revealed the causes of death in 112 patients with COPD in Japan. The leading cause of death was malignant disease, and lung cancer was the most common malignant disease. Respiratory disease was the second leading cause of death, and cardiovascular disease came in third [24].

Some results contradicted each other. Generally, the causes of death are influenced by sex, age, economic status in countries, and disease-specific comorbidities. In Japan, more than 85% of patients were aged ≥70 years. Increased aging might contribute to the increased prevalence of comorbidity-related deaths. The causes of death originate from views of these factors below.

4.1 Age- and Country-Associated Causes of Death

The World Health Organization has reported the leading causes of death worldwide. At a global level, the leading causes of death are ischemic heart disease, stroke, COPD, lower respiratory conditions, neonatal conditions, lung cancers, Alzheimer's disease (AD), diarrheal diseases, diabetes mellitus, and kidney diseases. It is summarized that circulatory system diseases and cancer are the two leading causes of death in most countries. Causes of death vary significantly between countries; non-communicable diseases, including cardiovascular disease (including stroke), cancers, diabetes, and chronic respiratory disease, dominate in rich countries, whereas the prevalence rates of infection disease, malnutrition, nutritional deficiencies, and neonatal and maternal diseases remain high in lower-income countries.

Increased aging contributes to AD being more prevalent as a cause of death. In Japan, as more than 85% of patients are aged ≥70 years, AD contributes to the cause of death.

4.2 Comorbidity-Associated Cause of Death

A risk factor for disease-specific comorbidities is determined to be the cause of death. For example, Jurevičienė et al. reported that there is an association between COPD and six-fold higher odds of developing lung cancer (odds ratio [OR], 6.66), a two-fold higher rate of heart failure (OR, 2.61), and CVD (OR, 1.83) [25].

In patients with asthma, COPD, or ACO, comorbidities influence mortality and are related to the cause of death. According to a 2012 Behavioral Risk Factor Surveillance System study, patients with ACO had a higher occurrence frequency of an additional comorbidity than those with COPD or asthma alone [26]. Comorbidities are widespread in both patient categories, and a more significant number of comorbidities may reduce the chances of survival in patients with ACO and COPD [27]. ACO is associated with more comorbidities than asthma, and some of these comorbidities affect mortality and are related to the cause of death [28].

4.2.1 IHD and Coronary Heart Disease as Comorbidity

IHD includes angina, acute myocardial infarction, ischemic heart failure, and lethal arrhythmia due to ischemic heart failure. The risk factors for ischemic heart disease are smoking, hypertension, diabetes, obesity, and hyperlipidemia. Several investigations have been conducted to see if there is a link between ischemic heart disease and obstructive pulmonary disease. In a Korean study, the odds ratio for IHD was significantly greater in patients with asthma than in non-asthmatic individuals [29]. In that study, an association between IHD and asthma was observed in older patients (>53 years) and patients not receiving treatment. In the Copenhagen General Population Study, obstructive respiratory diseases, including asthma, COPD, coronary heart disease, and IHD, were also linked with ACO. ACO with late-onset asthma, which is characterized by <50% of the predicted forced expiratory volume in the first second (GOLD 3 and 4), is the highest risk factor for coronary heart disease and heart failure [30]. Furthermore, in patients with asthma and ACO (GOLD 1 and 2), allergy was found to be a risk factor for hospital admission for coronary heart disease and heart failure [30]. Patients with asthma, COPD, or ACO had a higher risk of coronary heart disease and heart failure. The largest risks of coronary heart disease and heart failure were reported in patients with ACO who had late-onset asthma and a FEV1 of 50%; the hazard ratios (HR) were 2.2 (95% confidence interval (CI) 1.6 to 3.0) and 2.9 (95% CI 2.0 to 4.3), respectively [31]. After adjusting for several confounding variables—age, gender, comorbidities, and medication use—ACO was significantly related to an increased risk of CVDs [32].

4.2.2 Stroke as Comorbidity

Stroke is the second leading cause of death globally, and its risk factors include cardiovascular disease, atherosclerosis, hypertension, dyslipidemia, diabetes mellitus, older age, cigarette smoking, obesity, depression, and male sex. Several studies have demonstrated a relationship between stroke and obstructive lung diseases, including asthma, COPD, and ACO. In a Korean study, it has been reported that asthma is not associated with stroke incidence [22]. However, in a systematic review including 524,637 participants and 6031 cases, patients with asthma showed a risk of developing stroke, with an HR of 1.32 [33]. The review also found that the association between stroke and asthma was more robust in women than in men.

The risk of stroke is 1.2 times higher in patients with COPD than in healthy controls. Furthermore, the risk is seven-fold higher in patients with an acute exacerbation of COPD than in those with stable COPD. Shared risk factors for COPD and stroke are aging and smoking. Poor lung function is also related to an increased risk of stroke, and similar results have been observed for asthma [34]. In addition to these factors, systemic inflammation and oxidative stress may be related to an increased risk of stroke via the promotion of cerebral vascular dysfunction and insufficiency. During the acute exacerbation of COPD by viral or bacterial infections, systemic inflammation is further enhanced, and platelet activation and coagulation are induced; this increases the risk of stroke [35]. Asthma exacerbation is also associated with stroke. The accumulation of platelets, neutrophils, and fibrinogen during inflammation, hypoxemia, and oxidative stress is assumed to be the reason for the increased risk of stroke during asthma exacerbation [34]. However, the relationship between the frequency of acute exacerbation and stroke has not been observed in patients with COPD [36]. Stroke, however, is a comorbidity that occurs more frequently in patients with ACO than in those with asthma or COPD alone. Stroke was more frequently observed in patients with ACO than those without ACO in a cohort study [37]. A cohort study from Denmark, comprising 57,053 individuals, showed interesting results. Age, current smoking, unemployment, and divorce were associated with a high incidence of ACO, and stroke was associated with a higher risk of COPD [38].

4.2.3 AD and Other Dementias as Comorbidity

AD and other dementias are the seventh largest cause of mortality worldwide and the second leading cause in high-income countries. Dementia is classified into several disorders, with AD, Levy body dementia, cerebrovascular dementia, and frontotemporal dementia being four significant primary dementias that account for 90% of all dementia cases. Because asthma and COPD are common comorbidities in patients with dementia, several studies have reported the risks of dementia or cognitive impairment in patients with obstructive pulmonary diseases. Although the relationship between asthma or COPD and dementia is controversial, a recent cohort study revealed that neither asthma nor COPD is a risk factor for the development of dementia [39, 40]. However, a national cohort study in Taiwan showed that patients with ACO are at a high risk of developing dementia. Nevertheless, the use of ICS at a dose >0.13 g per year was found to decrease the risk of dementia [37]. The factors causing dementia development in persons with obstructive lung disease remain unknown. Aging, smoking, inflammation, the coexistence of cardiovascular disease, hypoxemia, and hypercapnia may be involved in the pathogenesis of cognitive impairment. Controlling eosinophilic inflammation and hypoxia may prevent the development of dementia and cognitive impairment.

5 Cause of Death with COVID-19 as a Concomitant Disease

COVID-19 is caused by SARS-CoV-2. Men, the elderly, and patients with comorbidities, including heart disease, cancer, obesity, and diabetes, experience worse clinical outcomes, including death. Respiratory diseases are also independent risk factors for an increased risk of SARS-CoV-2 infection and greater disease severity. The current literature on asthma, ACO, and COVID-19 is summarized in this section.

5.1 *Asthma with COVID-19*

Patients with asthma are more susceptible to common viral respiratory infections. They have a higher frequency and severity of lower respiratory tract infections than healthy individuals; therefore, it seems reasonable that they would be at an increased risk of SARS-CoV-2 infection and more severe COVID-19 manifestations. According to Li et al., the incidence of COVID-19 is low in patients with asthma, and there is no evidence of an increased risk of SARS-CoV-2 infection in these patients [41]. Nonetheless, the incidence of COVID-19 in individuals with asthma varies significantly across different countries [42].

Similarly, various epidemiological studies have investigated whether asthma is a risk factor for severe COVID-19. The results are controversial because asthma has diverse phenotypes, severities, and background therapies. Liu et al. found no link between asthma and a greater risk of severe COVID-19 infection and death in a thorough investigation and meta-analysis. Furthermore, patients with asthma had a lower mortality risk than patients without asthma, and mechanical ventilation use was not associated with an increased risk of mortality [43]. According to a report by Schultze et al., patients with asthma who were administered high-dose ICS had a greater risk of death from COVID-19; patients prescribed low- or medium-dose ICS were excluded from the study [44].

One noteworthy finding is that individuals with non-type 2 asthma have a greater probability of developing severe COVID-19. Jackson et al. found that angiotensin-converting enzyme 2 (ACE2) expression dramatically decreased in nasal and bronchial epithelial cells in patients with allergy and asthma [45]. The expression of the ACE2 gene is negatively correlated with type 2 biomarkers. Consequently, ACE2 gene expression is downregulated in individuals with asthma and Th2-type inflammation. These data imply that asthma patients, particularly those with Th2-type inflammation, may exhibit decreased susceptibility to SARS-CoV-2 infection, severe illness, and poor clinical outcomes of COVID-19. According to Peters et al., patients with asthma treated with ICS exhibit a considerably decreased expression of ACE2 and transmembrane protease serine 2, which may limit SARS-CoV-2 replication [46]. According to Solis et al., the percentage of non-hospitalized asthma patients who used ICS was significantly higher than that of patients requiring hospitalization for COVID-19. It seems that ICS may have a beneficial effect on SARS-CoV-2 infectivity and COVID-19 severity.

5.2 COPD with COVID-19

Some initial studies have suggested that patients with COPD are at increased risk of poor outcomes of COVID-19, including mortality [47, 48]. In a systematic study of patients with COPD affected by COVID-19, the pooled prevalence rates of COPD and smoking were 2% and 9%, respectively, whereas the crude case fatality rate was 7.4% [47]. Current smokers had a larger risk of serious complications and a higher mortality rate than non-smokers among patients with COPD affected by COVID-19.

5.3 ACO with COVID-19

As previously stated, patients with the Th2-high endotype are protected from SARS-CoV-2 infection and the onset of severe illness. In contrast, patients with COPD have a higher risk of severe COVID-19. According to Maes et al., ACE2 mRNA expression in the lung tissue of patients with ACO was not different from that in the lung tissue of individuals in the control group [49]. Wang et al., however, investigated a possible risk factor for hospitalization and death in COVID-19-affected asthma patients and found that COPD and hospitalization combined may be a significant risk factor for hospitalization [50]. According to a population-based prospective cohort study from the UK Biobank, patients with ACO had a greater risk of severe COVID-19 than patients with asthma [42]. Thus, patients with ACO appear to be at a higher risk of SARS-CoV-2 infection and experience severe COVID-19 symptoms. However, there is inadequate evidence regarding ACO as a risk factor for SARS-CoV-2 infection and severe COVID-19 outcomes; therefore, further research is warranted.

6 Conclusions

ACO is a condition that lies at the middle of a spectrum, with asthma and COPD at either end. ACO has some phenotypes such as smoke-related asthma or COPD with blood eosinophilia and bronchodilation. The mortality rate and cause of death in ACO patients are considered to be independent of both phenotypes. Emerging infectious diseases, including COVID-19, require further research to clarify their impact on ACO and asthma prognoses.

References

1. Diseases GBD, Injuries C. Global burden of 369 diseases and injuries in 204 countries and territories, 1990–2019: a systematic analysis for the Global Burden of Disease Study 2019. Lancet. 2020;396(10258):1204–22. https://doi.org/10.1016/S0140-6736(20)30925-9.
2. Moorman JE, Akinbami LJ, Bailey CM, Zahran HS, King ME, Johnson CA, et al. National surveillance of asthma: United States, 2001–2010. Vital Health Stat 3. 2012;(35):1–58.
3. Tsai CL, Lee WY, Hanania NA, Camargo CA Jr. Age-related differences in clinical outcomes for acute asthma in the United States, 2006–2008. J Allergy Clin Immunol. 2012;129(5):1252–8.e1. https://doi.org/10.1016/j.jaci.2012.01.061.
4. Goldacre MJ, Duncan ME, Griffith M. Death rates for asthma in English populations 1979–2007: comparison of underlying cause and all certified causes. Public Health. 2012;126(5):386–93. https://doi.org/10.1016/j.puhe.2012.01.022.
5. Dunn RM, Busse PJ, Wechsler ME. Asthma in the elderly and late-onset adult asthma. Allergy. 2018;73(2):284–94. https://doi.org/10.1111/all.13258.
6. Tsugio Nakazawa KD. Current asthma deaths among adults in Japan. Allergol Int. 2004;53:205–9.
7. Hosseini M, Almasi-Hashiani A, Sepidarkish M, Maroufizadeh S. Global prevalence of asthma-COPD overlap (ACO) in the general population: a systematic review and meta-analysis. Respir Res. 2019;20(1):229. https://doi.org/10.1186/s12931-019-1198-4.
8. Baarnes CB, Andersen ZJ, Tjonneland A, Ulrik CS. Incidence and long-term outcome of severe asthma-COPD overlap compared to asthma and COPD alone: a 35-year prospective study of 57,053 middle-aged adults. Int J Chron Obstruct Pulmon Dis. 2017;12:571–9. https://doi.org/10.2147/COPD.S123167.
9. Kendzerska T, Sadatsafavi M, Aaron SD, To TM, Lougheed MD, FitzGerald JM, et al. Concurrent physician-diagnosed asthma and chronic obstructive pulmonary disease: A population study of prevalence, incidence and mortality. PLoS One. 2017;12(3):e0173830. https://doi.org/10.1371/journal.pone.0173830.
10. Diaz-Guzman E, Khosravi M, Mannino DM. Asthma, chronic obstructive pulmonary disease, and mortality in the U.S. population. COPD. 2011;8(6):400–7. https://doi.org/10.3109/15412555.2011.611200.
11. Kobayashi S, Hanagama M, Ishida M, Ono M, Sato H, Yamanda S, et al. Clinical characteristics and outcomes of patients with asthma-COPD overlap in Japanese patients with COPD. Int J Chron Obstruct Pulmon Dis. 2020;15:2923–9. https://doi.org/10.2147/COPD.S276314.
12. Sorino C, Pedone C, Scichilone N. Fifteen-year mortality of patients with asthma-COPD overlap syndrome. Eur J Intern Med. 2016;34:72–7. https://doi.org/10.1016/j.ejim.2016.06.020.
13. Harada T, Yamasaki A, Fukushima T, Hashimoto K, Takata M, Kodani M, et al. Causes of death in patients with asthma and asthma-chronic obstructive pulmonary disease overlap syndrome. Int J Chron Obstruct Pulmon Dis. 2015;10:595–602. https://doi.org/10.2147/COPD.S77491.

14. Yamauchi Y, Yasunaga H, Matsui H, Hasegawa W, Jo T, Takami K, et al. Comparison of in-hospital mortality in patients with COPD, asthma and asthma-COPD overlap exacerbations. Respirology. 2015;20(6):940–6. https://doi.org/10.1111/resp.12556.
15. Fu JJ, Gibson PG, Simpson JL, McDonald VM. Longitudinal changes in clinical outcomes in older patients with asthma, COPD and asthma-COPD overlap syndrome. Respiration. 2014;87(1):63–74. https://doi.org/10.1159/000352053.
16. Leung JM, Sin DD. Asthma-COPD overlap syndrome: pathogenesis, clinical features, and therapeutic targets. BMJ. 2017;358:j3772. https://doi.org/10.1136/bmj.j3772.
17. Peltola L, Patsi H, Harju T. COPD comorbidities predict high mortality—asthma-COPD-overlap has better prognosis. COPD. 2020;17(4):366–72. https://doi.org/10.1080/15412555.2020.1783647.
18. Soto-Campos JG, Plaza V, Soriano JB, Cabrera-Lopez C, Almonacid-Sanchez C, Vazquez-Oliva R, et al. Causes of death in asthma, COPD and non-respiratory hospitalized patients: a multicentric study. BMC Pulm Med. 2013;13:73. https://doi.org/10.1186/1471-2466-13-73.
19. Kumbhare S, Strange C. Mortality in asthma-chronic obstructive pulmonary disease overlap in the United States. South Med J. 2018;111(5):293–8. https://doi.org/10.14423/SMJ.0000000000000807.
20. Australian Institute of Health and Welfare PL, Cooper SJ, Ampon R, Reddel HK and Marks, GB. Mortality from asthma and COPD in Australia. 2014. p. Cat. no. ACM 30. Canberra: AIHW.
21. Young RP, Hopkins RJ, Christmas T, Black PN, Metcalf P, Gamble GD. COPD prevalence is increased in lung cancer, independent of age, sex and smoking history. Eur Respir J. 2009;34(2):380–6. https://doi.org/10.1183/09031936.00144208.
22. Charokopos A, Braman SS, Brown SAW, Mhango G, de-Torres JP, Zulueta JJ, et al. Lung cancer risk among patients with asthma-chronic obstructive pulmonary disease overlap. Ann Am Thorac Soc. 2021;18(11):1894–900. https://doi.org/10.1513/AnnalsATS.202010-1280OC.
23. Suissa S, Dell'Aniello S, Gonzalez AV, Ernst P. Inhaled corticosteroid use and the incidence of lung cancer in COPD. Eur Respir J. 2020;55(2) https://doi.org/10.1183/13993003.01720-2019.
24. Makita H, Suzuki M, Konno S, Shimizu K, Nasuhara Y, Nagai K, et al. Unique mortality profile in Japanese patients with COPD: an analysis from the hokkaido COPD cohort study. Int J Chron Obstruct Pulmon Dis. 2020;15:2081–90. https://doi.org/10.2147/COPD.S264437.
25. Jureviciene E, Burneikaite G, Dambrauskas L, Kasiulevicius V, Kazenaite E, Navickas R, et al. Epidemiology of chronic obstructive pulmonary disease (COPD) Comorbidities in lithuanian national database: a cluster analysis. Int J Environ Res Public Health. 2022;19(2) https://doi.org/10.3390/ijerph19020970.
26. Kumbhare S, Pleasants R, Ohar JA, Strange C. Characteristics and prevalence of asthma/chronic obstructive pulmonary disease overlap in the United States. Ann Am Thorac Soc. 2016;13(6):803–10. https://doi.org/10.1513/AnnalsATS.201508-554OC.
27. Llanos JP, Ortega H, Germain G, Duh MS, Lafeuille MH, Tiggelaar S, et al. Health characteristics of patients with asthma, COPD and asthma-COPD overlap in the NHANES database. Int J Chron Obstruct Pulmon Dis. 2018;13:2859–68. https://doi.org/10.2147/COPD.S167379.
28. Wang W, Dou S, Dong W, Xie M, Cui L, Zheng C, et al. Impact of COPD on prognosis of lung cancer: from a perspective on disease heterogeneity. Int J Chron Obstruct Pulmon Dis. 2018;13:3767–76. https://doi.org/10.2147/COPD.S168048.
29. Wee JH, Park MW, Min C, Byun SH, Park B, Choi HG. Association between asthma and cardiovascular disease. Eur J Clin Investig. 2021;51(3):e13396. https://doi.org/10.1111/eci.13396.
30. Danieli GA, Barbujani G. On the estimation of the proportion of sporadic cases in Duchenne muscular dystrophy. Am J Hum Genet. 1988;42(1):182–4.
31. Ingebrigtsen TS, Marott JL, Vestbo J, Nordestgaard BG, Lange P. Coronary heart disease and heart failure in asthma, COPD and asthma-COPD overlap. BMJ Open Respir Res. 2020;7(1) https://doi.org/10.1136/bmjresp-2019-000470.

32. Yeh JJ, Wei YF, Lin CL, Hsu WH. Association of asthma-chronic obstructive pulmonary disease overlap syndrome with coronary artery disease, cardiac dysrhythmia and heart failure: a population-based retrospective cohort study. BMJ Open. 2017;7(10):e017657. https://doi.org/10.1136/bmjopen-2017-017657.
33. Wen LY, Ni H, Li KS, Yang HH, Cheng J, Wang X, et al. Asthma and risk of stroke: a systematic review and meta-analysis. J Stroke Cerebrovasc Dis. 2016;25(3):497–503. https://doi.org/10.1016/j.jstrokecerebrovasdis.2015.11.030.
34. Corlateanu A, Stratan I, Covantev S, Botnaru V, Corlateanu O, Siafakas N. Asthma and stroke: a narrative review. Asthma Res Pract. 2021;7(1):3. https://doi.org/10.1186/s40733-021-00069-x.
35. Austin V, Crack PJ, Bozinovski S, Miller AA, Vlahos R. COPD and stroke: are systemic inflammation and oxidative stress the missing links? Clin Sci (Lond). 2016;130(13):1039–50. https://doi.org/10.1042/CS20160043.
36. Windsor C, Herrett E, Smeeth L, Quint JK. No association between exacerbation frequency and stroke in patients with COPD. Int J Chron Obstruct Pulmon Dis. 2016;11:217–25. https://doi.org/10.2147/COPD.S95775.
37. Yeh JJ, Wei YF, Lin CL, Hsu WH. Effect of the asthma-chronic obstructive pulmonary disease syndrome on the stroke, Parkinson's disease, and dementia: a national cohort study. Oncotarget. 2018;9(15):12418–31. https://doi.org/10.18632/oncotarget.23811.
38. Baarnes CB, Andersen ZJ, Tjonneland A, Ulrik CS. Determinants of incident asthma-COPD overlap: a prospective study of 55,110 middle-aged adults. Clin Epidemiol. 2018;10:1275–87. https://doi.org/10.2147/CLEP.S167269.
39. Kim SY, Min C, Oh DJ, Choi HG. Risk of neurodegenerative dementia in asthma patients: a nested case-control study using a national sample cohort. BMJ Open. 2019;9(10):e030227. https://doi.org/10.1136/bmjopen-2019-030227.
40. Siraj RA, McKeever TM, Gibson JE, Gordon AL, Bolton CE. Risk of incident dementia and cognitive impairment in patients with chronic obstructive pulmonary disease (COPD): a large UK population-based study. Respir Med. 2020;177:106288. https://doi.org/10.1016/j.rmed.2020.106288.
41. Li X, Xu S, Yu M, Wang K, Tao Y, Zhou Y, et al. Risk factors for severity and mortality in adult COVID-19 inpatients in Wuhan. J Allergy Clin Immunol. 2020;146(1):110–8. https://doi.org/10.1016/j.jaci.2020.04.006.
42. Zhu Z, Hasegawa K, Ma B, Fujiogi M, Camargo CA Jr, Liang L. Association of asthma and its genetic predisposition with the risk of severe COVID-19. J Allergy Clin Immunol. 2020;146(2):327–9. e4. https://doi.org/10.1016/j.jaci.2020.06.001.
43. Liu S, Cao Y, Du T, Zhi Y. Prevalence of comorbid asthma and related outcomes in COVID-19: a systematic review and Meta-analysis. J Allergy Clin Immunol Pract. 2021;9(2):693–701. https://doi.org/10.1016/j.jaip.2020.11.054.
44. Schultze A, Walker AJ, MacKenna B, Morton CE, Bhaskaran K, Brown JP, et al. Risk of COVID-19-related death among patients with chronic obstructive pulmonary disease or asthma prescribed inhaled corticosteroids: an observational cohort study using the OpenSAFELY platform. Lancet Respir Med. 2020;8(11):1106–20. https://doi.org/10.1016/S2213-2600(20)30415-X.
45. Jackson DJ, Busse WW, Bacharier LB, Kattan M, O'Connor GT, Wood RA, et al. Association of respiratory allergy, asthma, and expression of the SARS-CoV-2 receptor ACE2. J Allergy Clin Immunol. 2020;146(1):203–6. e3. https://doi.org/10.1016/j.jaci.2020.04.009.
46. Peters MC, Sajuthi S, Deford P, Christenson S, Rios CL, Montgomery MT, et al. COVID-19-related Genes in sputum cells in asthma. Relationship to demographic features and corticosteroids. Am J Respir Crit Care Med. 2020;202(1):83–90. https://doi.org/10.1164/rccm.202003-0821OC.
47. Alqahtani JS, Oyelade T, Aldhahir AM, Alghamdi SM, Almehmadi M, Alqahtani AS, et al. Prevalence, severity and mortality associated with COPD and smoking in patients with COVID-19: a rapid systematic review and meta-analysis. PLoS One. 2020;15(5):e0233147. https://doi.org/10.1371/journal.pone.0233147.

48. Sanchez-Ramirez DC, Mackey D. Underlying respiratory diseases, specifically COPD, and smoking are associated with severe COVID-19 outcomes: a systematic review and meta-analysis. Respir Med. 2020;171:106096. https://doi.org/10.1016/j.rmed.2020.106096.
49. Maes T, Bracke K, Brusselle GG. COVID-19, asthma, and inhaled corticosteroids: another beneficial effect of inhaled corticosteroids? Am J Respir Crit Care Med. 2020;202(1):8–10. https://doi.org/10.1164/rccm.202005-1651ED.
50. Wang L, Foer D, Bates DW, Boyce JA, Zhou L. Risk factors for hospitalization, intensive care, and mortality among patients with asthma and COVID-19. J Allergy Clin Immunol. 2020;146(4):808–12. https://doi.org/10.1016/j.jaci.2020.07.018.

Part III
Pathophysiology of ACO

Chapter 8
Inflammatory Phenotypes and Potential Bio-markers of ACO: What Is the Specific Feature of ACO?

Keita Hirai

Abstract Asthma-chronic obstructive pulmonary disease (COPD) overlap (ACO) is a chronic obstructive airway disease subtype. Therefore, it is essential to elucidate the phenotype and endotype of patients with ACO to develop personalized or stratified medicine in patients with asthma and COPD. Furthermore, clarification of these aspects could contribute to the development of useful biomarkers for identifying ACO patients. Many previous studies have focused on the contribution of inflammatory markers, including eosinophil, fractional exhaled nitric oxide (FeNO), and serum IgE levels, to ACO identification. Moreover, recent studies have attempted to develop specific markers for ACO using several analysis approaches, such as genomics, epigenetics, transcriptomics, and metabolomics. Therefore, it is highly anticipated that the multidimensional characterization of the pathophysiology of ACO would lead to the development of biomarkers that would be helpful in the discrimination of ACO.

Keywords Biomarkers · Cytokines · MicroRNA · Transcriptome · Metabolomics

1 Introduction

Patients with asthma and chronic obstructive pulmonary disease (COPD) can be divided into several subgroups. Characterization of each subgroup by phenotype and endotype analysis is critically needed to realize a "Treatable traits approach" in patients with chronic obstructive airway disease. Therefore, the development of biomarkers that reflect treatable traits is desirable. Asthma-COPD overlap (ACO) has

K. Hirai (✉)
Department of Clinical Pharmacology and Therapeutics, Shinshu University Graduate School of Medicine, Matsumoto, Nagano, Japan
e-mail: hiraik@shinshu-u.ac.jp

H. Nagase et al. (eds.), *Asthma-COPD Overlap*, Respiratory Disease Series: Diagnostic Tools and Disease Managements,
https://doi.org/10.1007/978-981-96-0217-9_8

the potential to be one of the treatable traits for optimizing the treatment of patients with asthma and COPD. Although the characteristics of ACO have not been sufficiently elucidated, various studies have attempted to understand the ACO phenotype through multidirectional analysis approaches.

2 Type 2 Inflammatory Phenotype

The disease burden associated with airway type-2 inflammation in ACO patients has been studied. Hiles et al. demonstrated that 51% of ACO patients had blood eosinophil counts above 300 cells/μL [1]. This phenotype was most common in ACO subjects, followed by severe asthma alone (44%) and COPD alone (29%). The frequencies of eosinophilic inflammation phenotype were similar using sputum eosinophils thresholds of 3%. In addition, another study investigated the associations of increased FeNO and blood eosinophil counts with chronic airway disease [2]. Inflammatory phenotype represented by increased FeNO (≥25 ppb) and blood eosinophil (≥300 cells/μL) was found to be associated with the pathophysiology of ACO as well as those of asthma. However, the sensitivity and specificity of these two biomarkers in the discrimination of ACO subjects from COPD subjects were not high. Moreover, Lee et al. evaluated the clinical and demographic differences between ACO and non-ACO groups in the severe asthma cohort [3]. This study demonstrated that 23.7% of subjects with severe asthma were classified into the ACO group. ACO patients had lower peripheral blood eosinophil percentages and higher neutrophil percentages than the non-ACO group. There were no significant differences in sputum cell counts between the two groups. These results suggested that airway type-2 inflammation is one of the significant phenotypes of ACO but is not specific to ACO.

The utility of total serum IgE and specific IgE for diagnostic criteria of ACO was also evaluated. Among 2870 participants with COPD, ACO was defined by self-reported asthma [4]. ACO patients had higher total IgE levels and a higher proportion of positive results for at least one or more specific IgE than patients with COPD alone. When atopy was defined by total IgE levels >100 IU/mL or at least one positive specific IgE, there was no significant difference in exacerbation risk between ACO patients with and without atopy. These results concluded that the usefulness of IgE measurements in ACO diagnosis was not demonstrated. However, IgE levels may help identify the subgroup of ACO and understand different pathophysiological mechanisms of ACO.

3 Cytokines and Inflammatory Mediators

Several inflammatory mediators have been implicated in the distinct phenotypes of asthma and COPD (Table 8.1). In a single-center study, Ding et al. [5] attempted to investigate the markers for discrimination of ACO from asthmatic patients using serum cytokines levels. They analyzed interleukins and vascular endothelial growth

Table 8.1 Candidate biomarkers for ACO

Study	Subjects	Biological sample	Measurement procedure	Candidate biomarker for ACO
Ding et al. [5]	ACO 21, asthma 69	Serum	Targeted 15 cytokines (IL-3, IL-4, IL-8, IL-9, IL-13, IL-17A, IL-27, VEGFA, VEGFC, VEGFD, bFGF, Fit-1 PIGF, Tie-2, TGF-β) by immunoassay	*ACO vs. asthma* IL-8, VEFGA
Shirai et al. [6, 7]	ACO 115, asthma 177, COPD 61	Serum	Periostin, EDN, YKL-40 by immunoassay	*ACO vs. asthma* YKL-40 *ACO vs. COPD* Periostin, EDN
Wang et al. [8]	ACO 102, asthma 124, COPD 147	Serum	Periostin, TSLP, YKL-40, NGAL by immunoassay	*ACO vs. asthma* NGAL *ACO vs. COPD* YKL-40
Huang et al. [9]	ACO 68, asthma 87, COPD 73	Sputum supernatants	Targeted 5 DAMPs (HMGB1, HSP70, LL-37, S100A8, galectin-3) by immunoassay	*ACO vs. asthma* HMGB1
Asensio et al. [10]	Discovery cohort: 10 subjects each in groups Validation cohort: Smoking asthma 44, non-smoking asthma 85, eosinophilic COPD 61, non-eosinophilic COPD 84	Serum	miRNA array (2578 human mature miRNAs can be measured)	*Eosinophilic COPD vs. other groups* miR-619-5p, miR-4486
Hirai et al. [11]	Discovery cohort: 6 subjects each in ACO, asthma Validation cohort: 30 subjects each in ACO, asthma, COPD	Plasma	qPCR based miRNA PCR array (84 human mature miRNAs can be measured)	*ACO vs. other groups* miR-15b-5p, miR-148a-3p, miR-223-3p, miR-23a-3p, miR-26b-5p
Ghosh et al. [12]	Discovery cohort: ACO 35, asthma 34, COPD 30 Validation cohort: ACO 40, asthma 32, COPD 32	Serum	NMR based metabolomics	*ACO vs. other groups* citric acid, glutamate, valine

(continued)

Table 8.1 (continued)

Study	Subjects	Biological sample	Measurement procedure	Candidate biomarker for ACO
Ghosh et al. [13]	Same above	Serum	GC-MS based metabolomics	*ACO vs. other groups* glucose, 2-palmitoylglycerol, D-mannose, succinic acid
Ghosh et al. [14]	Same above	Exhaled breath condensates	NMR based metabolomics	*ACO vs. other groups* fatty acid, propionate, isopropanol, lactate, acetone, valine, methanol, for-mate
Oh et al. [15]	ACO 37, asthma 32, COPD 38	Urine	Q-ToF/MS-based metabolomics	*ACO vs. other groups* L-histidine
Cai et al. [16]	ACO 29, COPD 27	Serum	Targeted metabolites of eicosanoids by Q-ToF/MS	*ACO vs. COPD* 15(S)-HETE, 12(S)-HETE, 8(S)-HETE

factor (VEGF) family cytokines. The ACO group had significantly higher serum levels of IL-9, VEGFA, and placental growth factors and significantly lower levels of IL-8 and IL-17A than the non-ACO group (asthma alone). The receiver operating characteristics (ROC) analysis for discrimination of ACO patients from asthmatic patients indicated that serum levels of IL-8 and VEFGA had the highest sensitivity and specificity, respectively. Among clinical characteristics, lung function was correlated positively with IL-8 and negatively with VEGFA.

Another study [17] addressed the inflammatory phenotypes in chronic obstructive airway disease and whether they contribute to differences in the pathophysiology of asthma, COPD, and ACO. Subjects aged 40 years and over with airway obstruction were included, and they were classified into asthma, COPD, and ACO. In three groups, serum levels of type 2 markers (IL-5, IL-13, and periostin) and non-type 2 markers (IL-6, IL-8, IL-17, TNF-α) were analyzed. Patients with asthma had significantly higher serum IL-5 than patients with COPD. ACO patients had serum IL-5 levels intermediate between asthmatic and COPD patients. Among non-type 2 markers, serum IL-8 levels were significantly elevated in COPD and ACO patients. The inflammatory phenotype of ACO may be a mixture of type 2 and non-type 2. Although there were no biomarkers that reliably demonstrated the difference in the pathophysiology of asthma, COPD, and ACO, it was demonstrated that serum periostin was a more predictor for type 2 high inflammation (blood eosinophil count ≥300 cells/μL or sputum eosinophil ≥3%). Another study analyzed serum levels of IL-17, IL-18, and TNF-α in patients with asthma, ACO, and COPD [18]. These cytokines levels were higher in patients with asthma, ACO, and COPD than in healthy nonsmokers; however, there were no significant markers for ACO discrimination from asthma and COPD. It may be challenging to characterize the pathophysiology of patients with ACO using only cytokine levels in the blood as a biomarker.

However, in addition to cytokines, various inflammatory mediators are involved in the pathophysiologic development of asthma and COPD. Our previous study focused on periostin and chitinase-3-like protein 1 (YKL-40) and evaluated their utility in differentiating ACO patients [6]. Periostin is implicated in type-2 inflammation in asthma, while YKL-40 is associated with airway inflammation and remodeling in COPD. Serum periostin levels were significantly higher in patients with asthma and ACO than in COPD patients, whereas serum YKL-40 levels were significantly higher in patients with ACO and COPD than asthmatic patients. ACO patients had a higher proportion of high serum periostin and YKL-40 levels, and these criteria could identify patients with ACO with 38% sensitivity and 81% specificity. In addition, we examined the feasibility of eosinophil-derived neurotoxin (EDN) instead of periostin in a later investigation using the same cohort [7]. Interestingly, serum EDN levels were significantly elevated in patients with ACO than in both asthma and COPD. Therefore, the combined evaluation of serum EDN and YKL-40 was beneficial in identifying ACO with 45% sensitivity and 82% specificity.

Wang et al. [8] evaluated the plasma levels of inflammatory mediators that are previously reported to be associated with asthma and COPD, including periostin, TSLP, YKL-40, and NGAL. YKL-40 serum levels in ACO patients were significantly higher than in healthy subjects but were similar to those in asthmatics and significantly lower than in COPD patients. In addition, serum NGAL levels were significantly higher in COPD and ACO patients than in asthma and healthy subjects. In contrast, there were no significant differences in serum levels of periostin and TSLP among asthma, COPD, and ACO patients. The ROC analysis revealed that ACO patients could be distinguished from COPD patients by serum YKL-40 and asthmatic patients by serum NGAL.

Other inflammation-associated molecules have been suggested to be relevant in the inflammatory response of asthma and COPD. Damage-associated molecular patterns (DAMPs) are involved in innate and adaptive immune responses. Huang et al. [9] attempted to investigate that ACO patients have distinct expression profiles of sputum DAMPs, including HMGB1, HSP70, LL-37, S100A8, and galectin-3. The percentages of eosinophils in induced sputum cells were higher in asthma and ACO patients than in COPD, and those of neutrophils were higher in COPD and ACO patients than in asthma. Compared to patients with asthma, COPD and ACO patients had higher sputum levels of HMGB1, which is reported to be associated with airway neutrophilic inflammation. The expression levels of sputum LL-37, known as the antimicrobial peptides, were upregulated in COPD and ACO patients compared to asthma, and those levels in COPD patients were significantly higher than in ACO patients. Meanwhile, COPD and AOC patients had lower sputum levels of galectin-3 compared to asthmatic patients. Galectin-3 levels were also downregulated in healthy smokers. This study demonstrated that sputum HMGB1 is a potentially useful marker for discrimination of ACO in asthmatic patients. However, a valuable marker for differentiating ACO from COPD was not found.

Furthermore, a recent study evaluated the difference in plasma NET levels, measured by flow cytometry-based method, in chronic inflammatory lung disease [19]. However, there was no significant difference in plasma NET levels in any comparisons among 46 adult asthmatic patients, 6 with COPD, 6 with ACO, and 12 with adult control. At the same time, the severity of asthma and worse lung function (%FEV1 < 80%) were significantly associated with higher levels of plasma NET. Because of the small sample size, further studies are needed to validate these results.

4 Transcriptional and Post-Transcriptional Profiling

Eosinophilic airway inflammation is one of the critical phenotypes of ACO. A transcriptome study [20] revealed the relationship between peripheral blood eosinophil counts and gene expression levels measured from bronchial brushings in patients with asthma and COPD. The asthma cohort consisted of 85 subjects from the U-BIOPRED study. In this asthma cohort, when Affymetrix microarrays evaluated gene expression levels, there were 1197 genes significantly associated with blood eosinophil counts in the regression analysis model (false discovery rate <0.01). While in the COPD cohort ($N = 283$) from the EvA study, gene expression analysis by RNA sequencing found only 12 genes significantly associated with blood eosinophil count. Although the proportion of subjects with eosinophilic inflammation (blood eosinophil count >200 cells/μL) was only slightly lower in the COPD cohort (35%) than in the asthma cohort (47%), the relationship between gene expression and blood eosinophil counts was very different in the two groups. CST1, which codes cystatin SN and is involved in type 2 inflammation, was the only gene associated with blood eosinophil counts in both asthma and COPD cohorts.

In another study, Christenson et al. [21] investigated whether COPD patients had gene expression profiles similar to asthmatic patients with type-2 inflammation. They evaluated the expression levels of three genes, including *POSTN*, *CLCA1*, and *SERPINB2*, as a signature of airway type-2 inflammation. There were similar gene expression alterations in airway epithelial in asthma and COPD cohorts. COPD subjects with asthma-related type-2 gene signatures had increased eosinophil count and reasonable response to inhaled corticosteroid treatment. Common genetic alterations in asthma and COPD are likely to be essential findings in understanding the pathogenesis of ACO.

Micro RNAs (miRNAs), short-length non-coding RNAs, are attracting attention as a new biomarker. One miRNA is responsible for regulating multiple gene expressions, and multiple miRNAs regulate one gene. In addition, inflammatory and immunological responses are implicated in the post-transcriptional regulation of miRNAs. Therefore, it might be possible to characterize the pathophysiology of ACO by miRNA (Table 8.1). Asensio et al. [10] subdivided ACO patients into smoking asthma and eosinophilic COPD and tried to identify distinctive serum miRNAs signatures among patients with smoking asthma, non-smoking asthma, eosinophilic COPD, and non-eosinophilic COPD. In the discovery phase, they performed a comprehensive measurement of miRNAs using a microarray system in 10 subjects in each of the four groups. They found 30 significant differentially expressed miRNAs among any group, and two miRNAs had distinct expression patterns in patients with eosinophilic COPD. Then, candidate miRNAs, including miR-619-5p and miR-4486, were validated by qPCR in the complete cohort of 44 smoking asthma, 85 non-smoking asthma, 61 eosinophilic COPD, and 84 non-eosinophilic COPD. The study result indicated that serum expression levels of miR-619-5p and miR-4486 were downregulated in eosinophilic COPD compared with other groups. Therefore, it was suggested that these miRNAs could be a valuable marker for distinguishing eosinophilic COPD patients from asthma and COPD. Interestingly, this study demonstrated distinct pathophysiological mechanisms in smoking asthma and eosinophilic COPD, even though ACO patients are recognized as one subtype in many studies.

In another study, Lacedonia et al. [22] performed a targeted quantitative polymerase chain reaction (qPCR) to evaluate the association of miRNAs in sputum and serum with ACO phenotype. Two miRNAs, including miR-145 and miR-338, were measured in 13 patients with asthma, 31 patients with COPD, eight patients with ACO, and seven with healthy controls. ACO patients had significantly higher expression levels of miR-338 in sputum supernatant than healthy controls. However, miR-338 levels were also elevated in asthma and COPD patients. In contrast, miR-338 levels in serum significantly decreased in ACO patients compared to healthy controls, but there were no significant differences in miR-338 levels in serum among patients with AOC, asthma, and COPD. In addition, miR-145 in sputum and serum was also not helpful in discriminating patients with ACO from asthma and COPD.

Our previous study [11] also attempted to identify miRNAs capable of characterizing the ACO phenotype. We measured expression levels of miRNAs in plasma using a qPCR array. In the discovery cohort of 6 patients with ACO and 6 patients with asthma, qPCR array measurements found nine differentially expressed miRNAs between patients with ACO and asthma. Next, the expression levels of these nine candidate miRNAs were validated in another cohort of 30 patients each with asthma, COPD, and ACO. Of these miRNAs, eight miRNAs, including miR-148a-3p, miR-15b-5p, miR191-5p, miR-223-3p, miR-23a-3p, miR-24-3p, miR-26a-5p, and miR-26b-5p, were significantly decreased in patients with ACO compared to asthmatic patients. In addition, among these miRNAs, the following five miRNAs were also downregulated in ACO patients compared to COPD patients: miR-148a-3p, miR-15b-5p, miR-223-3p, miR-23a-3p, and miR-26b-5p. The pathway analysis demonstrated the association of these five miRNAs with inflammatory pathways such as the MAPK signaling pathway, PI3K/Akt signaling pathway, and TGF-β signaling pathway. Moreover, we recognized that miR-15b-5p was the most valuable biomarker for identifying patients with ACO in asthma and COPD by the random forest machine-learning algorithm.

5 Metabolomics Profiling

Various inflammatory responses may alter metabolite profiles. Several recent studies have attempted to elucidate the heterogeneity of chronic obstructive airway diseases using a metabolomics approach (Table 8.1). Ghosh et al. [12] studied metabolomic profiles in patients with asthma, ACO, and COPD using nuclear magnetic resonance (NMR) based metabolomics. Metabolites including asparagine, citric acid, glucose, glutamate, isoleucine, l-leucine, lysine, N-acetylglycoproteins, phenylalanine, and valine were downregulated in patients with ACO than both asthma and COPD. Histidine was elevated in patients with ACO, and the expression level of lipids in ACO patients was higher than in COPD and lower than in asthma. Moreover, ROC curves analysis revealed that citric acid, glutamate, and valine could be distinct serum metabolites for identifying ACO in asthma and COPD patients.

Oh et al. [15] examined the potential role of urinary metabolites as a biomarker for ACO. They performed a urine metabolomics study using liquid chromatography coupled with high-resolution quadrupole time-of-flight mass spectrometry. When urinary metabolites in ACO patients were compared with those of asthma and COPD, there was a significant difference in 223 metabolites between ACO and asthma patients and 215 metabolites between ACO and COPD patients. Among these metabolites, urinary levels of L-histidine, a precursor of histamine involved in the inflammatory response, were specificity increased in ACO patients than in asthma and COPD patients. Moreover, elevated levels of L-histidine were associated with a high value of blood eosinophil counts, bronchodilator response, and risk for exacerbation.

In another study, Ghosh et al. [13] performed non-targeted metabolomic profiling of serum using gas chromatography coupled with mass spectrometry (GC-MS). In the discovery phase, they were able to identify a total of 145 metabolites, and 11 metabolites showed distinct expression patterns in ACO patients compared to asthma and COPD patients. Serum metabolites, including serine, threonine, ethanolamine, glucose, D-mannose, and succinic acid, were decreased in ACO patients compared to those with asthma and COPD. Serum levels of cholesterol, 2-palmitoylglycerol, and lactic acid in ACO patients were upregulated compared to asthmatic patients and down-regulated compared to COPD patients. Stearic acid and linoleic acid were lower in ACO patients than asthma patients and higher in COPD patients. Moreover, the expression profiles of these 11 serum metabolites showed similar trends in the validation cohort. ROC analysis showed that glucose, 2-palmitoylglycerol, D-mannose, and succinic acid helped distinguish ACO from asthma and ACO from COPD. Furthermore, this study evaluated the correlations between candidate serum metabolites for ACO and immunological mediators such as Th1- and Th2-associated cytokines, MCP-1, YKL-40, and NGAL. Glucose, D-mannose, and succinic acid had significant negative correlations with Th1 cytokines such as INF-γ and IL-1β, Th2 cytokines such as IL-5, and other immunological markers such as IL-6 and YKL-40.

In a further study, Ghosh et al. [14] attempted to discriminate subjects with ACO from asthma and COPD using expression patterns of eight metabolites (fatty acid, propionate, isopropanol, lactate, acetone, valine, methanol, and formate) in exhaled breath condensate. Exhaled breath condensate is a non-invasive method to evaluate airway inflammation by collecting exhaled air. They indicated that acetone, isopropanol, and propionate expression levels were significantly higher, and valine was significantly lower in patients with ACO than in patients with asthma and COPD. They also validated these results in another cohort and found a similar expression profile of metabolites in exhaled breath condensate. This study indicated the potential of metabolomics of exhaled breath condensate as a non-inverse biomarker for ACO.

Cai et al. [16] attempted to discover specific serum metabolites of eicosanoids among patients with ACO ($N = 29$) and COPD ($N = 27$) using quadrupole time-of-flight mass spectrometry. ACO patients had a higher expression of lipoxygenase metabolites of arachidonic acids, such as hydroxyeicosatetraenoic acids (HETEs), hydroperoxyeicosatetraenoic acids (HPETEs), and hydroperoxyoctadecadienoic acid (HPODEs) compared to COPD and healthy control. The metabolite with the highest accuracy in the discrimination of ACO from COPD was 15(S)-HETE, followed by 12(S)-HETE and 8(S)-HETE. Meanwhile, serum metabolites in cyclooxygenase pathway, such as prostaglandins and thromboxanes, were not identified as useful markers.

6 Genetic Markers

Various studies have reported several genes associated with developing asthma and COPD individually. Therefore, the pathophysiologies of asthma and COPD are expected to be influenced to a certain degree by genetic variants. However, few studies have performed the genome association study to find specific gene variants involved in ACO. Smolonska et al. [23] conducted a genome-wide association study to discover genetic variants involved in disease susceptibility common to both asthma and COPD in nine independent cohorts. In the discovery cohort (921 asthma, 3246 asthma control, 1030 COPD, and 1808 COPD control) and first replication cohort (534 asthma, 2568 asthma control, 711 COPD, and 1854 COPD control), three genomic locations were suggested as common loci in asthma and COPD. The chromosome 2p24.3, 5q23.1, and 13q14.2 locus contained single nucleotide polymorphism (SNP) rs1477253 in the *DDX1* gene, rs254149 in the *COMMD10* gene, and rs9534578 in the *GNG5P5* gene, respectively, and only SNP rs9534578 was reached the genome-wide significance threshold. However, in the second replication phase using seven other independent cohorts, none of the SNPs replicated the association with asthma and COPD.

Hardin et al. [24] performed a genome-wide association analysis and investigated the genetic markers for identifying ACO in COPD patients. In the COPDGene study, subjects included non-Hispanic whites and African Americans aged

45–80 years with a smoking history (≥10 pack-years). A comparison between 450 patients with ACO and 3120 patients with COPD alone demonstrated that no SNPs reached the genome-wide significance threshold in either non-Hispanic whites or African Americans. The top-ranked SNPs in non-Hispanic whites were rs11779254 in the *CSMD1* gene, followed by rs59569785 in the *SOX5* gene, and those in African Americans were rs2686829 in the *PKD1L1* gene. The top two SNPs identified in the non-Hispanic white cohort were not validated in the African American cohort. Furthermore, a meta-analysis of two independent cohorts suggested that three SNPs (rs6574987, rs8004567, and rs14418089) with linkage disequilibrium in the *GPR65* gene were associated with ACO. *GPR65*, one of the G-protein coupled receptors, has reported an association with eosinophil activation. However, further studies are needed to validate the influences of candidate genes on the inflammatory phenotypes of ACO.

In contrast, Park et al. [25] performed a genome-wide association study to identify SNPs associated with ACO compared to asthma. In Korea's Cohort for Reality and Evolution of Adult Asthma, both ACO and asthma alone patients had similar profiles of serum total IgE, blood eosinophil count, induced sputum cell count, and C-reactive protein. The proportion of positive atopic tests (skin prick test) was lower in ACO patients than in asthma alone patients. From this cohort, GWAS data of 77 patients with ACO and 1356 patients with asthma were compared to find specific gene variants associated with ACO. However, no significant genetic markers discriminate ACO from asthmatic patients.

COPDGene study included 10,199 adult smokers and demonstrated that childhood asthma contributes to the risk of developing COPD in smokers [26]. In addition, it is well known the genetic influence on childhood asthma. Therefore, Hayden et al. analyzed the association of well-recognized polymorphisms related to childhood asthma in the COPDGene study. Five genes, including *IL1RL1*, *IL13*, *LINC01149*, near *GSDMB*, and C11orf39-LRRC32 region, contributed to childhood asthma in adult smokers. Therefore, genetic variants may be associated with the disease susceptibility of ACO.

7 Conclusion

Several studies have elucidated the inflammatory phenotypes of ACO using differential analysis approaches, such as transcriptomics, epigenetics, metabolomics, and genetics, to establish biomarkers of ACO. These studies have illustrated that several biomarkers can be beneficial in discriminating ACO from patients with asthma and COPD; however, they have not provided consensus findings. Although it is also important to standardize the diagnostic criteria for ACO, further studies would be desirable to validate the findings of previous studies and to establish specific biomarkers of ACO.

References

1. Hiles SA, Gibson PG, McDonald VM. Disease burden of eosinophilic airway disease: comparing severe asthma, COPD and asthma-COPD overlap. Respirology. 2021;26:52–61. https://doi.org/10.1111/resp.13841.
2. Çolak Y, Afzal S, Nordestgaard BG, Marott JL, Lange P. Combined value of exhaled nitric oxide and blood eosinophils in chronic airway disease: the Copenhagen General Population Study. Eur Respir J. 2018;52:1800616. https://doi.org/10.1183/13993003.00616-2018.
3. Lee H, Kim S-H, Kim B-K, Lee Y, Lee HY, Ban G, et al. Characteristics of specialist-diagnosed asthma-COPD overlap in severe asthma: observations from the Korean Severe Asthma Registry (KoSAR). Allergy. 2021;76:223–32. https://doi.org/10.1111/all.14483.
4. Hersh CP, Zacharia S, Prakash Arivu Chelvan R, Hayden LP, Mirtar A, Zarei S, et al. Immunoglobulin e as a biomarker for the overlap of atopic asthma and chronic obstructive pulmonary disease. Chronic Obstr Pulm Dis (Miami, Fla). 2020;7:1–12. https://doi.org/10.15326/jcopdf.7.1.2019.0138.
5. Ding Q, Sun S, Zhang Y, Tang P, Lv C, Ma H, et al. Serum IL-8 and VEGFA are two promising diagnostic biomarkers of asthma-COPD overlap syndrome. Int J Chron Obstruct Pulmon Dis. 2020;15:357–65. https://doi.org/10.2147/COPD.S233461.
6. Shirai T, Hirai K, Gon Y, Maruoka S, Mizumura K, Hikichi M, et al. Combined assessment of serum periostin and YKL-40 may identify asthma-COPD overlap. J allergy Clin Immunol Pract. 2019;7:134–145.e1. https://doi.org/10.1016/j.jaip.2018.06.015.
7. Shirai T, Hirai K, Gon Y, Maruoka S, Mizumura K, Hikichi M, et al. Combined assessment of serum eosinophil-derived neurotoxin and YKL-40 may identify asthma-COPD overlap. Allergol Int. 2021;70:136–9. https://doi.org/10.1016/j.alit.2020.05.007.
8. Wang J, Lv H, Luo Z, Mou S, Liu J, Liu C, et al. Plasma YKL-40 and NGAL are useful in distinguishing ACO from asthma and COPD. Respir Res. 2018;19:47. https://doi.org/10.1186/s12931-018-0755-6.
9. Huang X, Tan X, Liang Y, Hou C, Qu D, Li M, et al. Differential DAMP release was observed in the sputum of COPD, asthma and asthma-COPD overlap (ACO) patients. Sci Rep. 2019;9:19241. https://doi.org/10.1038/s41598-019-55502-2.
10. Asensio VJ, Tomás A, Iglesias A, de Llano LP, Del Pozo V, Cosío BG, et al. Eosinophilic COPD patients display a distinctive serum miRNA profile from asthma and non-eosinophilic COPD. Arch Bronconeumol. 2020;56:234–41. https://doi.org/10.1016/j.arbres.2019.09.020.
11. Hirai K, Shirai T, Shimoshikiryo T, Ueda M, Gon Y, Maruoka S, et al. Circulating microRNA-15b-5p as a biomarker for asthma-COPD overlap. Allergy. 2021;76:766–74. https://doi.org/10.1111/all.14520.
12. Ghosh N, Choudhury P, Subramani E, Saha D, Sengupta S, Joshi M, et al. Metabolomic signatures of asthma-COPD overlap (ACO) are different from asthma and COPD. Metabolomics. 2019;15:87. https://doi.org/10.1007/s11306-019-1552-z.
13. Ghosh N, Choudhury P, Kaushik SR, Arya R, Nanda R, Bhattacharyya P, et al. Metabolomic fingerprinting and systemic inflammatory profiling of asthma COPD overlap (ACO). Respir Res. 2020;21:126. https://doi.org/10.1186/s12931-020-01390-4.
14. Ghosh N, Choudhury P, Joshi M, Bhattacharyya P, Roychowdhury S, Banerjee R, et al. Global metabolome profiling of exhaled breath condensates in male smokers with asthma COPD overlap and prediction of the disease. Sci Rep. 2021;11:16664. https://doi.org/10.1038/s41598-021-96128-7.
15. Oh JY, Lee YS, Min KH, Hur GY, Lee SY, Kang KH, et al. Increased urinary l-histidine in patients with asthma-COPD overlap: a pilot study. Int J Chron Obstruct Pulmon Dis. 2018;13:1809–18. https://doi.org/10.2147/COPD.S163189.
16. Cai C, Bian X, Xue M, Liu X, Hu H, Wang J, et al. Eicosanoids metabolized through LOX distinguish asthma-COPD overlap from COPD by metabolomics study. Int J Chron Obstruct Pulmon Dis. 2019;14:1769–78. https://doi.org/10.2147/COPD.S207023.

17. de Llano LP, Cosío BG, Iglesias A, de Las CN, Soler-Cataluña JJ, Izquierdo JL, et al. Mixed Th2 and non-Th2 inflammatory pattern in the asthma-COPD overlap: a network approach. Int J Chron Obstruct Pulmon Dis. 2018;13:591–601. https://doi.org/10.2147/COPD.S153694.
18. Kubysheva N, Boldina M, Eliseeva T, Soodaeva S, Klimanov I, Khaletskaya A, et al. Relationship of serum levels of IL-17, IL-18, TNF-α, and lung function parameters in patients with COPD, asthma-COPD overlap, and bronchial asthma. Mediat Inflamm. 2020;2020:4652898. https://doi.org/10.1155/2020/4652898.
19. Gál Z, Gézsi A, Pállinger É, Visnovitz T, Nagy A, Kiss A, et al. Plasma neutrophil extracellular trap level is modified by disease severity and inhaled corticosteroids in chronic inflammatory lung diseases. Sci Rep. 2020;10:4320. https://doi.org/10.1038/s41598-020-61253-2.
20. George L, Taylor AR, Esteve-Codina A, Soler Artigas M, Thun GA, Bates S, et al. Blood eosinophil count and airway epithelial transcriptome relationships in COPD versus asthma. Allergy. 2020;75:370–80. https://doi.org/10.1111/all.14016.
21. Christenson SA, Steiling K, van den Berge M, Hijazi K, Hiemstra PS, Postma DS, et al. Asthma-COPD overlap. Clinical relevance of genomic signatures of type 2 inflammation in chronic obstructive pulmonary disease. Am J Respir Crit Care Med. 2015;191:758–66. https://doi.org/10.1164/rccm.201408-1458OC.
22. Lacedonia D, Palladino GP, Foschino-Barbaro MP, Scioscia G, Carpagnano GE. Expression profiling of miRNA-145 and miRNA-338 in serum and sputum of patients with COPD, asthma, and asthma-COPD overlap syndrome phenotype. Int J Chron Obstruct Pulmon Dis. 2017;12:1811–7. https://doi.org/10.2147/COPD.S130616.
23. Smolonska J, Koppelman GH, Wijmenga C, Vonk JM, Zanen P, Bruinenberg M, et al. Common genes underlying asthma and COPD? Genome-wide analysis on the Dutch hypothesis. Eur Respir J. 2014;44:860–72. https://doi.org/10.1183/09031936.00001914.
24. Hardin M, Cho M, McDonald M-L, Beaty T, Ramsdell J, Bhatt S, et al. The clinical and genetic features of COPD-asthma overlap syndrome. Eur Respir J. 2014;44:341–50. https://doi.org/10.1183/09031936.00216013.
25. Park S, Jung H, Kim J, Seo B, Kwon OY, Choi S, et al. Longitudinal analysis to better characterize Asthma-COPD overlap syndrome: findings from an adult asthma cohort in Korea (COREA). Clin Exp Allergy. 2019;49:603–14. https://doi.org/10.1111/cea.13339.
26. Hayden LP, Cho MH, Raby BA, Beaty TH, Silverman EK, Hersh CP, et al. Childhood asthma is associated with COPD and known asthma variants in COPDGene: a genome-wide association study. Respir Res. 2018;19:209. https://doi.org/10.1186/s12931-018-0890-0.

Chapter 9
Role of Nitrosative Stress: What Is the Potential Clinical Implication?

Tomohiro Ichikawa and Hisatoshi Sugiura

Abstract In the airways of COPD and asthma, NO is excessively produced by inducible NO synthesis (iNOS) during inflammation, which can react with concurrently produced superoxide, leading to the formation of peroxynitrite, a highly reactive nitrogen species (RNS). Peroxynitrite can cause tissue injury, lipid peroxidation and the nitration of tyrosine residues. Thus, RNS induces nitrosative stress in lung tissue and contributes to the pathophysiology such as airway remodeling, enhanced airway inflammation and corticosteroid resistance in severe asthma and COPD. Asthma-COPD overlap (ACO) has the physiological and clinical features of both asthma and COPD. It has been demonstrated that RNS is more enhanced in the airways of ACO than in asthma or COPD as confirmed by the formation of nitrotyrosine, a marker of nitrosative stress. Furthermore, the degree of nitrotyrosine in the airways is also known to be associated with the clinical course of patients with ACO. This chapter describes the basic mechanism of RNS formation and pathophysiological action of RNS in airway diseases. In addition, the clinical utility of nitrotyrosine as a biomarker for nirosative stress in ACO and the future potential of targeting nitrosative stress as a therapeutic strategy for ACO are discussed.

Keywords Inducible NO synthesis · Reactive nitrogen species · Nitrotyrosine · Oxidative stress

T. Ichikawa (✉) · H. Sugiura
Department of Respiratory Medicine, Tohoku University Graduate School of Medicine, Sendai, Japan
e-mail: tomohiro.ichikawa.d1@tohoku.ac.jp

H. Nagase et al. (eds.), *Asthma-COPD Overlap*, Respiratory Disease Series: Diagnostic Tools and Disease Managements,
https://doi.org/10.1007/978-981-96-0217-9_9

1 Introduction

Nitric oxide (NO) is an important endogenous signaling molecule that modulates miscellaneous biological functions. The physiological roles of NO include the regulation of vascular and bronchial tone, neurotransmission or immune defense [1, 2]. NO is usually produced through the conversion of L-arginine to L-citrulline by three main isoforms of NO synthases (NOS) including the neuronal (nNOS), endothelial (eNOS) and inducible (iNOS) isoforms [3]. nNOS and eNOS are constitutively expressed and categorized as constitutive NOS (cNOS). Their activation is dependent on the intracellular calcium concentration. Meanwhile, iNOS is expressed mainly in epithelial cells and macrophages and induced by inflammatory cytokines, interferon, and lipopolysaccharide (LPS) during inflammation and infection, independently of the calcium concentration [4, 5]. Furthermore, in contrast to nNOS and eNOS, the induction of iNOS produces excessive NO, which is considered one of the host defense mechanisms against bacterial infection and also causes shock and tissue damage [6]. In the context of inflammation, reactive oxygen species (ROS) are concurrently overproduced in a pathological condition mediated by NADPH oxidase or xanthine oxidase [7, 8], and oxidative stress occurs when ROS production exceeds antioxidant capacity in a variety of inflammatory diseases. Commonly formed ROS include superoxide, hydroxyl radical and hydrogen peroxide ($O_2.-$, .OH and H_2O_2.). Consequently, excessively produced NO by iNOS up-regulation can react with superoxide anions, leading to the formation of highly reactive nitrogen species (RNS) including peroxynitrite ($ONOO^-$). This is the main process of RNS production in a pathological condition. Furthermore, RNS are also generated through the H_2O_2/peroxidase-dependent nitrite oxidation pathway [9]. These RNS can cause damage due to active protease or toxic moieties released by stimulated inflammatory cells. RNS also augment plasma leakage and alter the function of several proteins by the nitration of tyrosine residues, resulting in nitrotyrosine [7, 10]. The formation of 3-nitrotyrosine (3-NT) represents a biomarker for RNS, as described below.

Nitrosative stress describes the indiscriminate nitrosation of biological nucleophiles that can lead to cell death and/or pathophysiological conditions [11] and is characterized by the overproduction of nitric oxide (·NO). The term "nitrosative stress" biochemcally should not be used to refer to the toxicity of nitrogen oxide including NO_2 and peroxynitrite because they are potent oxidants rather than nitrogen agents. However, in basic and clinical medical research, the term 'nitrosative stress' generally describes the increased production of reactive nitrogen species and the consequent amplified inflammation and changes in the tissue structure. Thus, in this chapter, the term "nitorsative stress" comprises the overall NO-related nitrosative action as well as the toxicity of RNS as proinflammatory agents with the potential for tissue damage. Taken together, under the condition of nitrosative stress, the reaction of the body tissues to nitric oxide, nitrous oxide or similar species at levels greater than can be neutralized and is often complicated by the simultaneous production of superoxide anions, resulting in the formation of peroxynitrite and other reactive nitrogen species.

2 Source of RNS in Respiratory Tract

2.1 Cellular Source of NO in Airway

The primary source of RNS in biological systems is the free radical NO generated from L-arginine by three related nitric oxide synthase isoforms, eNOS, nNOS and iNOS as described above. All of the isoforms are expressed in the airways [12]. In airways of normal human subjects, NO is thought to originate by local synthesis from both constitutive and inducible NOS located in several cell types within the respiratory tract, including the airway and alveolar epithelial cells, macrophages, neutrophils, mast cells, and vascular endothelial and smooth muscle cells [13]. eNOS is constitutively expressed in human bronchial epithelium, type II human alveolar epithelial cells, and endothelial cells of the pulmonary blood vessels. NO from eNOS regulates the regional blood pressure, platelet aggregation, leukocyte adhesion and smooth muscle cell proliferation. NO produced from eNOS has been shown to be isolated in the respiratory epithelium and is suggested to play a role in ciliary movement and mucus ejection [14]. nNOS is expressed in airway nerves. The nerve fibers are present in airway smooth muscle and NO-derived nNOS regulates the neural smooth muscle relaxation [15]. In the respiratory tract, iNOS expression is located in alveolar type II epithelial cells, lung fibroblasts, airway and vascular smooth muscle cells, airway epithelial cells, mast cells, endothelial cells, neutrophils, and chondrocytes [15]. NO derived from iNOS is mainly involved in the formation of RNS in airways, and a wide range of stimuli can cause transcriptional activation of iNOS in these cells.

2.2 Mechanisms Regulating RNS Production

Several molecular mechanisms that induce iNOS expression and the consequent RNS formation have been demonstrated in a pathophysiological condition. Excessive NO is generated in human airway epithelial cells, neutrophils and macrophages by iNOS and several inflammatory mediators, and cytokines such as interlukin(IL)-1β, lipopolysaccharide (LPS), and type I cytokines like interferon(IFN)-γ and tumor necrosis factor (TNF)-α has been shown to be involved in the up-regulation of iNOS [16, 17]. Upon allergen challenge and virus infection, the production of IFN-γ is increased in human airway epithelial cells and lung fibroblasts, leading to iNOS formation [18, 19]. IFN-γ also regulates NADPH oxidase activity and expression in human macrophages. RNS formation by IFN-γ/LPS stimulation depends on NADPH oxidase. This suggests that IFN-γ could be the connection between allergic airway inflammation or viral infection and both superoxide and NO release and, consequently, the formation of RNS [18].

TNF-α plays a key role in allergic reactions in the airways. It also mediates bronchial hyperresponsiveness in rats following exposure to aerosolized endotoxin and ozone. TNF-α production by alveolar macrophages is increased in experimental models of tissue injury induced by inhaled particulates and endotoxin. It is thought to be the major cytotoxic effector in bleomycin and silica-induced fibrosis by lung macrophages [17]. TNF-α activates a cascade of signaling molecules including phosphatidylinositol 3 (PI3)-kinase, p44/42 mitogen-activated protein (MAP) kinase, and the consequent activation of NF-κB, a transcription factor important in regulating many inflammatory genes including iNOS [17].

In addition to inflammatory mediators, allergens and cigarette smoke, the main causes of asthma and COPD are involved in the induction of nitrosative stress in the airways. After bronchial provocation to birch, FeNO and the expression of iNOS mRNA in the bronchial epithelial were increased in asthmatic patients compared to healthy controls [20]. In an animal model of COPD, cigarette smoke or elastase-induced iNOS expression and RNS production in the lungs of mice lead to the development of emphysema [21, 22].

Toll-like receptors (TLRs) are pattern recognition receptors (PRRs) that can recognize specific molecular structures on the surface of pathogens, apoptotic host cells, and damaged senescent cells and affect the process of immune responses [23]. TLR3 recognizes dsRNA from the virus. Respiratory viral infection is a major cause of exacerbation of asthma and COPD. During viral replication, rhinovirus and respiratory syncytial virus produce dsRNA. dsRNA activates TLR3 and stimulates the innate immune response by activating NF-KB and IRF-3, leading to inflammatory responses. We previously demonstrated that TLR3 activation induces iNOS expression and nitrotyrosine formation in lung fibroblasts, leading to the production and activation of MMPs [19]. House dust mite (HDM), a common aeroallergen for asthma, contains LPS and proteases that can be recognized by TLR4 and PAR2, respectively. We also reported that HDM induce iNOS expression in BEAS-2B cells [24]. These data suggest that the innate immune response contributes to RNS production and induces nitrative stress in the pathogenesis of airway disease.

3 Pathophysiological Role of RNS in Airway Diseases

RNS, such as nitrite and peroxynitrite, have been shown to amplify inflammation and structural changes in the airways. Peroxynitrite triggers signal transduction involving MAP kinases and, as a result, causes apoptosis and necrosis in the airways of asthmatic patients [14]. The fibrotic response and tissue remodeling are key pathological features of asthma and COPD. Peroxynitrite has been shown to enhance the production of TGF-β1, fibronectin, and vascular endothelial growth factor (VEGF) in lung fibroblasts [25]. Peroxynitrite also induces the differentiation of lung

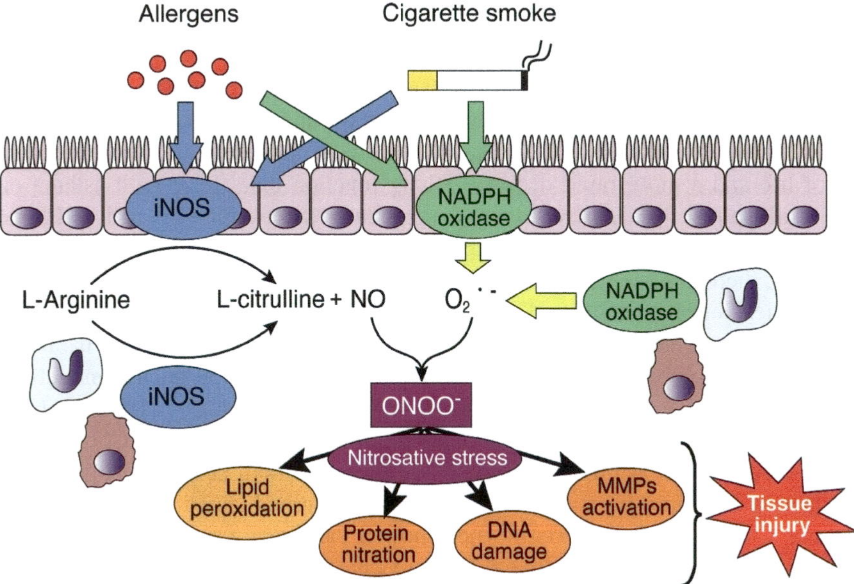

Fig. 9.1 Schematic illustration of the mechanisms by which peroxynitrite, a potent reactive nitrogen species (RNS) formation mediated by inducible nitric oxide synthase (iNOS), forms in the airways of asthma and COPD. Allergens or pathogens including house dust mite, pollen, viruses and fungus, and cigarette smoke can enhance the induction of iNOS and NADPH oxidase in the airway epithelium, and inflammatory cells such as macrophages and neutrophils in submucosa. iNOS produce NO through the conversion of L-ariginine to L-citrulline. NADPH oxidases produce reactive oxygen species such as superoxide (O2-). Excessively produced NO interacts with O2- leading to the formation of ONOO-. In the airways of ACO, both airborne pathogens and cigarette smoke are involved in the airway inflammation and peroxynitrite production might be more enhanced compared to asthma and COPD

fibroblasts to myofibroblasts through NF-kB activation [26]. Peroxynitrite activates matrix metalloproteinase (MMP)-2 and MMP-9, which are increased in patients with severe asthma and in those who smoke. RNS induces the recruitment of neutrophils into the airways, which generate more superoxide anions, producing more peroxynitrite and 3-NT. In the meantime, the release of neutrophil myeloperoxidase (MPO) generates an additional 3-NT, leading to persistent airway inflammation [27]. Peroxynitrite also causes DNA damage by the oxidation and nitration of guanine and induces DNA single-strand breaks [28]. This is related to peroxynitrite-mediated cytotoxicity and the induction of mitochondrial dysfunction, cell death and tissue inflammation. Finally, peroxynitrite contributes to the development of tissue damage (Fig. 9.1).

4 Role of Nitrative Stress in ACO

As described in other chapters, the overlap of asthma-chronic obstructive pulmonary disease (ACO) is defined as having both asthma and COPD's physiological and clinical features. Patients with ACO have more frequent exacerbations, poorer quality of life and a more rapid decline of lung function than those with asthma or COPD alone [29, 30]. Differences in clinical features between ACO and COPD or asthma are thought to be attributable to their pathophysiological differences. However, there has been only a quite small number of studies that investigated the pathological mechanisms of ACO. Because ACO is heterogeneous and patients have various combinations of asthma and COPD features, it is difficult to characterize the underlying pathogenic mechanisms and to establish experimental models of ACO that accurately reflect the key features of ACO in patients [31]. Meanwhile, there are several clinical studies that detected clinical biomarkers of ACO that distinguish ACO from asthma or COPD alone [32]. Iwamoto et al. investigated the production of various biomarkers in plasma and sputum obtained from the control, asthma, COPD, and ACO groups. They showed that there were significant differences in the amounts of plasma soluble receptors for advanced glycation end-products, plasma surfactant protein A, sputum myeloperoxidase, and sputum neutrophil gelatinase-associated lipocalin between the asthma and ACO groups [33]. It has been reported that patients with ACO had more neutrophils and higher amounts of IL-6 in the peripheral blood compared to those in patients with adult-onset asthma [34]. These markers might be useful for distinguishing ACO from asthma or COPD in a cross-sectional study. However, the role of these markers in the pathogenesis and the relationship between these markers and the clinical course of ACO have not been clarified.

4.1 Nitrosative Stress in COPD and Asthma

3-NT has been used as a marker for producing peroxynitrite in tissue. Peroxynitirte adds a nitro group to the 3-position adjacent to the hydroxyl group of tyrosine to produce the stable product 3-NT. Consequently, 3-NT reflects the local production of peroxynitrite. Thus, 3-NT as well as iNOS are widely used as nitrosative stress markers. We previously compared the production level of RNS in the airways of subjects with COPD to those in non-COPD with asthma and in healthy subjects using immunostaining for 3-NT and iNOS in induced sputum [35]. Cell counts of iNOS- and 3-NT-positive cells were significantly higher in both asthma and COPD than in healthy subjects. Furthermore, cell counts of 3-NT-positive cells were increased in patients with COPD compared to asthmatic patients. A negative correlation was observed between % FEV1 and 3-NT positive cell numbers in patients with COPD, but no significant correlation between them was observed in asthmatic patients. In contrast, exhaled NO levels were increased only in patients with asthma. Ricciardolo et al. expanded these studies to investigate the expressions of nitrative stress markers, including 3-NT, iNOS, eNOS, myeloperoxidase (MPO) and xanthine oxidase (XO) in bronchial biopsy samples and bronchoalveolar lavage fluid (BALF) from patients with mild to stable COPD. They compared them with non-COPD groups, including healthy smokers and nonsmokers [36]. They found that positive cell numbers of 3-NT and MPO were higher in the bronchial submucosa of patients with severe COPD than in patients with milder COPD or control subjects. In patients with COPD, the number of MPO-positive cells had a significant correlation with the number of neutrophils in the bronchial submucosa, and the numbers of 3-NT-positive cells and MPO-positive cells had a negative correlation with FEV1. These data suggest that MPO-mediated nitrative stress may be implicated in the pathogenesis of severe COPD. These results suggest that RNS may be involved in the pathogenesis of airway inflammation in asthma and COPD and that NO produced in airways mediated by iNOS is consumed by its reaction with superoxide anion, especially in COPD. Nitrosative stress may be highly mediated by iNOS in the airways of COPD.

RNS and nitrative stress have also been demonstrated to contribute to the pathogenesis of asthma, especially the severe phenotype. Hamid et al. demonstrated that iNOS immunopositivity was increased in the epithelium and inflammatory cells in biopsy samples from non-steroid-treated patients with asthma compared to controls [37]. Saleh et al. compared the immunoreactivity of nitrotyrosine in the airways of asthmatic patients with controls and also investigated the effect of inhaled budesonide on the formation of peroxynitrite [38]. Strong immunoreactivity to nitrotyrosine was observed in airway epithelium and inflammatory cells from patients with asthma, but there was weak or no immunoreacvitiy to nitrotyorsine in the airways of controls. The presence of nitrotyrosine in airway epithelium and inflammatory cells had a negative correlation with PC20 and FEV1. Budesonide reduced the formation of nitrotyrosine. This suggests that peroxynitrite can be involved in developing airway obstruction, airway hyperresponsiveness, and epithelial injury in asthmatic patients. We previously compared the number of 3-NT-positive cells in induced sputum from refractory asthma with that from well-controlled asthma [39]. Immunopositivity for 3-NT was enhanced in sputum from refractory asthma compared to well-controlled asthma, and the expression levels of nitrosative stress markers were negatively correlated with lung function. Thus, RNS, including peroxynitrite, cause lung inflammation, oxidative stress, activation of matrix metalloproteinase, and inactivation of antiprotease, which are involved in the pathophysiology of COPD and asthma. Furthermore, nitrative stress affects the disease severity and clinical course of the disease.

4.2 Nitrosative Stress in ACO

As discussed above, nitrative stress can affect both diseases, suggesting that nitrosative stress might be more strongly associated with ACO. To confirm the clinical contribution of nitrosative stress in ACO, we investigated nitrative stress in the airways of patients with ACO and compared the degree of nitrative stress in induced sputum from ICS-treated ACO patients with that of well-controlled asthmatic patients [40]. Immunoreactivity in sputum cells for iNOS was mainly observed in neutrophils and macrophages, and the percentages of iNOS-immunopositive cells were significantly higher in patients with ACO than those in healthy subjects and asthmatic patients. The percentage of iNOS-positive cells was negatively correlated with the baseline FEV1 percent predicted for all subjects. Similarly, immunopositivity for 3-NT was observed mainly in neutrophils and macrophages, and the percentage of 3-NT-positive cells in the sputum of patients with ACO significantly increased compared to those of healthy subjects and asthmatic patients. The percentage of 3-NT-positive cells had a positive correlation with the percentages of CBS and CSE-positive cells and was negatively correlated with the baseline FEV1 percent predicted values. In addition, the values of both iNOS- and 3-NT-immunopositive cells had a significant correlation with the frequency of exacerbations and the annual decline of FEV1. Furthermore, the values of 3-NT-positive cells were shown to have a positive correlation with the amounts of IL-8, MCP-1 and TNF-α. These data suggest nitrosative stress is more enhanced in the airways of ACO than in asthmatic patients, even when the patients with ACO were well-controlled with ICS and other appropriate treatment. Nitrative stress is a robust and common pathogenesis for both COPD and severe asthma and, therefore, can be a key mechanism that regulates the pathogenesis of ACO characterized by a more severe disease category compared to COPD and asthma alone. 3-NT might be a promising biomarker for predicting the risk for exacerbations and decline in lung function in ACO. Because it is difficult to obtain lung samples such as by bronchial biopsy or surgical lung dissection, further study is needed to characterize the degree of nitrative stress in the lungs of ACO and how nitrative stress affects the ACO pathogenesis using those pathological bronchial or lung samples from patients with ACO.

4.3 Antioxidant and Nitrosative Stress: Role of Reactive Persulfide Species in ACO

Oxidative stress arises from an imbalance between oxidants/antioxidants partly caused by the impaired production of endogenous antioxidants in the human body. Akaike et al. identified reactive persulfide and polysulfide species such as glutathione persulfide (GSSH), cysteine persulfide (CysSSH) and glutathione trisulfide (GSSSH) in human cells and plasmas using LC-ESI-MS/MS. They demonstrated that they are highly reactive and extremely powerful antioxidants that regulate oxidative stress and redox signaling mediated by various electrophiles [41]. Additionally, they showed that CysSSH is biosynthesized from cystine by cystathionine β-synthase (CBS) and cystathionine γ-lyase (CSE), which in turn may contribute to the production of GSSH and other CysSSH derivatives formed in human [41]. The antioxidant capacity and reactivity of GSSH and CysSSH are approximately 10–100 times greater than those of GSH and cysteine (CysSH) [41]. These data indicate that reactive persulfides and polysulfides could be potent antioxidants.

We first compared the levels of reactive persulfide species in the airways of patients with COPD with those of healthy subjects [42]. The GSSH, CySSH and GSSSH levels in primary bronchial cells and epithelial lining fluid (ELF) from COPD patients were significantly lower than in samples from healthy subjects. Meanwhile, the production of proinflammatory cytokines and chemokines including IL-8, IL-6, IL-1β and MCP-1 from bronchial epithelial cells of COPD patients was enhanced compared to cells of non-COPD subjects. The amounts of reactive persulfide species in the lung cells positively correlated to the degree of airflow limitation and negatively correlated with the levels of inflammatory mediators. These data suggest that the novel antioxidants reactive persulfide species can be a key player in regulating the redox balance and lung inflammation in the lungs of COPD patients.

As we discussed above, nitrosative stress occurs partly due to oxidative stress or concurrently arises with oxidative stress caused by aberrant reduction in endogenous antioxidants in the lungs, which might contribute to the development and/or pathogenesis of ACO. To clarify this, we investigated the levels of reactive persulfides and polysulfides in the induced sputum of patients with ACO, asthma, and healthy subjects (in the same cohort described above) using the sulfane sulfur probe (SSP)-4, a specific probe for reactive persulfide species [40]. We also measured the CBS and CSE expression levels in the sputum cells by immunostaining. The fluorescence intensity for SSP-4 was significantly lower in sputum in the patients with ACO compared to that of healthy subjects and patients with asthma, and it was significantly correlated to the baseline FEV1 percent predicted. In contrast to the SSP-4 levels, the percentages of CBS- and CSE-positive cells were significantly higher in patients with ACO compared to healthy subjects and asthmatics. Furthermore, the percentage of 3-NT-positive cells had a negative correlation with the intensity of SSP-4 but had a positive correlation with percentages of CBS- and CSE-positive cells. To investigate the contribution of RNS in the production of reactive persulfides, THP-1 cells were treated with peroxynitrite, and the expression of CBS and CSE and the amount of intracellular reactive persulfide were measured. Peroxynitrite increased the expression of CBS and CSE without affecting their enzymatic activity. The SSP-4 intensity in the cells was reduced after treatment with peroxynitrite. These clinical and in vitro data suggest that excessive nitrosative stress occurs in the airways of patients with ACO and can stimulate the expression of synthases of reactive persulfides. At the same time, RNS might consume the reactive persulfides produced by the synthases. Crosslinking of nitrosative stress and

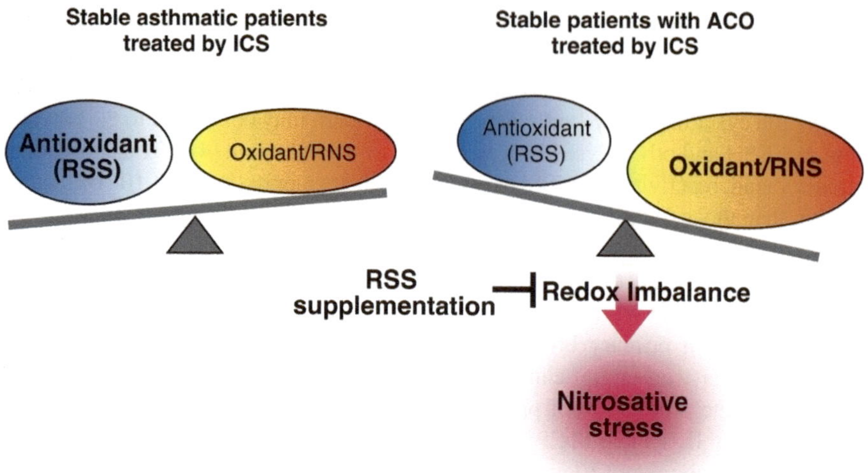

Fig. 9.2 Suggested role of reactive persulfide species (RSS) in redox imbalance in the airways of asthma and ACO. In the airways of patients with stable asthma under ICS treatment, the balance between an antioxidant such as RSS and an oxidant including reactive nitrogen species (RNS) is maintained. In contrast, in the airways of patients with ACO, the production of RNS overwhelms the levels of endogenous antioxidant and continuous nitrative stress occurs even in the airways of stable ACO patients. Nitrosative stress-mediated-redox imbalance can be a novel target for ACO treatment. RSS supplementation might be a promising approach for this strategy

regulation of the production of reactive persulfide species could play a pivotal role in the airway of patients with ACO and may be involved in the pathophysiology of ACO, which could provide a target for a novel therapeutic strategy (Fig. 9.2).

5 Therapeutic Potential of Targeting Nitrosative Stress for ACO

As discussed above, regulating RNS formation might be a potential therapeutic target for ACO. To date, there have been no established pharmacological molecules available in clinical practice for the treatment of ACO. However, some molecules have been shown to possess a potential for decreasing RNS production in experimental models and in human tissues of patients with asthma and COPD.

5.1 Corticosteroids and iNOS Inhibitors

Inhaled corticosteroids or systemic administration of glucocorticoids reduce FeNO in patients with asthma and COPD. In contrast, Donnelly et al. demonstrated that dexamethasone and budesonide had no effect on the expression of iNOS mRNA and iNOS protein in human primary epithelial cells obtained from asthmatic patients [16]. Larsson-Callerfelt et al. investigated the iNOS expressions in lung fibroblasts obtained from distal lungs of patients with asthma and healthy subjects and the effect of selective iNOS inhibitor 1400W on proteoglycan synthesis in the cells [43]. There was a tendency for a higher expression in lung fibroblasts from asthmatic patients. 1400W inhibited iNOS expression and increased the synthesis of proteoglycan versican in lung fibroblasts from asthmatic patients. We reported that 1400W reduced TLR3-mediated MMP production and activation in human lung fibroblasts [19]. Fysikopoulos et al. demonstrated that oral administration of iNOS inhibitor N(6)-(1-iminoethyl)-L-lysine (L-NIL) improves porcine pancreatic elastase-induced emphysema and pulmonary hypertension in the lungs of C57BL/6J mice [44]. Furthermore, L-NIL has been shown to be very effective in reducing FeNO in patients with asthma but has not been tested in COPD patients [45]. Another iNOS inhibitor, aminoguanidine, was shown to block peroxinitrite formation and prevents bleomycin-induced injury and fibrosis in the lungs of mice by reducing NO derived from iNOS [46]. Aminoguanidine also reduced the exhaled NO level and, partially, NO metabolites including nitrite/nitrate and peroxynitrite in exhaled breath condensate and induced sputum from patients with COPD [47]. These data suggest the potential effect of iNOS inhibitors in reducing nitrosative stress. However, the effect is limited, and no studies have been conducted on ACO patients. In a future study, the effect of iNOS inhibitors in patients with ACO should be investigated.

Resistance to corticosteroid treatment is another clinical feature of severe asthma and COPD. Several molecular mechanisms involved in corticosteroid resistance have been demonstrated. Reduced histone deacetylase (HDAC) 2 expression in the airways of these diseases has been suggested [48]. HDAC2 regulates the action of steroids to switch off activated inflammation genes. HDAC2 activity and expression were decreased by oxidative and nitrosative stress. Peroxynitrite nitrates tyrosine residues on HDAC2, leading to its inactivation, ubiquitination and degradation [49]. This suggests that nitrative stress might contribute to corticosteroid resistance in severe asthma and COPD. It remains unknown whether the HDAC pathway is altered in patients with ACO. It should be determined how the HDAC pathway contributes to the pathogenesis of ACO. Furthermore, a pharmacological strategy other than corticosteroid needs to be established to target nitrative stress in inflammatory airway disease.

5.2 *Theophylline*

Theophylline has been regarded as an optional treatment for COPD and asthma in addition to corticosteroids and bronchodilators and is usually not used as the main drug. However, we demonstrated that theophylline reduces the numbers of 3-NT positive neutrophils in induced sputum from patients with COPD, whereas inhaled corticosteroids had no significant effect on the numbers of 3-NT positive cells [50].

Theophylline has anti-inflammatory properties partly through restoring HDAC activity. It has been demonstrated that peroxynitrite inactivates HDAC, which was recovered by treatment with theophylline in lung fibroblast. Theophylline suppressed peroxynitrite-mediated MMP release by inhibiting NF-kB activation and recovery of the HDAC activity [51].

5.3 *Other Drugs*

Several drugs used in managing chronic diseases other than airway diseases have been shown to have the potential for regulating nitrative stress. Inhibition of XO by oral allopurinol reduced 3-nitrotyrosine formation in the induced sputum from patients with COPD as well as FeNO [52]. Simvastatin is generally used as a cholesterol-lowering drug for the prevention of cardiovascular diseases. The effect of simvastatin on the clinical course of asthma and COPD has been investigated in clinical trials. Cowan et al. demonstrated that simvastatin has a minor beneficial effect on symptoms, lung function and sputum eosinophil counts in patients with eosinophilic asthma but has no steroid-sparing effect in the patients [53]. Several studies demonstrated the beneficial effects of simvastatin on lung function decline, rates and severity of exacerbations, and hospitalization [54]. Simvastatin was demonstrated to reduce iNOS expression and nitrotyrosine formation but increased eNOS expression in the lungs of OVA-challenged mice. As a result, nitric oxide metabolism improved, reducing airway inflammation, epithelial injury and hyperresponsiveness in a murine asthma model [55]. This suggests that the effect of simvastatin on asthma and COPD might be partly attributable to the reduction in nitrosative stress.

6 Conclusion

Nitrosative stress plays an important role in the pathogenesis of ACO because RNS contributes to the development of the pathophysiological features observed in both asthma and COPD. Clinically, nitrosative stress might be a cause of the severe phenotype of these diseases. Markers of nitrosative stress, such as iNOS and 3-NT, can be useful tools for diagnosing ACO and predicting the clinical course of patients with ACO. Finally, targeting nitrosative stress is a promising therapeutic approach for the management of ACO. Experimental in vitro and in vivo models of ACO need to be established to clarify the precise role of nitrosative stress and to determine novel mechanisms by which the NOS-RNS system affects the pathogenesis of ACO.

References

1. Gaston B, et al. The biology of nitrogen oxides in the airways. Am J Respir Crit Care Med. 1994;149(2 Pt 1):538–51.
2. Moncada S, Palmer RM, Higgs EA. Nitric oxide: physiology, pathophysiology, and pharmacology. Pharmacol Rev. 1991;43(2):109–42.
3. Fulton DJR, et al. Reactive oxygen and nitrogen species in the development of pulmonary hypertension. Antioxidants (Basel). 2017;6(3):54.
4. Bayarri MA, et al. Nitric oxide system and bronchial epithelium: more than a barrier. Front Physiol. 2021;12:687381.
5. Okamoto T, et al. A new paradigm for antimicrobial host defense mediated by a nitrated cyclic nucleotide. J Clin Biochem Nutr. 2010;46(1):14–9.
6. Wang Y, Wang K, Fu J. HDAC6 mediates macrophage iNOS expression and excessive nitric oxide production in the blood during endotoxemia. Front Immunol. 2020;11:1893.
7. Sugiura H, Ichinose M. Oxidative and nitrative stress in bronchial asthma. Antioxid Redox Signal. 2008;10(4):785–97.
8. Beckman JS, et al. Apparent hydroxyl radical production by peroxynitrite: implications for endothelial injury from nitric oxide and superoxide. Proc Natl Acad Sci U S A. 1990;87(4):1620–4.
9. Eiserich JP, et al. Formation of nitric oxide-derived inflammatory oxidants by myeloperoxidase in neutrophils. Nature. 1998;391(6665):393–7.
10. Pryor WA, Squadrito GL. The chemistry of peroxynitrite: a product from the reaction of nitric oxide with superoxide. Am J Phys. 1995;268(5 Pt 1):L699–722.
11. Heinrich TA, et al. Biological nitric oxide signalling: chemistry and terminology. Br J Pharmacol. 2013;169(7):1417–29.
12. Ricciardolo FL, et al. Effect of bradykinin on allergen induced increase in exhaled nitric oxide in asthma. Thorax. 2003;58(10):840–5.
13. van der Vliet A, et al. Reactive nitrogen species and tyrosine nitration in the respiratory tract: epiphenomena or a pathobiologic mechanism of disease? Am J Respir Crit Care Med. 1999;160(1):1–9.
14. Zuo L, Koozechian MS, Chen LL. Characterization of reactive nitrogen species in allergic asthma. Ann Allergy Asthma Immunol. 2014;112(1):18–22.
15. Ricciardolo FL, et al. Reactive nitrogen species in the respiratory tract. Eur J Pharmacol. 2006;533(1–3):240–52.
16. Donnelly LE, Barnes PJ. Expression and regulation of inducible nitric oxide synthase from human primary airway epithelial cells. Am J Respir Cell Mol Biol. 2002;26(1):144–51.
17. Laskin DL, et al. Macrophages, reactive nitrogen species, and lung injury. Ann N Y Acad Sci. 2010;1203:60–5.
18. Folkerts G, et al. Reactive nitrogen and oxygen species in airway inflammation. Eur J Pharmacol. 2001;429(1–3):251–62.
19. Ichikawa T, et al. TLR3 activation augments matrix metalloproteinase production through reactive nitrogen species generation in human lung fibroblasts. J Immunol. 2014;192(11):4977–88.
20. Roos AB, et al. Elevated exhaled nitric oxide in allergen-provoked asthma is associated with airway epithelial iNOS. PLoS One. 2014;9(2):e90018.
21. Boyer L, et al. Role of nitric oxide synthases in elastase-induced emphysema. Lab Investig. 2011;91(3):353–62.
22. Ning Y, et al. Attenuation of cigarette smoke-induced airway mucus production by hydrogen-rich saline in rats. PLoS One. 2013;8(12):e83429.
23. Li D, Wu M. Pattern recognition receptors in health and diseases. Signal Transduct Target Ther. 2021;6(1):291.
24. Saito T, et al. PGC-1alpha regulates airway epithelial barrier dysfunction induced by house dust mite. Respir Res. 2021;22(1):63.

25. Sugiura H, et al. Reactive nitrogen species augment fibroblast-mediated collagen gel contraction, mediator production, and chemotaxis. Am J Respir Cell Mol Biol. 2006;34(5):592–9.
26. Ichikawa T, et al. Peroxynitrite augments fibroblast-mediated tissue remodeling via myofibroblast differentiation. Am J Physiol Lung Cell Mol Physiol. 2008;295(5):L800–8.
27. Barnes PJ. Nitrosative stress in patients with asthma-chronic obstructive pulmonary disease overlap. J Allergy Clin Immunol. 2019;144(4):928–30.
28. Pacher P, Beckman JS, Liaudet L. Nitric oxide and peroxynitrite in health and disease. Physiol Rev. 2007;87(1):315–424.
29. Menezes AMB, et al. Increased risk of exacerbation and hospitalization in subjects with an overlap phenotype: COPD-asthma. Chest. 2014;145(2):297–304.
30. Kauppi P, et al. Overlap syndrome of asthma and COPD predicts low quality of life. J Asthma. 2011;48(3):279–85.
31. Tu X, et al. Asthma-COPD overlap: current understanding and the utility of experimental models. Eur Respir Rev. 2021;30(159):190185.
32. Mekov E, et al. Update on asthma-COPD overlap (ACO): a narrative review. Int J Chron Obstruct Pulmon Dis. 2021;16:1783–99.
33. Iwamoto H, et al. Differences in plasma and sputum biomarkers between COPD and COPD-asthma overlap. Eur Respir J. 2014;43(2):421–9.
34. Tommola M, et al. Differences between asthma-COPD overlap syndrome and adult-onset asthma. Eur Respir J. 2017;49(5):1602383.
35. Ichinose M, et al. Increase in reactive nitrogen species production in chronic obstructive pulmonary disease airways. Am J Respir Crit Care Med. 2000;162(2 Pt 1):701–6.
36. Ricciardolo FL, et al. Nitrosative stress in the bronchial mucosa of severe chronic obstructive pulmonary disease. J Allergy Clin Immunol. 2005;116(5):1028–35.
37. Hamid Q, et al. Induction of nitric oxide synthase in asthma. Lancet. 1993;342(8886–8887):1510–3.
38. Saleh D, et al. Increased formation of the potent oxidant peroxynitrite in the airways of asthmatic patients is associated with induction of nitric oxide synthase: effect of inhaled glucocorticoid. FASEB J. 1998;12(11):929–37.
39. Sugiura H, et al. Nitrative stress in refractory asthma. J Allergy Clin Immunol. 2008;121(2):355–60.
40. Kyogoku Y, et al. Nitrosative stress in patients with asthma-chronic obstructive pulmonary disease overlap. J Allergy Clin Immunol. 2019;144(4):972–83. e14
41. Ida T, et al. Reactive cysteine persulfides and S-polythiolation regulate oxidative stress and redox signaling. Proc Natl Acad Sci U S A. 2014;111(21):7606–11.
42. Numakura T, et al. Production of reactive persulfide species in chronic obstructive pulmonary disease. Thorax. 2017;72(12):1074–83.
43. Larsson-Callerfelt AK, et al. iNOS affects matrix production in distal lung fibroblasts from patients with mild asthma. Pulm Pharmacol Ther. 2015;34:64–71.
44. Fysikopoulos A, et al. Amelioration of elastase-induced lung emphysema and reversal of pulmonary hypertension by pharmacological iNOS inhibition in mice. Br J Pharmacol. 2021;178(1):152–71.
45. Barnes PJ. Oxidative stress-based therapeutics in COPD. Redox Biol. 2020;33:101544.
46. Chen C, et al. Exogenous nitric oxide enhances the prophylactic effect of aminoguanidine, a preferred iNOS inhibitor, on bleomycin-induced fibrosis in the lung: implications for the direct roles of the NO molecule in vivo. Nitric Oxide. 2017;70:31–41.
47. Brindicci C, et al. Effects of aminoguanidine, an inhibitor of inducible nitric oxide synthase, on nitric oxide production and its metabolites in healthy control subjects, healthy smokers, and COPD patients. Chest. 2009;135(2):353–67.
48. Barnes PJ. Histone deacetylase-2 and airway disease. Ther Adv Respir Dis. 2009;3(5):235–43.
49. Barnes PJ. Corticosteroid resistance in patients with asthma and chronic obstructive pulmonary disease. J Allergy Clin Immunol. 2013;131(3):636–45.

50. Hirano T, et al. Inhibition of reactive nitrogen species production in COPD airways: comparison of inhaled corticosteroid and oral theophylline. Thorax. 2006;61(9):761–6.
51. Sugiura H, et al. Inhibitory effects of theophylline on the peroxynitrite-augmented release of matrix metalloproteinases by lung fibroblasts. Am J Physiol Lung Cell Mol Physiol. 2012;302(8):L764–74.
52. Ichinose M, et al. Xanthine oxidase inhibition reduces reactive nitrogen species production in COPD airways. Eur Respir J. 2003;22(3):457–61.
53. Cowan DC, et al. Simvastatin in the treatment of asthma: lack of steroid-sparing effect. Thorax. 2010;65(10):891–6.
54. Schenk P, et al. Can simvastatin reduce COPD exacerbations? A randomised double-blind controlled study. Eur Respir J. 2021;58(1):2001798.
55. Ahmad T, et al. Simvastatin improves epithelial dysfunction and airway hyperresponsiveness: from asymmetric dimethyl-arginine to asthma. Am J Respir Cell Mol Biol. 2011;44(4):531–9.

Chapter 10
Radiographic Features of ACO: How Is the Feature Applied to Practice?

Masato Karayama and Naoki Inui

Abstract A novel concept of asthma–chronic obstructive pulmonary disease overlap (ACO) has been proposed as a practical clinical approach to the complexity of asthma and chronic obstructive pulmonary disease (COPD). From the diagnostic radiology aspect, ACO exhibits mixed asthma and COPD radiologic features. First, emphysema, a major hallmark of COPD, is less frequently observed in ACO. Several genetic factors were reportedly associated with the difference in the development of emphysema between ACO and COPD in a genome-wide association study. Second, the thickening of airway walls and narrowing of the intraluminal area of central airways are more advanced in ACO than in COPD. However, small airway disease is comparable between ACO and COPD. Based on the traditional concept that asthma is characterized by proximal airway disease, whereas COPD is characterized by distal/small airway disease, ACO has mixed airway features common to both asthma and COPD. According to real-world studies, patients with COPD who exhibit airway-dominant radiologic features reportedly have a substantial possibility of having ACO. Radiologic assessments have the potential to provide useful information for the diagnosis of ACO.

Keywords Airway disease · Airway remodeling · Bronchus · Emphysema · Radiologic phenotype

M. Karayama
Second Division, Department of Internal Medicine, Hamamatsu University School of Medicine, Hamamatsu, Japan

N. Inui (✉)
Second Division, Department of Internal Medicine, Hamamatsu University School of Medicine, Hamamatsu, Japan

Department of Clinical Pharmacology and Therapeutics, Hamamatsu University School of Medicine, Hamamatsu, Japan
e-mail: inui@hama-med.ac.jp

H. Nagase et al. (eds.), *Asthma-COPD Overlap*, Respiratory Disease Series: Diagnostic Tools and Disease Managements,
https://doi.org/10.1007/978-981-96-0217-9_10

1 Introduction

Both asthma and chronic obstructive pulmonary disease (COPD) have similar clinical and physiologic features that are caused by airflow limitation. Although the underlying mechanisms of airflow limitation are different between asthma and COPD, it is sometimes difficult to distinguish these two diseases by clinical manifestations, such as symptoms, pulmonary function tests, and especially radiographic assessments. This is because the differences between the two diseases are functional and pathological, preventing assessment by usual clinical examinations. Another reason for the difficulty distinguishing the two diseases is that some patients with airflow limitation have asthma and COPD clinical features. Therefore, a novel concept of asthma-COPD overlap (ACO) has been proposed as a practical clinical approach to the complexity of the two disease entities [1].

Radiologic assessments using chest computed tomography (CT) can provide information regarding emphysema and airway disease in patients with ACO. Recent advances in diagnostic radiology have facilitated quantifying the degree of emphysema and airway remodeling, reconstruction of airway trees by three-dimensional CT (3D-CT), and evaluation of small airway disease by expiratory CT using image analysis software. Possible applications of these radiologic data are the diagnosis, classification, or therapeutic stratification of ACO. This chapter describes the common and differential aspects of the radiologic features of asthma, COPD, and ACO.

2 Emphysema

Emphysema is a major pathologic hallmark of COPD. Pathologically, emphysema is defined as "a condition of the lung characterized by abnormal, permanent enlargement of the air spaces distal to the terminal bronchiole, accompanied by destruction of their walls" [2]. In chest CT, emphysema is characterized by areas of abnormally low attenuation that contrast the surrounding normal lung parenchyma [3]. Emphysema not only appears as a radiologic finding but is also associated with symptoms and impaired pulmonary function [4–13]. Thus, assessment of emphysema is crucial in the clinical management of smokers and/or patients with COPD.

The pathogenesis of emphysema is considered to involve complex mechanisms of oxidative stress, inflammation, extracellular matrix proteolysis, and apoptotic and autophagic cell death [14]. Although emphysema develops as a result of a complex sequence of these events, the triggering factor for lung destruction is indisputably inhaled noxious substances, mostly tobacco smoke [15]. Therefore, emphysema is the most distinctive radiographic feature of COPD, in contrast to asthma in nonsmokers. Elucidation of the features of emphysema in ACO will provide useful information for the diagnosis and management of ACO.

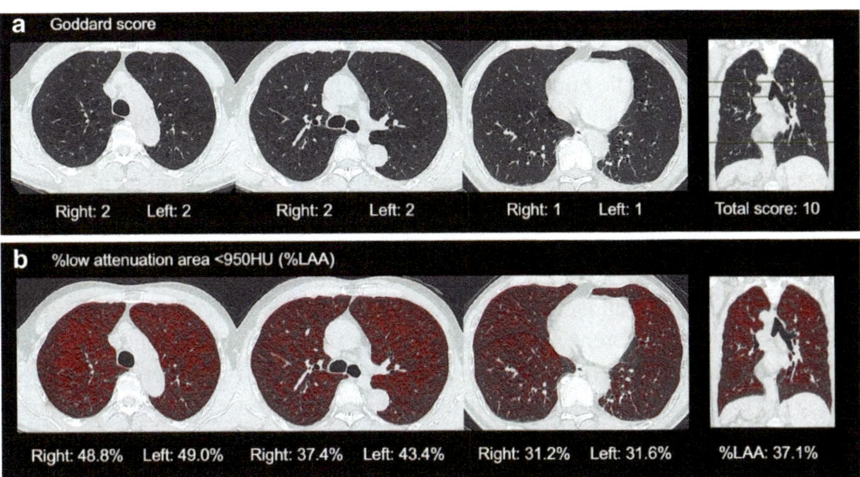

Fig. 10.1 Assessment of emphysema. Representative images of assessments of emphysema using the (**a**) Goddard score and (**b**) percentage low attenuation area of less than −950 HU

2.1 Assessment of Emphysema

Assessment of emphysema is broadly classified into two methods: a visual semi-quantitative method and an image analysis-based quantitative method. The representative method of the former is the Goddard classification [16]. In the Goddard classification, the extent of emphysema is scored from 0 to 4 (0, no emphysema; 1, <25%; 2, ≥25% to <50%; 3, ≥50% to <75%; and 4, ≥75%). These assessments are separately performed in the bilateral upper, middle, and lower lung fields, and the sum of the six lung fields represents the severity of emphysema (maximum of 24 points) (Fig. 10.1a). This method is easy and practicable; however, it has risks of both inter- and intra-observer differences. In contrast, image analysis-based methods facilitate quantitative and reproducible evaluation of the lung's CT density (Hounsfield unit, HU). The representative methods are the percentage of lung density less than −950 HU (percentage low attenuation area, %LAA) (Fig. 10.1b) and the 15th percentile of lung attenuation (Perc15) [4, 9, 11–13, 17]. These methods are not only quantitative and reproducible but can also detect low attenuation areas of the lungs that are not visually evaluable.

2.2 Emphysema in COPD

Naturally, emphysema is more frequent and severe in patients with COPD than in patients with asthma [18–20]. Even patients with severe asthma, whose degree of impairment in pulmonary function is similar to that of patients with COPD, have less frequent episodes and a smaller extent of emphysema than patients with COPD

[18, 20]. One study showed that patients who had asthma with airflow limitation [defined as a forced expiratory volume in 1 second (FEV_1)/forced vital capacity of <70% after inhalation of short-acting β_2-agonists] had a significantly smaller extent of emphysema as visually scored in high-resolution CT images than did patients with COPD [20]. Furthermore, another study showed that the extent of emphysema, as evaluated by image processing software, was significantly smaller in patients with asthma than in patients with COPD who had similar degrees of airflow limitation [18].

The difference in the existence and extent of emphysema between COPD and asthma is obvious and understandable; however, it can also offer important suggestions regarding the difference in the pathogenesis of airflow limitation between the two diseases. In addition to emphysema, airway narrowing is another key pathogenetic aspect of COPD and results in airflow limitation. Major mechanisms underlying airway narrowing in COPD are mucus hyperproduction, mucosal hyperplasia, and hypertrophy of airway smooth muscle [21, 22]. In addition, emphysema contributes to the development of airway narrowing. Lung alveoli are usually attached to the outside of the airway and help to maintain airway patency by tensional force [3, 23]. In patients with emphysema, the destruction of alveoli results in the loss of the supporting structure of the airway, which leads to airway collapse. Therefore, even if patients with and without emphysema demonstrate comparable airflow limitation as assessed by spirometry, the mechanisms of airflow limitation differ.

2.3 Emphysema in Asthma

Although visually detectable emphysema is not frequently observed, patients with asthma also have decreased lung attenuation when evaluated using image analysis-based methods [18, 20, 24]. In one study, an increased %LAA was observed in patients with asthma who had no history of smoking, and this increased %LAA was associated with the duration of the disease and correlated with airflow limitation [24]. The increased LAA observed in patients with asthma is presumably caused by overinflation of the lung parenchyma due to air trapping, and it is not completely identical to COPD-associated emphysema, which is pathologically accompanied by destruction of the lung parenchyma. Although an increased LAA observed in non-smoking patients with asthma is also an important radiologic finding that indicates severe airflow limitation accompanied by air trapping, it should be discriminated from emphysema, especially when diagnosing ACO.

2.4 Emphysema in ACO

Given the radiologic difference in the presence and extent of emphysema between asthma and COPD, it is possible that ACO and COPD also show some differences in emphysema. In the COPDGene study involving non-Hispanic White or

African-American patients with COPD, the characteristics of 3120 patients with COPD were compared with those of 450 patients with ACO (defined as a history of asthma diagnosed by a physician before the age of 40 years) [25]. The %LAA was significantly higher in patients with COPD than in those with ACO. Kitaguchi et al. [20] retrospectively evaluated 32 patients with ACO, defined as those with COPD who experienced asthmatic symptoms, such as episodic breathlessness, wheezing, coughing, and chest tightness that worsened at night or early morning. The patients with ACO demonstrated significantly lower emphysema scores (visually evaluated using the Goddard classification) than did 118 patients with COPD [20]. In a prospective study of 66 patients with COPD, the patients were divided into those with pure COPD ($n = 40$) and ACO ($n = 26$), defined as having a variable clinical history compatible with asthma (wheezing, chest tightness, shortness of breath, or coughing) and variable expiratory airflow limitation (post-bronchodilator improvement in FEV_1 of >12% and 200 mL) [26]. The patients with pure COPD had a significantly greater extent of emphysema, as evaluated by a %LAA of less than −950 HU, than did the patients with ACO.

However, the association between emphysema and ACO remains controversial. In a prospective multicenter study of COPD conducted in Japan (Hokkaido COPD cohort study), the clinical characteristics of 96 patients who had COPD with asthma-like features [defined as bronchodilator reversibility (FEV_1 of ≥12% or ≥200 mL), blood eosinophilia, and/or atopy] were compared with those of 135 patients without asthma-like features [27]. Among 96 patients with asthma-like features, 57 (59.4%), 52 (54.2%), and 67 (69.8%) had reversibility, eosinophilia, and atopy, respectively, and 96 (100%), 31 (32.3%), and 6 (6.3%) patients had one, two, and three asthma-like features, respectively. The emphysema score that was visually evaluated on chest CT was not different between COPD with and without asthma-like features, regardless of the types and/or numbers of asthma-like features. The patients' characteristics, including age, body mass index, pack-years of smoking, and FEV_1%, were comparable between patients with and without asthma-like features. In a prospective multicenter study of COPD conducted in Canada (CanCOLD study) [28], patients with ACO were defined as having post-bronchodilator reversibility, atopy, and/or a physician diagnosis of asthma. Among patients with COPD, the visually evaluated emphysema score was not different between those with and without ACO. Although the patients with and without ACO had comparable characteristics, those without ACO had a trend toward older age, more pack-years of smoking, and a significantly higher FEV_1% than those with ACO.

There are some possible limitations that make it difficult to reach a consensus regarding the difference in emphysema between ACO and COPD. First, the definitions of ACO differed among studies. Because COPD is a heterogeneous disease characterized by airflow limitation due to several different mechanisms, the characteristics of ACO differ according to the criteria employed in each study. Second, the methods of evaluating emphysema differed among studies; some employed visual semiquantitative scales, and others used image analysis-based quantitative scales. Notably, the two above-mentioned studies that showed no difference in emphysema between ACO and COPD used visual semiquantitative scales, which may have affected the measurement accuracy of emphysema. Lung density-based assessment by image analysis software can also be used to evaluate visually undetectable LAA. Such LAA without visible emphysema may represent an abnormal enlargement of alveoli due to overinflation or pathological but visually undetectable parenchymal destruction (as a sort of "preclinical emphysema"). Third, the patients' demographics between ACO and COPD were unmatched. The extent of emphysema is associated with age, sex, pack-years of smoking, and severity of airflow limitation [4, 8, 12, 29, 30]. Therefore, the differences in patients' demographics should be considered when comparing emphysema between COPD and ACO.

An observational study of matched patients with ACO and COPD showed radiological differences in emphysema using image analysis software. In that study, patients' demographics between COPD and ACO (defined as patients with COPD with a history of variable respiratory symptoms and variable expiratory airflow limitation) were matched for age, sex, and pack-years of smoking by propensity score-matched analysis [31]. Furthermore, the extent of emphysema was quantitatively assessed using the %LAA by image analysis software. Patients with COPD who had a history of variable respiratory symptoms and variable expiratory airflow limitation were defined as having ACO. The study showed that the %LAA was significantly lower in patients with ACO than in matched patients with COPD despite the fact that both groups had comparable demographics (including tobacco exposure) and airflow limitation [31].

Interesting findings regarding emphysema in ACO have been revealed in genome-wide association studies from the COPDGene study [25]. In that study, the %LAA was significantly higher in patients with COPD than in those with ACO. Among several single-nucleotide polymorphisms (SNPs) reported to be associated with ACO, SNPs in the *CSMD1* gene were the most significant variant in non-Hispanic Whites. Notably, the *CSMD1* gene is reportedly associated with emphysema [32]. Although the precise mechanisms underlying the association between SNPs in the *CSMD1* gene and the development of emphysema are unknown, patients with ACO may have different genetic susceptibility for emphysema even under similar tobacco exposure.

3 Airway Disease

Airflow limitation resulting from airway disease is a common physiological mechanism in both COPD and asthma. However, the underlying pathogenesis of airway disease is different between them. Generally, patients with asthma have distinctive pathologic features of damaged epithelium, thickening of the basement membrane, and hypertrophy and hyperplasia of smooth muscle, dominantly in proximal airways [33–35]. Eosinophils, mast cells, and $CD4^{+}$ T cells are responsible for airway inflammation in asthma. In contrast, the pathologic features of COPD are squamous cell metaplasia, goblet cell hyperplasia, and mucus hypersecretion in distal airways accompanied by increased numbers of neutrophils, macrophages, and $CD8^+$ T cells.

These pathogenic features of airways in asthma and COPD are well known; however, they are not completely disease-specific, and there are some shared features between the two disease entities. For example, neutrophils are considered to be associated with severe asthma [36, 37]. Goblet cell hyperplasia and increased mucus secretion are observed even in mild-to-moderate asthma. Conversely, eosinophilic inflammation is sometimes observed during acute exacerbations of COPD [38].

Although the pathologic features of ACO have not been well described, it is assumable that the airways of patients with ACO have mixed features of both asthma and COPD because of the nature of shared pathological features in asthma and COPD. Imaging techniques cannot facilitate direct observation of those pathological changes, but they can reveal abnormal changes in the airways in asthma, COPD, and ACO.

3.1 Assessment of Airway Disease

Some studies have focused on the evaluation of airway disease using chest CT. Visually assessable airways in chest CT are the central airways of fifth- or sixth-generation bronchi at maximum [31, 39–41]. The main site of the airflow limitation is considered to be small airways (<2 mm in diameter), which are not directly assessable in CT imaging. However, the morphological features of central airways are reportedly associated with airflow limitation and are therefore considered to be a surrogate for the changes in small airways [9, 11, 40–42]. Like the assessments of emphysema, manual semiquantitative assessments of airway disease in chest CT images by physicians have been performed [6, 13]. Recent advances in computational techniques have resulted in the development of several automatic quantitative methods to evaluate central airways using image analysis software [9, 11, 18, 40–42]. Despite some differences in the algorithms for detecting airways, most methods evaluate the thickness and/or area of the airway wall and caliber, which reflects airway remodeling [43] (Fig. 10.2a). Furthermore, reconstruction of the airway using 3D-CT enables the evaluation of cross-sectional images of arbitrary levels of intricate networks of airways (Fig. 10.2b–d) [11, 40–42].

Indirect assessments of small airways have also been performed by measuring air trapping using chest CT. In patients with small airway disease, air trapping occurs during the expiratory phase, which results in decreased lung attenuation. Therefore, the decreased lung voxels in the expiratory phase or the ratio of the expiratory to inspiratory phase is considered a surrogate for small airway dysfunction [44–46].

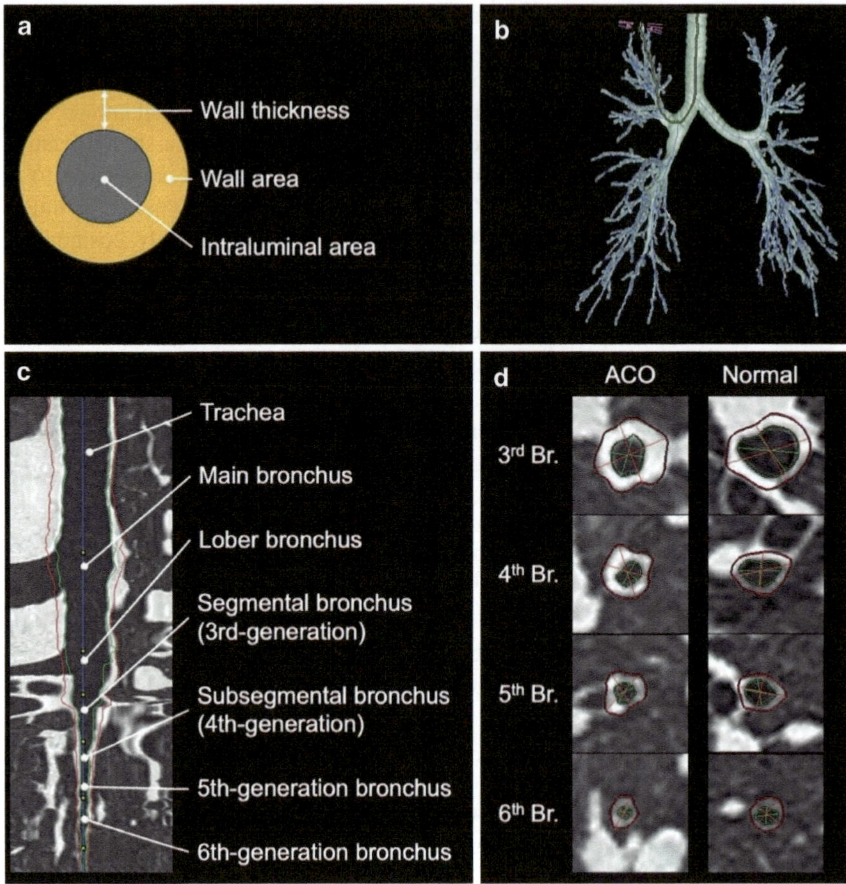

Fig. 10.2 Assessment of central airways. (**a**) Schema of evaluation of airway morphology. (**b**) Reconstructed image of airway tree. (**c**) Longitudinal section of reconstructed airway. (**d**) Representative cross-sectional images of airway from third- to sixth-generation bronchi in a patient with ACO and a normal subject. ACO, asthma–chronic obstructive pulmonary disease overlap

3.2 Airway Disease in COPD

In CT-based assessments of central airways, a decreased airway lumen area, increased airway wall thickness, and increased percentage wall area/total bronchial area in the central airways are associated with the disease severity and symptoms of COPD [6, 11, 13, 30, 40, 47–50]. The correlation between the morphological changes of airways and airflow limitation is strengthened when more peripheral airways are measured [11, 50]. Furthermore, the airway narrowing and/or airway wall thickening of the central airways reportedly improves after treatment with inhaled corticosteroids, beta-2 agonists, or anticholinergic agents, along with the improvement in airflow limitation [39, 40]. Pathologically, patients with COPD have an increased volume of tissue in the airway wall and accumulation of inflammatory mucous exudates in the airway lumen, which are associated with disease severity [22]. Although these pathological changes in small airways cannot be directly evaluated using chest CT, the morphological changes of central airways assessed by chest CT possibly reflect COPD-associated airway disease. Importantly, morphological changes in central airways are observed in smokers without COPD [51]. The thickness of the airway walls increases according to the amount of smoking and is associated with wheezing and dyspnea [5, 29].

3.3 Airway Disease in Asthma

Airway narrowing and airway wall thickening on chest CT are also observed in patients with asthma. The degree of the morphologic changes of the central airways is correlated with the disease duration, disease severity, airflow limitation, and symptoms [18, 24, 41, 52–60]. Furthermore, the airway narrowing and airway wall thickening of the central airways improves after effective inhaler treatment, along with improvements in airflow limitation and/or mucosal eosinophilic infiltration [61, 62]. The morphological changes of the central airway observed by chest CT are thought to reflect pathological findings of airway remodeling, such as basement membrane thickening and smooth muscle hypertrophy/hyperplasia [33, 63]. In fact, several studies have demonstrated correlations between CT-assessed wall thickening of the central airways with the pathological findings of epithelial thickening or reticular basement membrane thickening [56, 64, 65]. As in patients with COPD, CT-based assessment of the central airways has clinical utility for the evaluation of airway remodeling in patients with asthma.

The morphologic differences in the central airways between asthma and COPD are largely unknown. Shimizu et al. [66] compared the central airways using 3D-CT between patients with asthma and COPD. The airway luminal area in the third- to sixth-generation bronchi was significantly smaller in patients with asthma than in those with COPD. Hartley et al. [18] reported that patients with asthma who had a post-bronchodilator %FEV_1 of 50% to 80% had a significantly decreased airway luminal area and increased percent wall area than did patients with COPD who also had a %FEV_1 of 50–80%. These data support the widely accepted concept of the difference in disease sites between asthma (proximal airway-dominant disease) and COPD (peripheral airway-dominant disease) [33, 34]. However, the above-mentioned study also showed that when limited to patients with an %FEV_1 of <50%, there was no significant difference in the airway luminal area and percent wall area between the two diseases, suggesting that patients with severe COPD have proximal airway disease similar to patients with asthma [18].

The degree of airway remodeling is associated with several clinical factors including age, disease duration, and severity. Additionally, patients with asthma who have a history of smoking exhibit smoking-induced airway changes in addition to intrinsic airway changes due to asthma. Therefore, it is difficult to directly compare the differences between the two diseases with different patient demographics.

3.4 Airway Disease in ACO

It is natural to assume that the airways of patients with ACO have characteristics of the airways in both patients with asthma and those with COPD. However, the morphological features of airways in ACO are controversial.

Kitaguchi et al. [20] reported that patients with ACO demonstrated no significant difference in visually assessed bronchial wall thickening compared with patients with COPD. Lu et al. [26] compared the airways from the third- to sixth-generation bronchi in patients with COPD with and without ACO using 3D-CT analysis software. The two groups had no significant difference in the bronchial wall thickening or the airway luminal area. In both studies, the two groups were unmatched, and the differences were not adjusted by clinical factors. Because the degree of morphological changes in the airways is associated with age, the amount of smoking, and the severity of airflow limitation, the results of unadjusted and/or unmatched comparisons of ACO and COPD are difficult to interpret.

In the CanCOLD study, a significantly lower proportion of patients with ACO (especially those with a history of atopy) demonstrated a mild to severe bronchiolitis score compared with patients with COPD after adjusting for age, sex, race, and pack-years of smoking [28]. The limitation of the study was that the bronchiolitis score was visually and semiquantitatively assessed by radiologists [67]. In the COPDGene study, the square root of the wall area of a 10-mm luminal perimeter (Pi_{10}) and the percentage of the segmental and subsegmental wall area were quantified using image analysis software in patients with ACO. After adjustment for age, sex, pack-years of smoking, body mass index, and type of CT scanner, 450 patients with ACO had a significantly higher Pi_{10}, segmental wall area, and subsegmental wall area than 3120 patients with COPD who had comparable airflow limitation [25]. In a 3D-CT airway analysis, patients with ACO had significantly greater airway wall thickness in third- to fourth-generation bronchi and a smaller airway intraluminal area in fifth- to sixth-generation bronchi compared with propensity score-matched patients with COPD [31]. These data indicate that even when patients with ACO and COPD have comparable age, pack-years of smoking, and airflow limitation, those with ACO have greater morphological changes in the central airways.

Although controversy exists, it is reasonable to assume that patients with ACO have proximal airway-dominant changes similar to those of patients with asthma and therefore demonstrate greater morphological changes in the central airways than patients with COPD.

3.5 Small Airway Disease

In contrast to proximal airway-dominant disease in asthma, small airway disease is a hallmark of COPD [22, 33, 34, 68]. The CT-based assessment of air trapping is associated with airflow limitation of COPD [44]. Furthermore, one study showed that a small airway-dominant phenotype of COPD, as assessed by inspiratory and expiratory CT images, showed a greater association with FEV_1 decline than an emphysema-dominant phenotype [46]. CT-based assessment of small airway disease has the potential to provide information not only regarding the disease severity of COPD but also for differentiation between asthma and COPD. Research has shown that air trapping, measured by the lung density on expiratory and inspiratory chest CT images, is significantly greater in patients with COPD than in those with asthma [18, 69].

Given the presence of small airway disease in patients with COPD, it is assumed that patients with ACO also have small airway disease in addition to COPD. In fact, Hardin et al. [25] reported in the COPDGene study that there was no significant difference in gas trapping (defined as attenuation of less than −856 HU on expiratory CT images) between patients with ACO and COPD. Additionally, Lu et al. [26] reported that patients with ACO had small airway dysfunction (assessed by the expiration to inspiration rate of mean lung density) comparable with that in patients with COPD.

In contrast, Hwang et al. [70] reported a difference in the ventilation status between ACO and COPD using dual-energy CT with xenon ventilation imaging. Among three ventilation patterns, patients with COPD dominantly demonstrated the diffuse heterogeneous pattern (45.7%) and lobar/segmental/subsegmental defect pattern (43.5%), whereas patients with ACO demonstrated the peripheral wedge/diffuse defect pattern (66.7%). The latter pattern is frequently seen in patients with asthma, and the authors speculated that the characteristics of small airway disease in ACO may be similar to those of asthma [71, 72]. However, the remaining 33.3% of patients with ACO demonstrated a ventilation pattern similar to that of COPD. These data indicate that ACO is a heterogeneous disease entity and that the degree of overlap between the asthmatic and COPD-like components may differ among patients.

4 Distribution of ACO in Radiologic Phenotypes of COPD

Radiographic phenotypes of emphysema- and airway-dominant disease are well-known phenotypes of COPD. The two phenotypes have different demographics, airflow limitations, degrees of symptoms, comorbidities, and exacerbation frequencies [73]. Considering the above-described radiographic characteristics of ACO, it is assumed that a substantial proportion of patients with ACO have airway-dominant COPD.

In a prospective observational study of 189 patients with COPD conducted in Japan, the patients were categorized into 4 radiologic phenotypes according to the %LAA and percent wall area of the segmental bronchus: mild, airway-dominant, emphysema-dominant, and mixed [74]. In that study, 28% of patients with the airway-dominant phenotype had a history of asthma diagnosed before the age of 40 years, while 2%, 6%, and 14% of patients with the mild, emphysema-dominant, and mixed phenotypes, respectively, had such a history. Furthermore, when the criteria were applied in another prospective observational study of 93 patients with COPD conducted in Japan, patients with the airway-dominant phenotype had higher rates of a blood eosinophil count of ≥300/μL and a history of atopy [74]. We previously reported the radiographic phenotypes of COPD as determined by cluster analysis using 3D-CT data of the %LAA and airway intraluminal and wall area of the 3rd- to 6th-generation bronchi in 167 patients with COPD [75]. Four radiologic clusters were determined according to the radiologic features: Cluster I, mild emphysema with severe airway changes (severe airway-dominant phenotype); Cluster II, mild emphysema with moderate airway changes (moderate airway-dominant phenotype); Cluster III, severe emphysema with moderate airway changes (severe emphysema-dominant phenotype); and Cluster IV, moderate emphysema with mild airway changes (moderate emphysema-dominant phenotype). The severe airway-dominant phenotype had the highest exacerbation rate, and the severe emphysema-dominant phenotype was characterized by the most severe dyspnea. We employed a post-hoc analysis of the distribution of ACO among the four phenotypes (unpublished data). Patients with ACO were defined as having a history of variable respiratory symptoms and variable expiratory airflow limitation. The severe airway-dominant phenotype constituted the highest proportion of patients with ACO (53.3%), followed by the moderate airway-dominant phenotype (28.2%), the moderate emphysema-dominant phenotype (18.8%), and the severe emphysema-dominant phenotype (14.0%) (Fig. 10.3).

Although these data reveal an association between ACO and airway-dominant phenotypes in COPD, it should be emphasized that a certain proportion of patients with non-airway-dominant phenotypes also had characteristics associated with ACO. Radiographic findings may support the detection of ACO in patients with COPD; however, they should not be used to exclude ACO.

5 Conclusions

The three representative radiographic characteristics of ACO are less emphysema, greater airway wall thickening and airway luminal narrowing, and small airway disease comparable with that of COPD (Table 10.1). Physicians should consider the possibility of ACO in patients with COPD who have these radiologic characteristics. However, the absence of these radiographic features cannot be used to exclude ACO. Therefore, comprehensive assessments are important in the diagnosis of ACO.

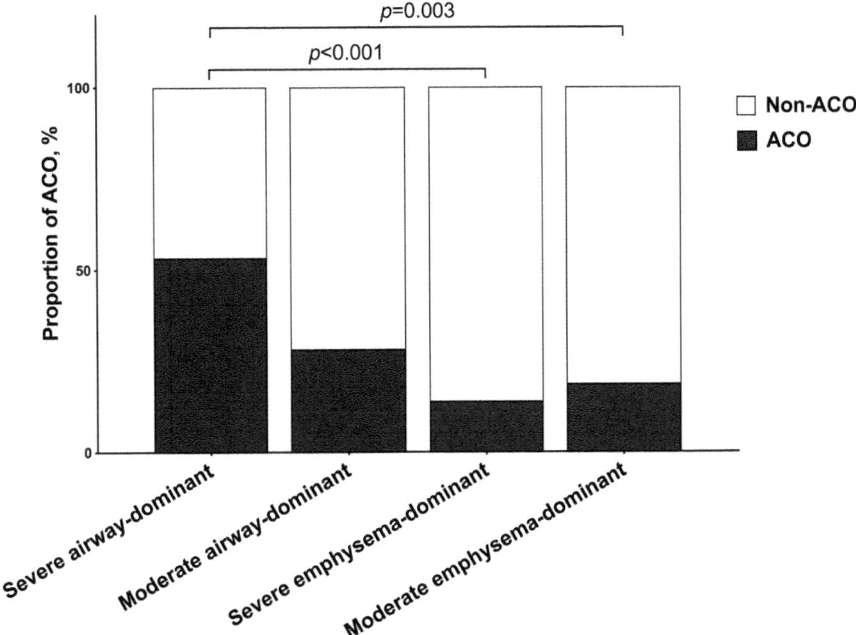

Fig. 10.3 Distributions of ACO in radiologic phenotypes of COPD. Four radiologic phenotypes of COPD were determined by cluster analysis using three-dimensional computed tomography data of the airways (post-hoc analysis of Reference [75]). *P*-values represent Fisher's exact test among the phenotypes. Gray and white bar indicates ACO and non-ACO, respectively. *COPD* Chronic obstructive pulmonary disease, ACO Asthma–chronic obstructive pulmonary disease overlap

Table 10.1 Radiologic characteristics of asthma, COPD, and ACO

Radiologic findings	Asthma	COPD	ACO
Emphysema	–	++	+
Central airway wall thickening	++	+	++
Central airway intraluminal area narrowing	++	+	++
Small airway disease	+	++	++

COPD Chronic obstructive pulmonary disease, *ACO* Asthma–chronic obstructive pulmonary disease overlap

References

1. Woodruff PG, van den Berge M, Boucher RC, Brightling C, Burchard EG, Christenson SA, Han MLK, Holtzman MJ, Kraft M, Lynch DA, Martinez FD, Reddel HK, Don and RAW. ATS/NHLBI Asthma–chronic obstructive pulmonary disease overlap workshop report. Am J Respir Crit Care Med. 2017;196:375–81.
2. Thurlbeck WM, Muller NL. Emphysema: definition, imaging, and quantification. Am J Roentgenol. 1994;163:1017–25.
3. Richard WW, Nester LM, Naidich PD, editors. Emphysema and chronic obstructive pulmonary disease. In: High-resolution CT lung. 5th ed. Wolters Kluwer Health: Philadelphia; 2015. p. 517–51.

4. Cerveri I, Dore R, Corsico A, Zoia MC, Pellegrino R, Brusasco V, Pozzi E. Assessment of emphysema in COPD: a functional and radiologic study. Chest. 2004;125:1714–8.
5. Grydeland TB, Dirksen A, Coxson HO, Eagan TML, Thorsen E, Pillai SG, Sharma S, Eide GE, Gulsvik A, Bakke PS. Quantitative computed tomography measures of emphysema and airway wall thickness are related to respiratory symptoms. Am J Respir Crit Care Med. 2010;181:353–9.
6. Aziz ZA, Wells AU, Desai SR, Ellis SM, Walker AE, MacDonald S, Hansell DM. Functional impairment in emphysema: contribution of airway abnormalities and distribution of parenchymal disease. Am J Roentgenol. 2005;185:1509–15.
7. Ostridge K, Gove K, Paas KHW, et al. Using novel computed tomography analysis to describe the contribution and distribution of emphysema and small airways disease in chronic obstructive pulmonary disease. Ann Am Thorac Soc. 2019;16:990–7.
8. Nakano Y, Muro S, Sakai H, et al. Computed tomographic measurements of airway dimensions and emphysema in smokers correlation with lung function. Am J Respir Crit Care Med. 2000;162:1102–8.
9. Schroeder JD, McKenzie AS, Zach JA, Wilson CG, Curran-Everett D, Stinson DS, Newell JD, Lynch DA. Relationships between airflow obstruction and quantitative CT measurements of emphysema, air trapping, and airways in subjects with and without chronic obstructive pulmonary disease. Am J Roentgenol. 2013;201:20894.
10. Diaz AA, Bartholmai B, San José Estépar R, Ross J, Matsuoka S, Yamashiro T, Hatabu H, Reilly JJ, Silverman EK, Washko GR. Relationship of emphysema and airway disease assessed by CT to exercise capacity in COPD. Respir Med. 2010;104:1145–51.
11. Karayama M, Inui N, Mori K, et al. Respiratory impedance is correlated with morphological changes in the lungs on three-dimensional CT in patients with COPD. Sci Rep. 2017;7:41709.
12. Pauls S, Gulkin D, Feuerlein S, Muche R, Krügger S, Schmidt SA, Dharaiya E, Brambs HJ, Hetzel M. Assessment of COPD severity by computed tomography: correlation with lung functional testing. Clin Imaging. 2010;34:172–8.
13. Nambu A, Zach J, Schroeder J, Jin G, Kim SS, Kim YIL, Schnell C, Bowler R, Lynch DA. Quantitative computed tomography measurements to evaluate airway disease in chronic obstructive pulmonary disease: relationship to physiological measurements, clinical index and visual assessment of airway disease. Eur J Radiol. 2016;85:2144–51.
14. Tuder RM, Petrache I. Pathogenesis of chronic obstructive pulmonary disease. J Clin Invest. 2012;122:2749–55.
15. Global Initiative for Chronic Obstructive Lung Disease Global strategy for the diagnosis, management, and prevention of chronic obstructive pulmonary disease: updated; 2016.
16. Goddard PR, Nicholson EM, Laszlo G, Watt I. Computed tomography in pulmonary emphysema. Clin Radiol. 1982;33:379–87.
17. Mohamed Hoesein FAA, Van Rikxoort E, Van Ginneken B, De Jong PA, Prokops M, Lammers JWJ, Zanen P. Computed tomography-quantified emphysema distribution is associated with lung function decline. Eur Respir J. 2012;40:844–50.
18. Hartley RA, Barker BL, Newby C, et al. Relationship between lung function and quantitative computed tomographic parameters of airway remodeling, air trapping, and emphysema in patients with asthma and chronic obstructive pulmonary disease: a single-center study. J Allergy Clin Immunol. 2016;137:1413–1422.e12.
19. Xie M, Wang W, Dou S, Cui L, Xiao W. Quantitative computed tomography measurements of emphysema for diagnosing asthma-chronic obstructive pulmonary disease overlap syndrome. Int J Chron Obstruct Pulmon Dis. 2016;11:953–61.
20. Kitaguchi Y. Comparison of pulmonary function in patients with COPD, asthma-COPD overlap syndrome, and asthma with airflow limitation. Int J COPD. 2016;11:991–7.
21. Kuwano K, Bosken CH, Pare PD, Bai TR, Wiggs BR, Hogg JC. Small airways dimensions in asthma and in chronic obstructive pulmonary disease. Am Rev Respir Dis. 1993;148:1220–5.
22. Hogg JC, Chu F, Utokaparch S, et al. The nature of small-airway obstruction in chronic obstructive pulmonary disease. N Engl J Med. 2004;350:2654–3.

23. Scichilone N, Battaglia S, Taormina S, Modica V, Pozzecco E, Bellia V. Alveolar nitric oxide and asthma control in mild untreated asthma. J Allergy Clin Immunol. 2013;131:1513–7.
24. Donohue KM, Hoffman EA, Baumhauer H, Guo J, Ahmed FS, Lovasi GS, Jacobs DR, Enright P, Barr RG. Asthma and lung structure on computed tomography: the Multi-Ethnic Study of Atherosclerosis Lung Study. J Allergy Clin Immunol. 2013;131:361–8.
25. Hardin M, Cho M, McDonald M-L, et al. The clinical and genetic features of COPD-asthma overlap syndrome. Eur Respir J. 2014;44:341–50.
26. Lu D, Chen L, Fan C, Zeng W, Fan H, Wu X, Yu H. The value of impulse oscillometric parameters and quantitative HRCT parameters in differentiating asthma–COPD overlap from COPD. Int J Chron Obstruct Pulmon Dis. 2021;16:2883–94.
27. Suzuki M, Makita H, Konno S, Shimizu K, Kimura H, Kimura H, Nishimura M. Asthma-like features and clinical course of chronic obstructive pulmonary disease: an analysis from the Hokkaido COPD cohort study. Am J Respir Crit Care Med. 2016;194:1358–65.
28. Barrecheguren M, Pinto L, Mostafavi-Pour-Manshadi SMY, et al. Identification and definition of asthma–COPD overlap: the CanCOLD study. Respirology. 2020;25:836–49.
29. Grydeland TB, Dirksen A, Coxson HO, Pillai SG, Sharma S, Eide GE, Gulsvik A, Bakke PS. Quantitative computed tomography: emphysema and airway wall thickness by sex, age and smoking. Eur Respir J. 2009;34:858–65.
30. Patel BD, Coxson HO, Pillai SG, et al. Airway wall thickening and emphysema show independent familial aggregation in chronic obstructive pulmonary disease. Am J Respir Crit Care Med. 2008;178:500–5.
31. Karayama M, Inui N, Yasui H, et al. Physiological and morphological differences of airways between COPD and asthma–COPD overlap. Sci Rep. 2019;9:1–8.
32. Kong X, Cho MH, Anderson W, et al. Genome-wide association study identifies BICD1 as a susceptibility gene for emphysema. Am J Respir Crit Care Med. 2011;183:43–9.
33. Sköld CM. Remodeling in asthma and COPD—Differences and similarities. Clin Respir J. 2010;4:20–7.
34. Sarkar S. Asthma and chronic obstructive pulmonary disease. J Assoc Chest Physicians. 2017;5:26–30.
35. Athanazio R. Airway disease: similarities and differences between asthma, COPD and bronchiectasis. Clinics. 2012;67:1335–43.
36. The ENFUMOSA Study. The ENFUMOSA cross-sectional European multicentre study of the clinical phenotype of chronic severe asthma. Eur Respir J. 2003;22:470–7.
37. Jeffery PK. Remodeling and inflammation of bronchi in asthma and chronic obstructive pulmonary disease. Proc Am Thorac Soc. 2004;1:176–83.
38. Brightling CE, Monteiro W, Ward R, Parker D, Morgan MDL, Wardlaw AJ, Pavord ID. Sputum eosinophilia and short-term response to prednisolone in chronic obstructive pulmonary disease: a randomised controlled trial. Lancet. 2000;356:1480–5.
39. Yasui H, Inui N, Furuhashi K, Nakamura Y, Uto T, Sato J, Yasuda K, Takehara Y, Suda T, Chida K. Multidetector-row computed tomography assessment of adding budesonide/formoterol to tiotropium in patients with chronic obstructive pulmonary disease. Pulm Pharmacol Ther. 2013;26:336–41.
40. Hasegawa M, Makita H, Nasuhara Y, Odajima N, Nagai K, Ito Y, Betsuyaku T, Nishimura M. Relationship between improved airflow limitation and changes in airway calibre induced by inhaled anticholinergic agents in COPD. Thorax. 2009;64:332–8.
41. Karayama M, Inui N, Mori K, et al. Respiratory impedance is correlated with airway narrowing in asthma using three-dimensional computed tomography. Clin Exp Allergy. 2018;48:278–87.
42. Nakano Y, Wong JC, De Jong PA, Buzatu L, Nagao T, Coxson HO, Elliott WM, Hogg JC, Paré PD. The prediction of small airway dimensions using computed tomography. Am J Respir Crit Care Med. 2005;171:142–6.
43. Richard WW, Nester ML, Naidich PD, editors. Airway diseases. In: High-resolution CT lung. 5th ed. Wolters Kluwer Health: Philadelphia, 2015. p. 552–621.

44. Matsuoka S, Kurihara Y, Yagihashi K, Hoshino M, Watanabe N, Nakajima Y. Quantitative assessment of air trapping in chronic obstructive pulmonary disease using inspiratory and expiratory volumetric MDCT. Am J Roentgenol. 2008;190:762–9.
45. Galbán CJ, Han MK, Boes JL, et al. Computed tomography-based biomarker provides unique signature for diagnosis of COPD phenotypes and disease progression. Nat Med. 2012;18:1711–5.
46. Bhatt SP, Soler X, Wang X, et al. Association between functional small airway disease and FEV1 decline in chronic obstructive pulmonary disease. Am J Respir Crit Care Med. 2016;194:178–84.
47. Matsuoka S, Kurihara Y, Yagihashi K, Hoshino M, Nakajima Y. Airway dimensions at inspiratory and expiratory multisection CT in chronic obstructive pulmonary disease: correlation with airflow limitation. Radiology. 2008;248:1042–9.
48. Ohara T, Hirai T, Sato S, Sato A, Nishioka M, Muro S, Mishima M. Comparison of airway dimensions in different anatomic locations on chest CT in patients with COPD. Respirology. 2006;11:579–85.
49. Yamashiro T, Matsuoka S, Estépar RSJ, et al. Quantitative assessment of bronchial wall attenuation with thin-section CT: an indicator of airflow limitation in chronic obstructive pulmonary disease. AJR Am J Roentgenol. 2010;195:363–9.
50. Hasegawa M, Nasuhara Y, Onodera Y, Makita H, Nagai K, Fuke S, Ito Y, Betsuyaku T, Nishimura M. Airflow limitation and airway dimensions in chronic obstructive pulmonary disease. Am J Respir Crit Care Med. 2006;173:1309–15.
51. Berger P, Perot V, Desbarats P, Tunon-de-Lara JM, Marthan R, Laurent F. Airway wall thickness in cigarette smokers: quantitative thin-section CT assessment. Radiology. 2005;235:1055–64.
52. Bumbacea D, Campbell D, Nguyen L, Carr D, Barnes PJ, Robinson D, Chung KF. Parameters associated with persistent airflow obstruction in chronic severe asthma. Eur Respir J. 2004;24:122–8.
53. Marchac V, Emond S, Mamou-Mani T, Le Bihan-Benjamin C, Le Bourgeois M, De Blic J, Scheinmann P, Brunelle F. Thoracic CT in pediatric patients with difficult-to-treat asthma. Am J Roentgenol. 2002;179:1245–52.
54. Siddiqui S, Gupta S, Cruse G, Haldar P, Entwisle J, Mcdonald S, Whithers PJ. Airway wall geometry in asthma and nonasthmatic eosinophilic bronchitis. Allergy. 2009;64:951–8.
55. Lee Y, Park J, Hwang J, Park S, Uh S, Kim Y, Park C. High-resolution CT findings in patients with near-fatal asthma: comparison of patients with mild-to-severe asthma and normal control subjects and changes. Chest. 2004;126:1840–8.
56. Aysola RS, Hoffman EA, Gierada D, et al. Airway remodeling measured by multidetector CT is increased in severe asthma and correlates with pathology. Chest. 2008;134:1183–91.
57. Kurashima K, Kanauchi T, Hoshi T, Takaku Y, Ishiguro T, Takayanagi N, Ubukata M, Sugita Y. Effect of early versus late intervention with inhaled corticosteroids on airway wall thickness in patients with asthma. Respirology. 2008;13:1008–13.
58. Awadh N, Müller NL, Park CS, Abboud RT, Fitzgerald JM. Airway wall thickness in patients with near fatal asthma and control groups: assessment with high resolution computed tomographic scanning; 1998. p. 248–253.
59. Hoshino M, Matsuoka S, Handa H, Miyazawa T, Yagihashi K. Correlation between airflow limitation and airway dimensions assessed by multidetector CT in asthma. Respir Med. 2010;104:1817–24.
60. Gupta S, Siddiqui S, Haldar P, Entwisle JJ, Mawby D, Wardlaw AJ, Bradding P, Pavord ID, Green RH, Brightling CE. Quantitative analysis of high-resolution computed tomography scans in severe asthma subphenotypes. Thorax. 2010;65:775–81.
61. Capraz F, Kunter E, Cermik H, Ilvan A, Pocan S. The effect of inhaled budesonide and formoterol on bronchial remodeling and HRCT features in young asthmatics. Lung. 2007;185:89–96.
62. Niimi A, Matsumoto H, Amitani R, et al. Effect of short-term treatment with inhaled corticosteroid on airway wall thickening in asthma. Am J Med. 2004;116:725–31.

63. Carroll N, Elliot J, Morton A, James A. The structure of large and small airways in nonfatal and fatal asthma. Am Rev Respir Dis. 1993;147:405–10.
64. Kasahara K, Shiba K, Ozawa T, Okuda K, Adachi M. Correlation between the bronchial subepithelial layer and whole airway wall thickness in patients with asthma. Thorax. 2002;57:242–6.
65. de Blic J, Tillie-Leblond I, Emond S, Mahut B, Duy TLD, Scheinmann P. High-resolution computed tomography scan and airway remodeling in children with severe asthma. J Allergy Clin Immunol. 2005;116:750–4.
66. Shimizu K, Hasegawa M, Makita H, Nasuhara Y, Konno S, Nishimura M. Comparison of airway remodelling assessed by computed tomography in asthma and COPD. Respir Med. 2011;105:1275–83.
67. Tan WC, Hague CJ, Leipsic J, et al. Findings on thoracic computed tomography scans and respiratory outcomes in persons with and without chronic obstructive pulmonary disease: a population-based cohort study. PLoS One. 2016;11:1–14.
68. McDonough JE, Yuan R, Suzuki M, et al. Small-airway obstruction and emphysema in chronic obstructive pulmonary disease. N Engl J Med. 2011;365:1567–75.
69. Choi S, Haghighi B, Choi J, et al. Differentiation of quantitative CT imaging phenotypes in asthma versus COPD. BMJ Open Respir Res. 2017;4:1–8.
70. Hwang HJ, Lee SM, Seo JB, Lee JS, Kim N, Lee SW, Oh YM. Visual and quantitative assessments of regional xenonventilation using dual-energy CT in asthma-chronic obstructive pulmonary disease overlap syndrome: a comparison with chronic obstructive pulmonary disease. Korean J Radiol. 2020;21:1104–13.
71. Chae EJ, Seo JB, Lee J, Kim N, Goo HW, Lee HJ, Lee CW, Ra SW, Oh YM, Cho YS. Xenon ventilation imaging using dual-energy computed tomography in asthmatics: initial experience. Investig Radiol. 2010;45:354–61.
72. Altes TA, Powers PL, Knight-Scott J, Rakes G, Platts-Mills TAE, De Lange EE, Alford BA, Mugler JP, Brookeman JR. Hyperpolarized 3He MR lung ventilation imaging in asthmatics: preliminary findings. J Magn Reson Imaging. 2001;13:378–84.
73. Han MK, Kazerooni EA, Lynch DA, et al. Chronic obstructive pulmonary disease exacerbations in the COPDGene study: associated radiologic phenotypes. Radiology. 2011;261:274–82.
74. Tanabe N, Shimizu K, Terada K, et al. Central airway and peripheral lung structures in airway disease-dominant COPD. ERJ Open Res. 2021; https://doi.org/10.1183/23120541.00672-2020.
75. Karayama M, Inui N, Yasui H, et al. Clinical features of three-dimensional computed tomography-based radiologic phenotypes of chronic obstructive pulmonary disease. Int J COPD. 2019;14:1333–42.

Chapter 11
Pulmonary Function of ACO: What Is the Role of the Forced Oscillation Technique?

Toshihiro Shirai

Abstract ACO patients had an intermediate degree of airflow obstruction, as measured by spirometry, between asthma and COPD patients, although it depended on the studied population. Reversible airflow limitation was more common in ACO patients than in COPD patients. ACO patients had more severe airway obstruction measured by the forced oscillation technique (FOT), expiratory flow limitation, and emphysema than asthma patients. Although the difference between ACO and COPD patients was modest, recursive partitioning analysis revealed that the combined assessment of respiratory system resistance (Rrs) and respiratory system reactance (Xrs) enabled the differentiation between ACO and asthma or COPD with high specificity. Colored 3-dimensional images of ACO patients showed an intermediate pattern between asthma and COPD patients. The annual changes in FOT parameters, especially Xrs, correlated with the annual changes in FEV1 in asthma, ACO, and COPD patients. Reversible airflow limitation measured by spirometry was predicted by the FOT in asthma and ACO patients but not in COPD patients. Most FOT parameters changed in linkage with spirometry after treatment. Although the interpretation of the FOT parameters, especially the difference between Rrs at 5 Hz and 20 Hz (R5−R20), is controversial, there is a trend toward using R5−R20 and Xrs as small airway dysfunction.

Keywords Forced oscillation technique · Recursive partitioning analysis · Respiratory system reactance · Respiratory system resistance · Small airway dysfunction

---

T. Shirai (✉)
Department of Respiratory Medicine, Shizuoka General Hospital, Shizuoka, Japan
e-mail: toshihiro-shirai@i.shizuoka-pho.jp

H. Nagase et al. (eds.), *Asthma-COPD Overlap*, Respiratory Disease Series: Diagnostic Tools and Disease Managements,
https://doi.org/10.1007/978-981-96-0217-9_11

1 Introduction

The forced oscillation technique (FOT) is used worldwide for physiological research and the management of obstructive lung diseases, including asthma and chronic obstructive pulmonary disease (COPD) [1]. In Japan, MostGraph (Chest M.I. Co. Ltd., Tokyo, Japan) and Impulse Oscillometry (IOS) (MasterScreen IOS; Jaeger, Hoechberg, Germany) have been commercially available for more than a decade, and more than 500 units of MostGraph and approximately 100 units of IOS are used now. Recently, the European Respiratory Society task force of international experts published the technical standards of the FOT and advocated using the term 'oscillometry' [2]. In the past, the interpretation of the difference between respiratory system resistance (Rrs) at 5 Hz and 20 Hz (R5−R20), a marker of frequency dependence, has been controversial, whether it may reflect peripheral airway resistance. In this regard, recent studies indicated that R5−R20 and respiratory system reactance (Xrs), including Xrs at 5 Hz (X5), resonant frequency (Fres), and low-frequency reactance area (ALX), are markers of small airways dysfunction [3, 4]. The usefulness of the FOT in managing asthma and COPD is currently established. However, there are limited reports concerning the FOT in ACO [5–8]. In this chapter, the author describes the pulmonary function of ACO, especially the role of the FOT in the diagnosis and management of ACO.

2 Spirometry in ACO

Although the Global Initiative for Chronic Obstructive Lung Disease (GOLD) stated in the preface in 2020 that they no longer refer to ACO [9], the Global Initiative for Asthma (GINA) devotes a whole chapter of the report to ACO [10]. Table 11.1 shows the spirometric measures in asthma, ACO, and COPD with modifications. ACO patients have reduced post-bronchodilator (BD) forced expiratory volume in 1 second (FEV1)/forced vital capacity (FVC) <0.7 and higher or lower post-BD FEV1. If post-BD FEV1 values are ≥80% predicted, patients have mild persistent airflow limitation. If post-BD FEV1 values are <80% predicted, patients have risk factors for exacerbations or mortality. Reversible airflow limitation (Post-BD increase in FEV1 ≥12% and 200 mL from baseline) is common and more likely when FEV1 is low.

2.1 Comparison of Spirometry Between Asthma, ACO, and COPD

Our previous report compared the spirometry between asthma, ACO, and COPD patients (Table 11.2) [5]. The study subjects included 344 adult patients who visited outpatient clinics at Shizuoka General Hospital or Nihon University Itabashi

Table 11.1 Spirometry in asthma, ACO, and COPD described in Global Initiative for Asthma 2021 with modifications

Spirometric variable	Asthma	ACO	COPD
Normal FEV1/FVC pre- or post-BD	Compatible with asthma	Not compatible	Not compatible with COPD
Reduced post-BD FEV1/FVC (<0.7)	Indicates airflow limitation but may improve spontaneously or on treatment	Required for diagnosis of ACO	Required for diagnosis of COPD
Post-BD FEV1 ≥80% predicted	Compatible with diagnosis of asthma (good asthma control or interval between symptoms)	Compatible with mild persistent airflow limitation if post-BD FEV1/FVC is reduced	Compatible with mild persistent airflow limitation if post-BD FEV1/FVC is reduced
Post-BD FEV1 <80% predicted	Compatible with diagnosis of asthma. Risk factor for asthma exacerbations	As for asthma and COPD	An indicator of severity of airflow limitation and risk of future events (e.g. mortality and COPD exacerbations)
Post-BD increase in FEV1 ≥12% and 200 mL from baseline (reversible airflow limitation)	Usual at some time in course of asthma, but may not be present when well-controlled or on controller therapy	Common and more likely when FEV1 is low	Common and more likely when FEV1 is low

BD Bronchodilator, *FEV1* Forced expiratory volume in 1 second, *FVC* Forced vital capacity

Hospital for routine check-ups between February 2013 and August 2016 (ASCOPE cohort). The participants were classified into three groups: asthma (n = 170), COPD (n = 60), and ACO (n = 114). Asthma and COPD patients fulfilled the definition of the GINA [10] and the GOLD [9] reports, respectively. ACO was diagnosed if asthma patients were older than 40 years old, had post-BD FEV1/FVC <0.7, and fulfilled at least one of the following criteria, including more than 10 pack-years smoking history, less than 80% of diffusing capacity of the lung for carbon monoxide/alveolar volume, or a presence of low attenuation area (LAA) on high-resolution computed tomography (HRCT). In addition, ACO was diagnosed if COPD patients fulfilled at least two of the following criteria, including a history of asthma, blood eosinophil count ≥250 cells/μL, fractional exhaled nitric oxide (FeNO) >35 ppb, or serum total IgE >100 IU/mL [11].

The ACO patients were older and male-dominant and had more pack-years, lower FEV1, FEV1/FVC, and forced expiratory flow at 25–75% of FVC (FEF25-75) than the asthma patients. In addition, the ACO patients were younger and had a higher body mass index, FEV1, FEV1/FVC, and FEF25-75 than the COPD patients. These findings indicate that ACO patients had intermediate airflow obstruction between asthma and COPD patients, although it depends on the studied population.

Table 11.2 Spirometry and the FOT in asthma, ACO, and COPD patients in the ASCOPE cohort

	Asthma ($N = 170$)		ACO ($N = 114$)		COPD ($N = 60$)		Overall P-value	Asthma vs. ACO	Asthma vs. COPD	ACO vs. COPD
Age (years)	58	(42, 70)	69	(61, 75)	74	(69, 78)	<0.001	<0.001	<0.001	<0.001
Gender (male/female)	51/119		89/25		48/12		<0.001	<0.001	<0.001	0.847
Body mass index (kg/m^2)	23.1	(20.6, 25.8)	22.5	(20.9, 24.7)	21.4	(18.7, 23.3)	<0.001	0.308	<0.001	0.001
Pack-years	0	(0, 1)	30	(12, 48)	44	(26, 68)	<0.001	<0.001	<0.001	0.002
FEV_1 (L)	2.12	(1.63, 2.79)	1.69	(1.28, 2.23)	1.46	(1.07, 1.90)	<0.001	<0.001	<0.001	0.039
FEV1 (% predicted)	89.4	(77.0, 101.7)	66.6	(49.0, 81.1)	65.1	(46.6, 82.9)	<0.001	<0.001	<0.001	0.412
FVC (L)	2.79	(2.42, 3.55)	3.08	(2.49, 3.86)	2.98	(2.38, 3.69)	0.287	0.129	0.890	0.283
FVC (% predicted)	97.6	(85.9, 106.6)	93.3	(77.0, 106.0)	93.1	(80.1, 109.7)	0.199	0.075	0.363	0.722
FEV1/FVC (%)	73.8	(67.8, 79.7)	58.9	(45.9, 65.6)	50.8	(43.2, 59.1)	<0.001	<0.001	<0.001	0.004
FEF_{25-75}	1.53	(0.99, 2.09)	0.73	(0.41, 1.01)	0.46	(0.30, 0.77)	<0.001	<0.001	<0.001	0.031
$\%FEF_{25-75}$	52.3	(38.1, 63.5)	24.2	(14.4, 34.7)	17.6	(10.5, 29.5)	<0.001	<0.001	<0.001	0.076
R5 ($cmH_2O/L/s$)	3.58	(2.87, 4.34)	3.56	(2.92, 4.47)	3.30	(2.62, 4.03)	0.372	0.676	0.253	0.169
R20 ($cmH_2O/L/s$)	2.98	(2.43, 3.49)	2.83	(2.25, 3.37)	2.54	(1.97, 3.07)	0.011	0.292	0.003	0.043
R5−R20 ($cmH_2O/L/s$)	0.60	(0.30, 1.00)	0.81	(0.48, 1.12)	0.81	(0.53, 1.08)	0.008	0.008	0.017	0.789

R5–R20 >0.07 kPa/L/s (0.714 $cmH_2O/L/s$)	70	(41)	62	(54)	35	(58)	0.023	0.030	0.024	0.634
X5 ($cmH_2O/L/s$)	−0.63	(−1.30, −0.33)	−1.06	(−1.85, −0.39)	−1.04	(−2.45, −0.61)	0.001	0.008	<0.001	0.273
ΔX5	0.04	(−0.13, 0.30)	0.30	(−0.04, 1.02)	0.45	(0.08, 1.00)	<0.001	<0.001	<0.001	0.259
Fres (Hz)	8.50	(6.93, 12.96)	11.93	(7.42, 15.44)	12.72	(8.69, 17.4)	<0.001	<0.001	<0.001	0.097
ALX ($cmH_2O/L/s$ x Hz)	2.40	(1.07, 6.59)	5.35	(1.37, 12.13)	5.50	(2.22, 17.33)	<0.001	0.003	<0.001	0.217

Data are shown as median (interquartile range) or frequency (percentage). *ALX* Low-frequency reactance area, *Δ* the difference between the inspiratory and expiratory phases, *FEF25-75* Forced expiratory flow at 25–75% of FVC, *FEV1* Forced expiratory volume in 1 second;, *FOT* Forced oscillation technique, *Fres* Resonant frequency, *Rrs* Respiratory system resistance, *R5 and R20* Rrs at 5 Hz and 20 Hz, respectively, *R5-R20* The difference between R5 and R20, *X5* Xrs at 5 Hz, *Xrs* Respiratory system reactance

2.2 Reversible Airflow Limitation in Asthma, ACO, and COPD

We found reversible airflow limitation in 14% (30/209), 22% (13/59), and 6% (9/152) of asthma, ACO, and COPD patients, respectively, in a retrospective study [12]. In a previous study by Kitaguchi et al., the increase in FEV1 in response to short-acting β2-agonists was significantly greater in 32 ACO patients than in 118 COPD patients (229 ± 29 mL vs. 72 ± 10 mL) [7].

3 The FOT in ACO

The FOT measures Rrs and Xrs during tidal breathing and provides information that cannot be obtained by spirometry [1]. If reference values and proper interpretation of the measured data are established, this technique will be useful in older patients who experience difficulty performing spirometry and young children who cannot cooperate with the maneuver.

For the ASCOPE mentioned above study [5], we hypothesized that FOT could differentiate ACO from asthma and COPD and assessed the usefulness of FOT for diagnosing ACO in a cross-sectional design.

3.1 Comparison of the FOT Between Asthma, ACO, and COPD

As shown in Table 11.2, we found that the ACO patients had lower X5 and higher R5–R20, the difference between inspiratory and expiratory phases of X5 (ΔX5), Fres, and ALX than the asthma patients. In addition, the ACO patients had higher R20 than the COPD patients [5]. In general, Rrs and Xrs indices are markers of airflow obstruction and correlate weakly or moderately with FEV1 and FEV1/FVC in both asthma and COPD [13]. ΔX5 is a marker of expiratory flow limitation (EFL), a major determinant of dynamic hyperinflation and exercise limitation, and is common in severe COPD patients [14]. The predictors of higher ΔX5 included higher R5, degree of emphysema, functional residual capacity, and lower FEF25-75. A previous study using 3-dimensional (3D)-HRCT analyses revealed correlations between Xrs parameters and LAA in COPD patients [15]. Taken together, these results suggest that ACO patients had more severe airway obstruction during tidal breathing, EFL, and emphysema than asthma patients. However, the difference between ACO and COPD patients was modest. In this regard, Kitaguchi et al. found no difference in Rrs or Xrs between ACO and COPD patients [7]. As stated earlier, spirometry revealed that ACO patients had an intermediate degree of airflow obstruction between asthma and COPD patients. Isn't the FOT helpful for differentiating between ACO and COPD because both disorders have EFL and emphysema to varying degrees? Then, we performed a recursive partitioning analysis to assess the usefulness of FOT for diagnosing ACO.

3.2 *Recursive Partitioning Analysis to Differentiate ACO from Asthma and COPD*

Recursive partitioning analysis to create a classification tree revealed that ΔX5, R20, ALX, and Fres were the significant parameters (Fig. 11.1). Classes 3 and 4 consisted predominantly of ACO patients. The accuracy of ACO diagnosis (class 3 and class 4) was as follows: diagnostic odds ratio, 3.47 (95% confidence interval, 1.98–6.09); sensitivity, 32%; and specificity, 88%.

We previously reported that ΔX5 was useful for differentiating COPD and asthma [13]. As stated earlier, a significantly higher value of ΔX5 in ACO and COPD patients suggests the presence of EFL compared to asthma patients (Table 11.2). ACO patients showed an intermediate value of R20 between asthma and COPD patients. A previous study found that R20 had clinical significance,

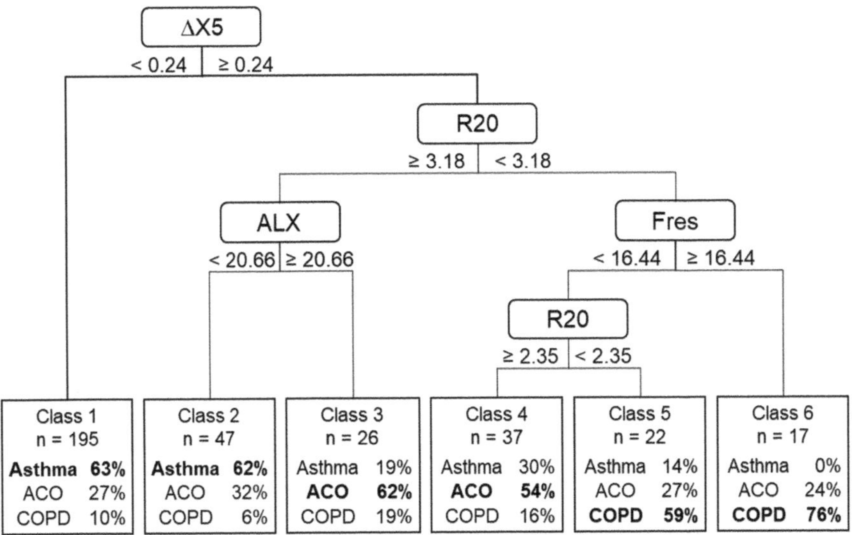

Fig. 11.1 Recursive partitioning analysis using FOT data to classify patients into asthma, ACO, or COPD. (Reproduced from reference 5). Rounded squares and squares represent the internal and terminal nodes, respectively. Values represent the number of patients with asthma, ACO, or COPD and the percentage in each node. Abbreviations: *ACO* Asthma-COPD overlap, *ALX* Low-frequency reactance area, *COPD* Chronic obstructive pulmonary disease, *ΔX5* The difference between inspiratory and expiratory phases of respiratory system reactance at 5 Hz, *Fres* Resonant frequency, *Rrs* Respiratory system resistance, *R20* Rrs at 20 Hz

including severity, impaired control, quality of life, and frequent asthma exacerbation [16]. R20 seems to reflect the characteristics of asthma rather than those of COPD. Previous studies indicated that Xrs values, including X5, Fres, and ALX, were higher in COPD patients than in asthma patients [1, 13]. Comparable levels of X5, Fres, and ALX between ACO and COPD patients, but higher than in asthma patients, suggest the presence of COPD components in ACO patients. Overall, the combined assessment of Rs and Xrs led to ACO identification with high specificity despite low sensitivity. The diagnostic accuracy of this study was comparable to that of the combined assessment of serum periostin and YKL-40 (both high levels): diagnostic odds ratio, 2.59 (95% confidence interval, 1.58–4.25); sensitivity, 38%; and specificity, 81% [11].

3.3 Colored 3D Images of Rrs and Xrs in Asthma, ACO, and COPD

MostGraph software visualizes the time course and the absolute values in colored 3D graphics; this approach is suitable for medical staff members and patients to understand various respiratory conditions, such as bronchoconstriction in asthma and COPD or the effects of treatment [17]. Based on the values of recursive partitioning analysis, typical colored 3D images of Rrs and Xrs for each representative patient are shown in Fig. 11.2. ACO patients generally showed an intermediate pattern between asthma and COPD patients.

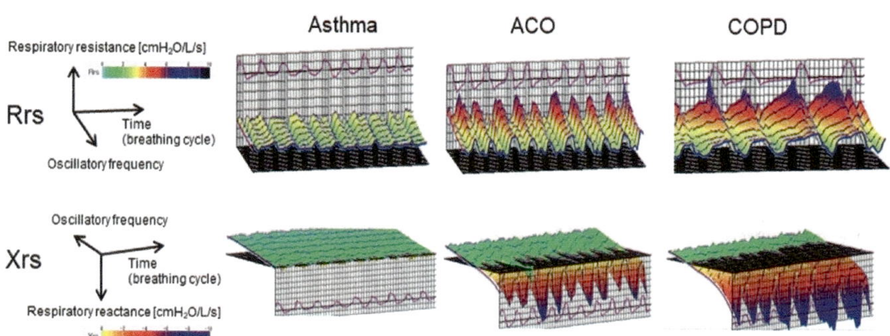

Fig. 11.2 Typical colored 3-dimensional images of Rrs and Xrs in each representative patient. ACO patients generally showed an intermediate pattern between asthma and COPD patients. (Reproduced from reference 5). Abbreviations: *ACO* Asthma-COPD overlap, *COPD* Chronic obstructive pulmonary disease, *Rrs* Respiratory system resistance, *Xrs* Respiratory system reactance

3.4 Annual Changes in FOT Parameters and Spirometry in Asthma, ACO, and COPD

Previous studies focused on the difference in annual FOT parameters and spirometry changes in asthma and COPD patients [18, 19]. Subsequently, we investigated the relationship between the annual changes in FOT parameters and FEV1 in ACO, asthma, and COPD patients [6]. This study is meaningful since spirometry, which requires forced expiration, burdens the patient in the advanced stages of each disease. Subjects included 75 adult patients with asthma ($n = 23$), ACO ($n = 29$), and COPD ($n = 23$). In this study, we made two important clinical observations. First, the annual changes in FOT parameters correlated with the annual changes in FEV1 in asthma, ACO, and COPD patients. Further, the annual changes in FEV1 exhibited a higher correlation with Xrs parameters than with Rrs parameters. Second, rapid declines in FEV1 (>30 mL/year) could be predicted by the annual changes in FOT parameters in asthma, ACO, and COPD patients.

3.5 The FOT as a Predictor of Reversible Airflow Limitation in Asthma, ACO, and COPD

In the retrospective study described earlier [12], we investigated whether the FOT would predict reversible airflow limitation measured by spirometry. Again, reversible airflow limitation was found in 14% (30/209), 22% (13/59), and 6% (9/152) of asthma, ACO, and COPD patients, respectively. The strongest Pearson's correlation was found between the change of Fres and that of FEV1 (absolute change: $r = -0.490, -0.505$; percentage change: $r = -0.572, -0.384$) in asthma and ACO patients, respectively. No correlation was observed in COPD patients. In univariate regression analysis, the changes of Fres corresponding to an increase in $FEV_1 \geq 12\%$ and 200 ml were 2.0 Hz and 13.5% for asthma and 4.2 Hz and 18.0% for ACO, respectively. In predicting reversible airflow limitation using Fres, sensitivity and specificity were 53.3% and 81.0% in asthma and 38.4% and 80.4% in ACO, respectively. Thus, the FOT helps predict reversible airflow limitation in asthma and ACO with high specificity. A strong correlation between Fres and FEV1 has been reported so far [13, 20, 21]. Interestingly, a previous study found a hyperbolic relationship between Fres and FEV1 and a linear relationship between a reciprocal Fres and FEV1 in airway reversibility tests [21].

3.6 Changes in the FOT Parameters After Treatment in Asthma, ACO, and COPD

The ability of FOT parameters to predict an improvement in FEV1 after inhaled corticosteroid (ICS)/long-acting β2-agonist (LABA) combination treatment was investigated in 31 untreated asthma patients [22]. In multivariate logistic regression analyses, >10% change in FEV1 was independently predicted by R5 (adjusted odds ratio 15.9). The ROC curve analyses also revealed that the area under the curve was higher for R5 (0.731) than for any other parameters.

The ability of FOT parameters to predict the COPD Assessment Test (CAT) score improvement (CAT score ≥2) after long-acting muscarinic antagonist (LAMA) or LAMA/LABA treatment was investigated in 65 untreated COPD patients [23]. Recursive partitioning analysis identified 3 improved classes, defined by R20, X5, and ΔX5, but not by spirometry. The accuracy of predicting CAT improvement was as follows: odds ratio, 25.3; 95% confidence interval, 6.1 to 104.1; sensitivity, 91.2%; specificity, 71.0%; positive likelihood ratio, 3.14; and negative likelihood ratio, 0.12. Thus, the FOT helps predict improved health status in untreated COPD patients.

Only a few reports assessed the changes in FOT parameters after treatment in ACO patients. A recent randomized, open-label, cross-over pilot study was conducted in 17 ACO patients to evaluate the effect of LAMA added-on to ICS/LABA [8]. After 4 weeks of triple therapy, FVC, FEV1, R5, R5−R20, X5, Fres, and ALX significantly improved. However, there was no improvement in R20, FeNO, CAT, or Asthma Control Test scores. R20 may be a less sensitive parameter to the improvement in ACO.

4 SAD in Asthma, ACO, and COPD

4.1 Interpretation of R5−R20

Among the FOT parameters, the interpretation of R5−R20 has been controversial. Basically, R5−R20 should be interpreted as a marker of frequency dependence of the FOT [24, 25]. Frequency dependence of Rrs means that Rrs is increased at the lower frequencies and decreased at higher frequencies, which is explained based on mechanical inhomogeneities of the lungs [24]. However, several researchers interpret R5−R20 as an indicator of peripheral airway resistance because they consider R5 and R20 to reflect the total and central airway resistance, respectively, in asthma [26, 27]. The IOS system adopts this interpretation. This hypothesis was based on experimental findings in animals that low oscillation frequencies (<15 Hz) were transmitted more distally in the lungs. In comparison, high oscillation frequencies (>20 Hz) were damped out in intermediate-sized airways [28]. Physiologically, high R5−R20 values are detected in children mainly due to upper airway mechanics [29] and clinically found in patients with tracheobronchial central airway obstruction, including malignant or benign diseases [30]. Thus, R5−R20 is not a specific parameter for peripheral airway resistance.

4.2 The FOT as SAD Parameters

However, a recent study demonstrated using computational modeling that R5 − R20 is a direct measure of anatomical narrowing in the small airways and that small airway narrowing has a marked impact on asthma control and quality of life [3]. In a recent large cohort asthma study to explore the relevance and extent of SAD (ATLANTIS), consisting of 773 asthma patients and 99 controls, the researchers focused on the spirometric indices, including FVC and FEF25-75, and the FOT parameters, including R5−R20 and Xrs [4]. Thus, there is a trend toward using R5−R20 and Xrs as SAD parameters, although still controversial. Some researchers advocated the cutoff value of 0.07 kPa/L/s (0.714 $cmH_2O/L/s$) for the presence of SAD [31]. Based on such interpretation, FEF25–75 in ACO patients was lower than in asthma patients but higher than in COPD patients (Table 11.2). R5−R20 and Xrs values were lower in ACO and COPD patients than in asthma patients. However, there was no difference between ACO and COPD patients.

4.3 Mucus Plugs and SAD in Asthma, ACO, and COPD

We evaluated the relationship between mucus plugs and pulmonary function in 49 asthma, 40 ACO, and 41 COPD patients and investigated the relevance to SAD and type 2 inflammation in a retrospective study [32]. Mucus plugs were detected on HRCT images in 29 (59%) asthma, 25 (65%) ACO, and 17 (41%) COPD patients, respectively. Patients with mucus plugs had reduced spirometry and larger FOT parameters, especially in COPD patients. Mucus scores correlated positively with IgE in ACO and FeNO in asthma patients but not in COPD patients. Multivariate logistic regression analysis revealed that SAD parameters, including FVC and Fres, were significantly associated with mucus plugs in the whole studied population. Thus, SAD was associated with mucus plugs in asthma, ACO, and COPD patients rather than large airway dysfunction.

5 Conclusion

The FOT assesses airway obstruction in ACO, asthma, and COPD. The FOT also reflects EFL and emphysema, the characteristics of COPD, causing some difficulty in the discrimination between ACO and COPD. However, since degrees of these characteristics are less severe in most ACO patients, combining the FOT parameters differentiates ACO from COPD with high specificity. Reversible airflow limitation, annual changes, and treatment effects measured by spirometry are predictable using the FOT in ACO as well as asthma and COPD. There is a trend toward using the FOT as SAD parameters in asthma, ACO, and COPD.

References

1. Shirai T, Kurosawa H. Clinical application of the forced oscillation technique. Intern Med. 2016;55(6):559–66. https://doi.org/10.2169/internalmedicine.55.5876.
2. King GG, Bates J, Berger KI, Calverley P, de Melo PL, Dellacà RL, et al. Technical standards for respiratory oscillometry. Eur Respir J. 2020;55:1900753. https://doi.org/10.1183/13993003.00753-2019.
3. Foy BH, Soares M, Bordas R, Richardson M, Bell A, Singapuri A, et al. Lung computational models and the role of the small airways in asthma. Am J Respir Crit Care Med. 2019;200:982–91. https://doi.org/10.1164/rccm.201812-2322OC.
4. Postma DS, Brightling C, Baldi S, Van den Berge M, Fabbri LM, Gagnatelli A, et al. Exploring the relevance and extent of small airways dysfunction in asthma (ATLANTIS): baseline data from a prospective cohort study. Lancet Respir Med. 2019;7:402–16. https://doi.org/10.1016/S2213-2600(19)30049-9.
5. Shirai T, Hirai K, Gon Y, Maruoka S, Mizumura K, Hikichi M, et al. Forced oscillation technique may identify asthma-COPD overlap. Allergol Int. 2019;68:385–7. https://doi.org/10.1016/j.alit.2019.01.002.
6. Tanaka Y, Hirai K, Nakayasu H, Tamura K, Masuda T, Takahashi S, et al. Annual changes in forced oscillation technique parameters correlate with FEV1 decline in patients with asthma, COPD, and asthma-COPD overlap. Allergol Int. 2020;69:626–7. https://doi.org/10.1016/j.alit.2020.03.013.
7. Kitaguchi Y, Yasuo M, Hanaoka M. Comparison of pulmonary function in patients with COPD, asthma-COPD overlap syndrome, and asthma with airflow limitation. Int J Chron Obstruct Pulmon Dis. 2016;11:991–7. https://doi.org/10.2147/COPD.S105988.
8. Ishiura Y, Fujimura M, Ohkura N, Hara J, Kasahara K, Ishii N, et al. Effect of triple therapy in patients with asthma-COPD overlap. Int J Clin Pharmacol Ther. 2019;57:384–92. https://doi.org/10.5414/CP203382.
9. Global Initiative for Chronic Obstructive Lung Disease. Global strategy for the diagnosis, management, and prevention of chronic obstructive pulmonary disease; 2020. Available from: https://goldcopd.org.
10. Global Initiative for Asthma. Global Strategy for Asthma Management and Prevention; 2021. Available from: www.ginasthma.org.
11. Shirai T, Hirai K, Gon Y, Maruoka S, Mizumura K, Hikichi M, et al. Combined assessment of serum periostin and YKL-40 may identify asthma-COPD overlap. J Allergy Clin Immunol Pract. 2019;7:134–45.e1. https://doi.org/10.1016/j.jaip.2018.06.015.
12. Nakayasu H, Akamatsu T, Tamura K, Masuda T, Takahashi S, Tanaka Y, et al. Usefulness of bronchodilator reversibility test using the forced oscillation technique in bronchial asthma, COPD, and asthma-COPD overlap. American Thoracic Society annual meeting; 2020. Philadelphia: A2981.
13. Mori K, Shirai T, Mikamo M, Shishido Y, Akita T, Morita S, et al. Colored 3-dimensional analyses of respiratory resistance and reactance in COPD and asthma. COPD. 2011;8:456–63. https://doi.org/10.3109/15412555.2011.626818.
14. Mikamo M, Shirai T, Mori K, Shishido Y, Akita T, Morita S, et al. Predictors of expiratory flow limitation measured by forced oscillation technique in COPD. BMC Pulm Med. 2014;14:23. https://doi.org/10.1186/1471-2466-14-23.

15. Karayama M, Inui N, Mori K, Kono M, Hozumi H, Suzuki Y, et al. Respiratory impedance is correlated with morphological changes in the lungs on three-dimensional CT in patients with COPD. Sci Rep. 2017;7:41709. https://doi.org/10.1038/srep41709.
16. Gonem S, Natarajan S, Desai D, Corkill S, Singapuri A, Bradding P, et al. Clinical significance of small airway obstruction markers in patients with asthma. Clin Exp Allergy. 2014;44:499–507. https://doi.org/10.1111/cea.12257.
17. Shirai T, Mori K, Mikamo M, Shishido Y, Akita T, Morita S, et al. Usefulness of colored 3D imaging of respiratory impedance in asthma. Allergy Asthma Immunol Res. 2013;5:322–8. https://doi.org/10.4168/aair.2013.5.5.322.
18. Kamada T, Kaneko M, Tomioka H. The relationship between respiratory system impedance and lung function in asthmatics: a prospective observational study. Respir Physiol Neurobiol. 2017;239:41–5. https://doi.org/10.1016/j.resp.2017.01.016.
19. Akita T, Shirai T, Akamatsu T, Saigusa M, Yamamoto A, Shishido Y, et al. Long-term change in reactance by forced oscillation technique correlates with FEV1 decline in moderate COPD patients. Eur Respir J. 2017;49(4):1601534. https://doi.org/10.1183/13993003.01534-2016.
20. Shirai T, Mori K, Mikamo M, Shishido Y, Akita T, Morita S, et al. Respiratory mechanics and peripheral airway inflammation and dysfunction in asthma. Clin Exp Allergy. 2013;43:521–6. https://doi.org/10.1016/j.anai.2012.02.007.
21. Shibasaki A, Kurosawa H, Tamura G. [Evaluation of airway narrowing by MostGraph and spirometry -examination using a reversibility test-]. Arerugi. 2013;62(5):566–73. Japanese.
22. Akamatsu T, Shirai T, Shimoda Y, Suzuki T, Hayashi I, Noguchi R, et al. Forced oscillation technique as a predictor of FEV1 improvement in asthma. Respir Physiol Neurobiol. 2017;236:78–83. https://doi.org/10.1016/j.resp.2016.11.013.
23. Takahashi S, Shirai T, Hirai K, Akamatsu T. Forced oscillatory parameters as predictors of COPD assessment test improvement in untreated COPD patients. Respir Physiol Neurobiol. 2022;296:103809. https://doi.org/10.1016/j.resp.2021.103809.
24. Oostveen E, Macleod D, Lorino H, Farré R, Hantos Z, Desager K, et al. The forced oscillation technique in clinical practice: methodology, recommendations and future developments. Eur Respir J. 2003;22:1026–41. https://doi.org/10.1183/09031936.03.00089403.
25. Shirai T. Is R5-R20 a marker of small airway function? Respir Investig. 2018;56:199–200. https://doi.org/10.1016/j.resinv.2018.02.003.
26. Shi Y, Aledia AS, Galant SP, George SC. Peripheral airway impairment measured by oscillometry predicts loss of asthma control in children. J Allergy Clin Immunol. 2013;131:718–23. https://doi.org/10.1016/j.jaci.2012.09.022.
27. Bickel S, Popler J, Lesnick B, Eid N. Impulse oscillometry. Interpretation and practical applications. Chest. 2014;146:841–7. https://doi.org/10.1378/chest.13-1875.
28. Goldman MD, Saadeh C, Ross D. Clinical applications of forced oscillation to assess peripheral airway function. Respir Physiol Neurobiol. 2005;148:179–94. https://doi.org/10.1016/j.resp.2005.05.026.
29. Murakami K, Habukawa C, Kurosawa H, Takemura T. Evaluation of airway responsiveness using colored three-dimensional analyses of a new forced oscillation technique in controlled asthmatic and nonasthmatic children. Respir Investig. 2014;52:57–64. https://doi.org/10.1016/j.resinv.2013.07.003.
30. Yasuo M, Kitaguchi Y, Kinota F, Kosaka M, Urushihata K, Ushiki A, et al. Usefulness of the forced oscillation technique in assessing the therapeutic result of tracheobronchial central airway obstruction. Respir Investig. 2018;56:222–9. https://doi.org/10.1016/j.resinv.2018.01.005.
31. Lipworth B, Manoharan A, Anderson W. Unlocking the quiet zone: the small airway asthma phenotype. Lancet Respir Med. 2014 Jun;2(6):497–506. https://doi.org/10.1016/S2213-2600(14)70103-1.
32. Tamura K, Shirai T, Hirai K, Nakayasu H, Takahashi S, Kishimoto Y, et al. Mucus plugs and small airway dysfunction in asthma, COPD, and asthma-COPD overlap. Allergy Asthma Immunol Res. 2022; (in press)

Chapter 12
Underlying Mechanism Suggested by the ACO Model: What Is the Lesson Learned from the Model?

Hirotaka Matsuzaki, Kensuke Fukuda, and Yoshihisa Hiraishi

Abstract The coexistence of asthma and chronic obstructive pulmonary disease (COPD) is known as asthma–COPD overlap (ACO). Because of the rapid disease progression, frequent and severe exacerbation, and increased comorbidities compared with asthma or COPD alone, the pathogenesis of ACO is believed to be different from each of these respiratory diseases. Because appropriate animal models are lacking, the pathogenesis of ACO including its exacerbation has not been elucidated. We previously developed a well-established murine model that showed the important clinical features of ACO via weekly intratracheal administration of papain in aerosol form in wild-type mice. In this chapter, we describe the phenotype of our single-agent-induced ACO mouse model and knowledge obtained from this model to date. Furthermore, we discuss what should be done in future research using this model to elucidate the pathological processes and identify the diagnostic markers or therapeutic targets of ACO.

Keywords ACO · Mouse model · Exacerbation

1 Introduction

Bronchial asthma and chronic obstructive pulmonary disease (COPD) are the most common chronic respiratory diseases and are among the leading causes of mortality and morbidity worldwide. Approximately 300 million people worldwide have asthma, and approximately 400 million people are expected to develop asthma

H. Matsuzaki (✉)
Center for Epidemiology and Preventive Medicine, The University of Tokyo Hospital, Tokyo, Japan

K. Fukuda · Y. Hiraishi
Department of Respiratory Medicine, Graduate School of Medicine, The University of Tokyo, Tokyo, Japan

H. Nagase et al. (eds.), *Asthma-COPD Overlap*, Respiratory Disease Series: Diagnostic Tools and Disease Managements,
https://doi.org/10.1007/978-981-96-0217-9_12

by 2025 [1]. According to the World Health Organization, COPD caused 3.23 million deaths (the third leading cause of death) in 2019.

Asthma is characterized by chronic airway inflammation, airway hyperresponsiveness, and airway remodeling. Meanwhile, COPD is a chronic respiratory disease accompanied by persistent neutrophilic inflammation and parenchymal lung tissue destruction, which are mainly associated with cigarette smoke (CS) exposure. Acute exacerbation is a significant predictor of poor quality of life and prognosis. Viral infection in the respiratory tract is the most common cause of acute exacerbation in patients with asthma and COPD [2].

1.1 Clinical Features of Asthma–COPD Overlap

The coexistence of asthma and COPD is known as asthma–COPD overlap (ACO) [3]. Patients with ACO show chronic airway inflammation, airway remodeling, and airflow obstruction. Although there is no international consensus regarding the definition of ACO and its prevalence can vary, the prevalence has been estimated in approximately 20% of patients with obstructive airway diseases, which indicates the high prevalence of ACO [4]. A previous study reported that patients with ACO show greater airway hyperresponsiveness, higher blood and sputum eosinophil counts, and increased levels of type 2 cytokines than those with COPD. Patients with ACO also show significantly high fractional exhaled nitric oxide (FeNO) levels and serum total/antigen-specific IgE [5].

1.1.1 Clinical Problem in the Diagnosis and Treatment of ACO

Recently, ACO was recognized as a separate disease from asthma or COPD. Because of the rapid disease progression [6], frequent and severe exacerbation [7], and increased comorbidities compared with asthma or COPD alone, the pathogenesis of ACO is believed to be different from each of these respiratory diseases. Several biomarkers for asthma, including eosinophils, IgE, FeNO, and periostin, have been clinically determined. However, the biomarkers for COPD or ACO have not been well established. Neutrophil gelatinase-associated lipocalin (NGAL), also known as lipocalin-2, is a marker of acute kidney injury. NGAL could be considered as a potential biomarker to distinguish ACO from asthma or COPD alone. Studies have shown that NGAL levels in the sputum [8] or serum [9] of patients with ACO were higher than those of patients with asthma or COPD. NGAL was originally identified as a neutrophil component and later also found to be expressed in low levels in the epithelia of the respiratory and alimentary tracts, prostate, and kidney. The mechanism of NGAL elevation in respiratory diseases has not been elucidated yet. Thus, elucidating the mechanism of NGAL elevation could lead to the practical use of NGAL as a biomarker in respiratory diseases. Furthermore, patients with ACO are excluded from the majority of asthma and COPD randomized control trials, which contributes to the lack of efficacy and safety data on effective therapies for patients with ACO [10].

Past Animal Models of Asthma, COPD, and ACO

There is accumulating knowledge about the clinical phenotype of ACO; however, the detailed molecular pathology of ACO and the reason for its frequent and severe exacerbation are not fully understood. The lack of an appropriate animal model has been a major impediment to the elucidation of appropriate biomarkers, pathogenesis, including its exacerbation, and identification of novel therapeutic targets in ACO. Generally, animal models are used to obtain new insights into the disease and its prevention, diagnosis, and treatment. In asthma, previous studies have used allergens to establish animal models and obtain new knowledge about the disease. In particular, mouse models of asthma have allowed us to understand the disease-causing processes, identify potential therapeutic targets, and develop novel biologics (e.g., anti-IL-5, anti-IL-13, and anti-IgE) [10]. The following allergens have been used to establish animal models of asthma: ovalbumin (OVA), house dust mite (*Dermatophagoides pteronyssinus* [Der p] or *D. farinae* [Der f]), mite allergens (Der p 1, Der f 1, Der p 23, etc.), fungi (*Aspergillus fumigatus*, *Alternaria alternata*), cockroach extracts, *Ascaris* antigens, cotton dust, ragweed, and latex (*Hevea brasiliensis*) [11]. In COPD, porcine pancreatic elastase (PPE) and CS have been used to establish the emphysema model.

A previous study induced allergic airway inflammation (AAI) and pulmonary emphysema in a murine model via OVA inhalation and surfactant protein-D (SP-D) knockout, respectively [12]. Although this model had features of asthma and COPD, SP-D knockout caused only slight emphysematous changes, which presented soon after birth. Moreover, SP-D knockout led to subpleural fibrosis that is not typically seen in clinical ACO. Thus, appropriate animal models that exhibit the features of patients with ACO are needed.

Previous Research Related to Papain

We first developed a well-established murine model that showed the important clinical features of ACO via weekly intratracheal administration of papain in aerosol form in wild-type mice [13].

Papain, a cysteine protease in papaya, breaks down polypeptides and is used for tenderizing meat or cephalopods; it is also used for beer clarification and producing pharmaceutical drugs and cosmetics. Occupational allergies to papain have been documented, and in the animal model, papain was found to induce acute/subacute AAI via type 2 response characterized by interleukin (IL)-5, IL-13, IL-33, and group 2 innate lymphoid cells [14]. Previous murine experiments showed that short-term intratracheal or intranasal exposure to papain induces emphysema [15].

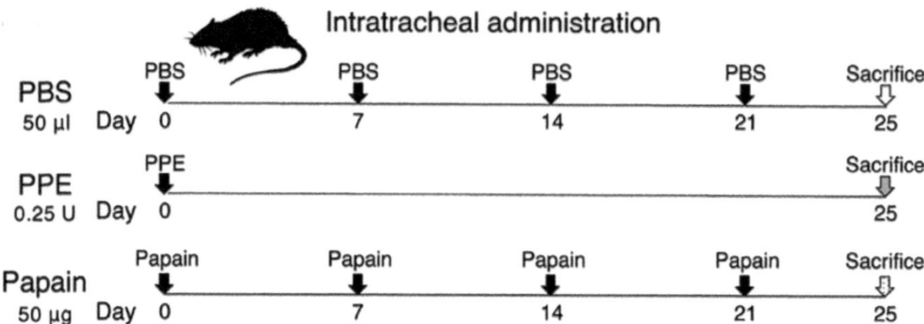

Fig. 12.1 Schematic diagram of the study design; 0.25 U of PPE on day 0 or 50 µg of papain on days 0, 7, 14, and 21 were intratracheally administered in aerosol form. Vehicles were 50 µl of PBS. Mice were sacrificed on day 25

Based on previous reports, we used papain to develop an appropriate animal model to reproduce the features in patients with ACO, including pulmonary emphysema, airway hyperresponsiveness, chronic airway eosinophilia, and increased levels of type 2 cytokines.

2 ACO Mouse Model by Weekly Intratracheal Papain Administration

In our ACO mouse model protocol, 5- to 6-week-old female C57BL/6N mice were housed in a specific-pathogen-free environment with free access to diet and water. Then, the mice were treated intratracheally with 50 µg of papain in 50 µl of PBS on days 0, 7, 14, and 21 (Fig. 12.1).

2.1 COPD and Asthmatic Features in Our ACO Model

To describe the features of this animal model, we first evaluated how papain administration reproduces COPD features compared with the PPE-induced emphysema model and control mice (PBS-treated mice). A COPD model was induced by treating mice intratracheally with 0.25 U of PPE in 50 µl of PBS on day 0 (Fig. 12.1). PPE- and papain-treated mice showed increased inspiratory capacity/weight and dynamic compliance, whereas airway resistance remained unchanged. The representative histology of hematoxylin and eosin (H&E)-stained lung sections of PPE- and papain-treated mice showed emphysema. The mean linear intercept (MLI), which is a common morphometric parameter used to assess emphysema in animal models, was significantly increased in the PPE- or papain-treated group compared with that in the control group. The PPE- and papain-treated groups did not show significantly different MLI. Thus, PPE and papain induced pulmonary emphysema. Furthermore, goblet cell hyperplasia was exclusively seen in the lung sections of the papain-treated group. Although it is not a specific feature of asthma, it is a feature of COPD. Only the papain-treated group showed increased mRNA expression of Muc5ac and Muc5b in whole lung homogenates, which are closely associated with mucus hypersecretion in the respiratory tract. These findings were consistent with those of Alcian blue and periodic acid-Schiff–stained histopathology; however, the results of Muc5b did not reach statistical significance.

Next, to describe the asthmatic features of this model, we conducted bronchoalveolar lavage fluid (BALF) analysis, airway hyperresponsiveness test, and quantitative polymerase chain reaction. The total number of cells, macrophages, and eosinophils in BALF was significantly increased in the papain-treated group. The papain-treated group exhibited higher airway responsiveness with increasing doses of methacholine than other groups. Whole lung homogenates of papain-treated mice showed increased expression levels of eotaxin-1 and eotaxin-2, which are induced by IL-5 and IL-13 and promote the recruitment and proliferation of eosinophils in the lungs [16]. Thus, our papain-treated model had COPD and asthmatic features and was considered to be an appropriate model for ACO.

2.1.1 Analysis of Multiple Cytokines/Chemokines in the ACO Model and Long-Term Effect of Papain Administration

Multiple cytokines/chemokines in BALF were quantitatively detected using cytokine arrays. Table 12.1 shows the cytokine array findings. Macrophage/neutrophil-related cytokines/chemokines were only detectable in papain-treated mice. Macrophage colony-stimulating factor (M-CSF), keratinocyte-derived chemokines (KC: CXCL1), and IL-6 were not detected in the PBS- or PPE-treated group. Regarding type 2 inflammation-associated cytokines, the RANTES (CCL5) levels were high in the papain-treated group; however, they failed to reach statistical significance. IL-4 levels were not significantly different among the groups, whereas IL-5 and IL-13 levels were detectable only in papain-treated mice. IL-33 concentrations in the serum and BALF were not significantly different among the groups. Total IgE levels, one of the serum markers of asthma endotypes, were significantly increased in papain-treated mice.

We further evaluated the long-term effect of papain administration. We analyzed the features of papain-treated mice on day 56 (35 days after the last papain treatment). Eosinophils were still significantly increased in the BALF of papain-treated mice sacrificed on day 56 (8 weeks), indicating prolonged eosinophilic inflammation after papain treatment. The respiratory mechanics was also determined. Similar to the 4-week group, the inspiratory capacity/weight and lung compliance were increased in the papain-treated group at 8 weeks. H&E-stained lung sections also showed papain-induced emphysema. Enzyme-linked immunosorbent assay of

Table 12.1 Cytokine array data

	PBS	PPE	Papain	PPE+Poly(I:C)	Papain+Poly(I:C)
GM-CSF	18.06 (±2.395)	15.08 (±1.970)	15.45 (±0.8398)	18.29 (±2.709)	13.64 (±2.463)
IFN-γ	25.36 (±6.080)	33.81 (±7.248)	26.08 (±4.268)	50.42 (±20.57)	30.16 (±5.597)
IL-1α	1.602 (±1.055)	3.063 (±1.134)	3.717 (±0.7083)	9.052 (±0.8196)	10.26 (±1.238)
IL-1β	15.27 (±4.282)	23.17 (±7.681)	14.20 (±1.665)	ND	ND
IL-2	17.71 (±2.586)	24.55 (±10.19)	10.72 (±3.905)	8.454 (±5.865)	8.915 (±1.934)
IL-3	2.168 (±0.2027)	2.085 (±0.2380)	2.032 (±0.1490)	2.160 (±0.1912)	1.863 (±0.09033)
IL-4	2.448 (±1.495)	1.968 (±0.8217)	2.401 (±1.317)	ND	4.411 (±0.4189)
IL-5	ND	ND	26.12 (±12.46)	ND	ND
IL-6	ND	ND	362.1 (±244.7)	1848 (±371.3)	731.2 (±298.0)
IL-9	95.93 (±38.63)	93.81 (±45.73)	92.39 (±40.30)	ND	ND
IL-10	ND	ND	ND	ND	ND
IL-12	7.216 (±2.439)	5.941 (±3.815)	5.554 (±2.330)	8.554 (±3.454)	4.997 (±1.615)
IL-13	ND	ND	173.6 (±82.79)	ND	291.1 (±116.8)
IL-17	4.496 (±1.583)	11.28 (±5.999)	9.658 (±0.8300)	ND	ND
KC	ND	ND	17.27 (±9.034)	14.21 (±6.342)	9.165 (±2.619)
MCP-1	20.75 (±2.047)	21.99 (±0.8488)	47.85 (±13.85)	610.5 (±43.70)	914.4 (±316.9)
M-CSF	ND	ND	13.03 (±6.842)	1.818 (±1.119)	3.344 (±0.7033)
RANTES	2.008 (±0.6949)	3.225 (±0.7369)	18.34 (±9.646)	456.9 (±110.8)	316.6 (±79.96)
TNF-α	14.72 (±6.985)	22.50 (±15.38)	37.25 (±9.076)	137.5 (±13.27)	52.06 (±13.90)
VEGF	35.15 (±4.788)	39.52 (±5.512)	48.96 (±7.898)	58.59 (±13.02)	10.70 (±2.302)

(pg/ml)

serum samples demonstrated elevated total and papain-specific IgE antibodies at 4 and 8 weeks. Thus, our papain-induced ACO model showed prolonged eosinophilic type 2 airway inflammation along with emphysema.

NGAL Levels in the ACO Mouse Model in the Serum and BALF

The levels of NGAL, a potential biomarker to distinguish ACO from asthma or COPD alone, were analyzed in this model. The papain-treated mice showed significantly elevated NGAL levels in BALF, but the levels in the serum did not significantly increase. In the 8-week model likewise, the papain-treated group exhibited higher NGAL levels in BALF samples. Thus, NGAL levels were elevated in the BALF of ACO models. Taken together, weekly intratracheal papain administration in mice resulted in emphysema, prolonged asthmatic features, and increased NGAL levels in BALF, which are similarly exhibited in patients with ACO.

The Phenotype of Our ACO Model

Pediatric asthma is a major predictor for the development of clinical ACO after middle age [17]. Since we started papain administration to mice at 5–6 weeks, our ACO model would correspond to patients with early-onset asthma during the growing process to the adult stage. Considering other features, our papain-induced mice could be considered an ACO model of early-onset, eosinophilic, high-IgE, and Th2-dominant phenotypes/endotypes. Eosinophilic inflammation accompanied by elevated serum total IgE and papain-specific IgE levels persisted even after 35 days from the last papain treatment. However, the half-lives of murine eosinophils and IgE antibodies are <36 and 12 h, respectively [18]. The presence of specific antibodies and prolonged AAI may indicate the presence of acquired immunity in our ACO model.

The clinical data of patients with COPD showed that ex-smokers have fewer inflammatory cells in the BALF than current smokers [19]. These reports support the validity of our models as clinical COPD and ACO, although the PPE- and papain-treated models (8 weeks) did not show increased neutrophil/macrophage levels. However, the papain-treated group (4 weeks) showed increased levels of macrophages, M-CSF, IL-6, CXCL-1, IL-5, and IL-13 in the BALF, which correspond to the clinical data of asthma or COPD [20–22]. This papain-induced ACO model reproduced the characteristics of asthmatic and COPD airway inflammation concurrently, together with airway hyperresponsiveness and emphysema.

3 Acute Exacerbation of the ACO Model via Poly (I:C) Administration

As described above, patients with ACO show frequent and severe exacerbation. Nevertheless, no studies have evaluated the acute exacerbation of ACO mouse model. Thus, the acute exacerbation models of PPE-induced COPD and papain-induced ACO were compared using poly(I:C) (Fig. 12.2). Poly(I:C) is a double-stranded RNA that acts as a TLR3 agonist, and it is frequently used to mimic viral infection. It has been used in acute exacerbation models of CS-induced COPD mouse models [23], OVA-induced asthmatic mouse models [24], etc. Neutrophils and lymphocytes were significantly increased in the poly(I:C)-induced exacerbation model and the increase in eosinophil count was sustained in the ACO exacerbation model. Lung histopathology showed alveolar wall destruction and inflammatory

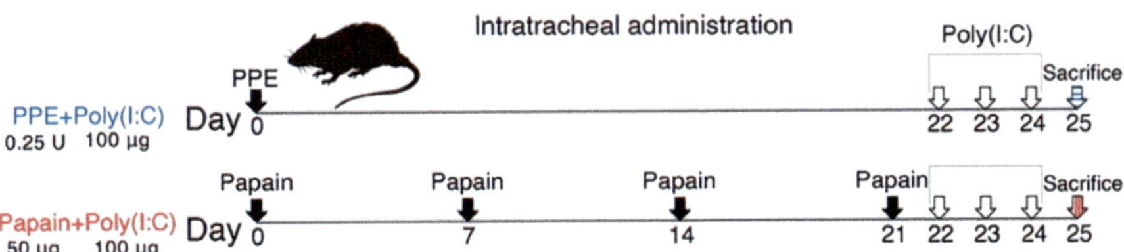

Fig. 12.2 Schematic diagram of the study design; 0.25 U of PPE on day 0 or 50 μg of papain on days 0, 7, 14, and 21 were intratracheally administered. 100 μg of poly(I:C) was administered on days 22, 23, and 24. Mice were sacrificed on day 25

cell infiltration around the blood vessels. Using a cytokine array kit, we quantitatively detected multiple cytokines/chemokines (Table 12.1). In the PPE-treated group, poly(I:C) induced significantly high levels of inflammatory cytokines such as monocyte chemotactic protein-1 (CCL2), IL-1α, tumor necrosis factor-alpha, keratinocyte chemoattractant, IL-6, and RANTES. Poly(I:C) had a similar effect on the papain-treated group, but the levels of some of these cytokines did not reach statistical significance. Although IL-5 levels were diminished by poly(I:C) treatment in the papain-treated group, IL-13 levels in the papain-treated group remained higher than those in the PPE-treated group even after poly(I:C) treatment. Thus, poly(I:C) caused similar inflammatory cytokine induction and inflammatory cell influx in the airways in the COPD and ACO models, whereas AAI was sustained only in the ACO model.

Next, we analyzed the levels of NGAL in the acute exacerbation model. Poly(I:C) induced elevated NGAL levels in the serum and BALF of the COPD and ACO models, although the elevation of NGAL levels in the BALF of the papain+poly(I:C)-treated group was not statistically significant compared with that in the papain-treated group. Thus, NGAL levels were elevated in the BALF of ACO models and the serum and BALF of exacerbation models.

4 Lesson of Our ACO Model

4.1 Speculated Mechanism of NGAL Elevation in the ACO and Exacerbation Models

Increased concentrations of NGAL have been reported in the sputum of subjects with ACO. In the ACO model, elevated levels of NGAL were observed in the BALF of papain-treated mice at the relatively early (4 weeks) and late (8 weeks) phases. To our knowledge, our study is the first to show NGAL levels in murine models of obstructive lung diseases, which showed the same trend as clinical data [13]. NGAL has two important functions in COPD pathogenesis: inhibition of bacterial growth and enhancement of matrix degradation [25]. NGAL also promotes airway remodeling via epithelial–mesenchymal transition and airway hyperreactivity via CD1d-restricted invariant natural killer T cells [26]. We found that poly(I:C) administration increased the NGAL levels in the serum and BALF, but papain administration only slightly increased the serum NGAL levels. Since NGAL is expressed not only in the neutrophils but also in the respiratory epithelial cells [27], the elevation of NGAL in the BALF could be attributed to activated neutrophils or inflammation-induced secretion from epithelial cells. Hence, we could infer that poly(I:C)-derived NGAL was largely from the neutrophils, whereas the papain-derived NGAL was predominantly from the epithelial cells. This hypothesis was reinforced by the fact that papain induced only a slight influx of neutrophils in the lungs, whereas NGAL levels in the BALF were elevated. Combined with the NGAL elevation in the late phase in the ACO model, the mechanism of NGAL elevation would be different between ACO and exacerbation models. Further studies are needed to clarify the mechanism of NGAL elevation.

4.1.1 Difference of COPD and ACO Exacerbation Models

Patients with ACO experience more frequent and severe exacerbations than those with COPD. Poly(I:C) triggered similar inflammatory cytokine induction and inflammatory cell influx in the airways of the COPD and ACO models. Moreover, IL-5 was not detected in our ACO exacerbation model. However, IL-13 levels remained higher in the papain-treated group than in the PPE-treated group even after poly(I:C) treatment. The damaged airway epithelium of an asthmatic patient was reported to be susceptible to viral infection, and eosinophilic airway inflammation was sufficiently maintained even in the absence of IL-5 [28]. The damaged airway epithelium and sustained AAI by type 2 cytokines other than IL-5, such as IL-13, may account for the difference between the clinical features of COPD and ACO exacerbation.

What Should Be Done in the Future Study

In *vivo* animal models are able to accommodate local and systemic interactions of multifaceted diseases, including ACO. Thus, they are essential for investigating the complex interplay between different molecular pathways and designing and testing preventive strategies and drug treatments [10]. In asthma and COPD, the inflammatory response involves innate immunity (eosinophils, neutrophils, macrophages, mast cells, natural killer cells, γδ-T cells, innate lymphoid cells, and dendritic cells) and adaptive immunity (T and B lymphocytes) [29]. Thus, we must further evaluate each cell's involvement (expression and functional analyses) in the ACO mouse model and conduct subsequent in vitro evaluation.

5 Limitations of Our ACO Model

There are various types of AAI and emphysema; therefore, ACO is a heterogeneous disease, and our ACO model cannot cover all ACO types, which is a potential limitation. However, type 2 AAI is the most common and clinically important in asthma. The development of emphysema during the growing process might be too early to mimic the clinical pulmonary emphysema induced by CS. Moreover, although PPE, papain, and CS produce emphysema through a proteolytic attack on the lung matrix, the mechanisms that actually occur with smoke exposure remain unclear [30]. Despite these limitations, our rapidly inducible model could be useful as the first well-established murine model for ACO. This model is simpler and easier to use than most smoking models as it does not require several months of daily procedures and special equipment.

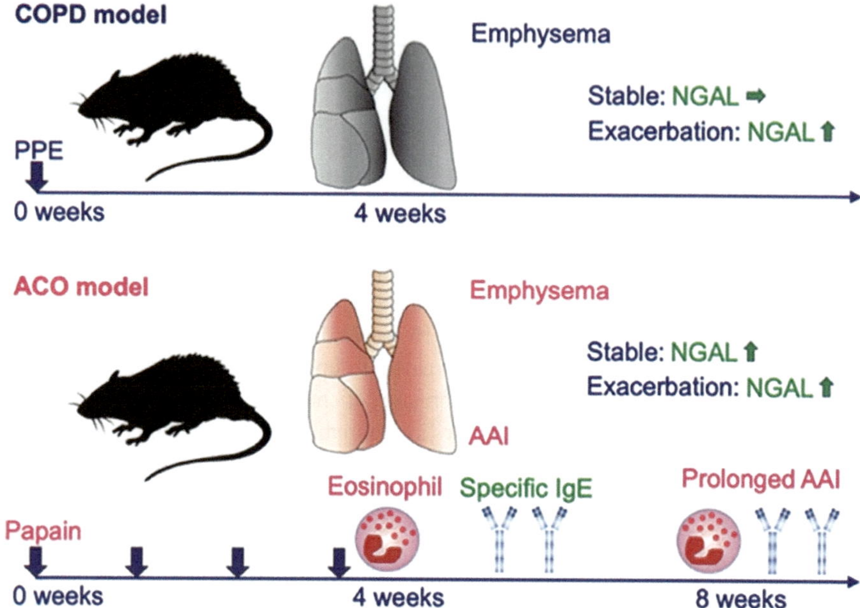

Fig. 12.3 Papain-induced asthma–COPD overlap murine model. Weekly intratracheal papain administration induced pulmonary emphysema and allergic airway inflammation (AAI), whereas porcine pancreatic elastase induced only emphysema. AAI and papain-specific IgE antibodies persisted even after 5 weeks of last papain treatment. This mice model's features were identical to those of patients with asthma–COPD overlap, including airway hyper-responsiveness, mucus hypersecretion, type 2 cytokine elevation, and NGAL increase

6 Conclusions

Weekly intratracheal papain administration in mice results in emphysema, prolonged asthmatic features, and increased NGAL levels, which are similarly exhibited in patients with ACO (Fig. 12.3). Our single-agent-induced model may be used in the future to clarify the underlying pathogenesis of and develop novel treatments for ACO.

References

1. Dharmage SC, Perret JL, Custovic A. Epidemiology of asthma in children and adults. Front Pediatr. 2019;7:246. https://doi.org/10.3389/fped.2019.00246. eCollection 2019
2. Jackson DJ, Sykes A, Mallia P, Johnston SL. Asthma exacerbations: origin, effect, and prevention. J Allergy Clin Immunol. 2011;128(6):1165–74. https://doi.org/10.1016/j.jaci.2011.10.024.
3. Yanagisawa S, Ichinose M. Definition and diagnosis of asthma-COPD overlap (ACO). Allergol Int. 2018;67(2):172–8. https://doi.org/10.1016/j.alit.2018.01.002. Epub 2018 Feb 9.

4. Gibson PG, McDonald VM. Asthma-COPD overlap 2015: now we are six. Thorax. 2015;70(7):683–91. https://doi.org/10.1136/thoraxjnl-2014-206740. Epub 2015 May.
5. Toyota H, Sugimoto N, Kobayashi K, Suzuki Y, Takeshita Y, Ito A, et al. Comprehensive analysis of allergen-specific IgE in COPD: mite-specific IgE specifically related to the diagnosis of asthma-COPD overlap. Allergy Asthma Clin Immunol. 2021;17(1):13. https://doi.org/10.1186/s13223-021-00514-9.
6. Lange P, Parner J, Vestbo J, Schnohr P, Jensen G. A 15-year follow-up study of ventilatory function in adults with asthma. N Engl J Med. 1998;339(17):1194–200. https://doi.org/10.1056/NEJM199810223391703.
7. Hardin M, Silverman EK, Barr RG, Hansel NN, Schroeder JD, Make BJ, et al. The clinical features of the overlap between COPD and asthma. Respir Res. 2011;12(1):127. https://doi.org/10.1186/1465-9921-12-127.
8. Gao J, Iwamoto H, Koskela J, Alenius H, Hattori N, Kohno N, et al. Characterization of sputum biomarkers for asthma–COPD overlap syndrome. Int J Chron Obstruct Pulmon Dis. 2016;11:2457–65. https://doi.org/10.2147/COPD.S113484.
9. Jo YS, Kwon SO, Kim J, Kim WJ. Neutrophil gelatinase-associated lipocalin as a complementary biomarker for the asthma-chronic obstructive pulmonary disease overlap. J Thorac Dis. 2018;10(8):5047–56.
10. Tu X, Donovan C, Kim RY, Wark PAB, Horvat JC, Hansbro PM. Asthma-COPD overlap: current understanding and the utility of experimental models. Eur Respir Rev. 2021;30(159):190185. https://doi.org/10.1183/16000617.0185-2019.
11. Aun MV, Bonamichi-Santos R, Arantes-Costa FM, Kalil J, Giavina-Bianchi P. Animal models of asthma: utility and limitations. J Asthma Allergy. 2017;10:293–301. https://doi.org/10.2147/JAA.S121092. eCollection 2017.
12. Tamura K, Matsumoto K, Fukuyama S, Keiko K-O, Ishii Y, Tonai K, et al. Frequency-dependent airway hyperresponsiveness in a mouse model of emphysema and allergic inflammation. Physiol Rep. 2018;6(2):e13568. https://doi.org/10.14814/phy2.13568.
13. Fukuda K, Matsuzaki H, Mikami Y, Makita K, Miyakawa K, Miyashita N, et al. A mouse model of asthma-chronic obstructive pulmonary disease overlap induced by intratracheal papain. Allergy. 2021;76(1):390–4. https://doi.org/10.1111/all.14528. Epub 2020 Aug 19.
14. Oboki K, Ohno T, Kajiwara N, Arae K, Morita H, Ishii A, et al. IL-33 is a crucial amplifier of innate rather than acquired immunity. Proc Natl Acad Sci U S A. 2010;107(43):18581–6. Published online 2010 Oct 11.
15. Secher T, Maillet I, Mackowiak C, Le Bérichel J, Philippeau A, Panek C, et al. The probiotic strain Escherichia coli Nissle 1917 prevents papain-induced respiratory barrier injury and severe allergic inflammation in mice. Sci Rep. 2018;8:11245. https://doi.org/10.1038/s41598-018-29689-9. Published online 2018 Jul 26.
16. Nussbaum JC, Van Dyken SJ, von Moltke J, Cheng LE, Mohapatra A, Ari B. Molofsky, et al. Type 2 innate lymphoid cells control eosinophil homeostasis. Nature. 2013;502(7470):245–8. https://doi.org/10.1038/nature12526. Published online 2013 Sep 15.
17. Melén E, Guerra S, Hallberg J, Jarvis D, Stanojevic S. Linking COPD epidemiology with pediatric asthma care: implications for the patient and the physician. Pediatr Allergy Immunol. 2019;30(6):589–97. https://doi.org/10.1111/pai.13054. Epub 2019 Jun 2.
18. Carlens J, Wahl B, Ballmaier M, Bulfone-Paus S, Förster R, Pabst O. Common gamma-chain-dependent signals confer selective survival of eosinophils in the murine small intestine. J Immunol. 2009;183(9):5600–7. https://doi.org/10.4049/jimmunol.0801581.
19. Tanino M, Betsuyaku T, Takeyabu K, Tanino Y, Yamaguchi E, Miyamoto K, et al. Increased levels of interleukin-8 in BAL fluid from smokers susceptible to pulmonary emphysema. Thorax. 2002;57(5):405–11. https://doi.org/10.1136/thorax.57.5.405.
20. Bai Y, Zhou Q, Fang Q, Song L, Chen K. Inflammatory cytokines and T-lymphocyte subsets in serum and sputum in patients with bronchial asthma and chronic obstructive pulmonary disease. Med Sci Monit. 2019;25:2206–10. https://doi.org/10.12659/MSM.913703. Published online 2019 Mar 25.

21. Ghebre MA, Pang PH, Diver S, Desai D, Bafadhel M, Haldar K, et al. Biological exacerbation clusters demonstrate asthma and chronic obstructive pulmonary disease overlap with distinct mediator and microbiome profiles. J Allergy Clin Immunol. 2018;141(6):2027–2036.e12. https://doi.org/10.1016/j.jaci.2018.04.013. Epub 2018 Apr 28.
22. Culpitt SV, Rogers DF, Shah P, De Matos C, Russell REK, Donnelly LE, et al. Impaired inhibition by dexamethasone of cytokine release by alveolar macrophages from patients with chronic obstructive pulmonary disease. Am J Respir Crit Care Med. 2003;167(1):24–31. https://doi.org/10.1164/rccm.200204-298OC. Epub 2002 Sep 17.
23. Mebratu YA, Smith KR, Agga GE, Tesfaigzi Y. Inflammation and emphysema in cigarette smoke-exposed mice when instilled with poly (I:C) or infected with influenza A or respiratory syncytial viruses. Respir Res. 2016;17(1):75. https://doi.org/10.1186/s12931-016-0392-x.
24. Lunding LP, Webering S, Vock C, Behrends J, Wagner C, Hölscher C. Poly(inosinic-cytidylic) acid-triggered exacerbation of experimental asthma depends on IL-17A produced by NK cells. Poly(inosinic-cytidylic) acid-triggered exacerbation of experimental asthma depends on IL-17A produced by NK cells. J Immunol. 2015;194(12):5615–25. https://doi.org/10.4049/jimmunol.1402529. Epub 2015 May 13.
25. Yan L, Borregaard N, Kjeldsen L, Moses MA. The high molecular weight urinary matrix metalloproteinase (MMP) activity is a complex of gelatinase B/MMP-9 and neutrophil gelatinase-associated lipocalin (NGAL). Modulation of MMP-9 activity by NGAL. J Biol Chem. 2001;276(40):37258–65. https://doi.org/10.1074/jbc.M106089200. Epub 2001 Aug 2.
26. Karisola P, Lehto M, Kinaret P, Ahonen N, Haapakoski R, Anthoni M. Invariant natural killer T cells play a role in chemotaxis, complement activation and mucus production in a mouse model of airway hyperreactivity and inflammation. PLoS One. 2015;10(6):e0129446. https://doi.org/10.1371/journal.pone.0129446. Published online 2015 Jun 12.
27. Cowland JB, Borregaard N. Molecular characterization and pattern of tissue expression of the gene for neutrophil gelatinase-associated lipocalin from humans. Genomics. 1997;45(1):17–23. https://doi.org/10.1006/geno.1997.4896.
28. Nakagome K, Nagata M. Involvement and possible role of eosinophils in asthma exacerbation. Front Immunol. 2018;9:2220. https://doi.org/10.3389/fimmu.2018.02220. eCollection 2018.
29. Barnes PJ. Cellular and molecular mechanisms of asthma and COPD. Clin Sci (Lond). 2017;131(13):1541–58. https://doi.org/10.1042/CS20160487.
30. Wright JL, Cosio M, Churg A. Animal models of chronic obstructive pulmonary disease. Am J Physiol Lung Cell Mol Physiol. 2008;295(1):L1–15. https://doi.org/10.1152/ajplung.90200.2008. Epub 2008 May 2

Part IV
Diagnosis of ACO

Chapter 13
Comparison of Diagnostic Criteria of ACO: What Is the Point of Difference?

Akira Koarai

Abstract Now, patients with both features of asthma and chronic obstructive pulmonary disease (COPD) are demonstrated to have greater respiratory symptoms, frequent exacerbations, and poor quality of life compared to those with asthma or COPD alone and are widely recognized as asthma-COPD overlap (ACO). Until recently, various diagnostic algorithms of ACO have been proposed around the world, but there is no single universally accepted definition for ACO. In this chapter, we describe the diagnostic criteria of ACO in the recent literature, including Japanese Respiratory Society's proposal and compare them to clarify how they differ. There are variations in the diagnostic criteria based on only the symptoms or, additionally, employing several objective diagnostic tests including the bronchodilator response in forced expiratory volume in 1 s, blood or sputum eosinophil count, serum IgE levels, and fractioned exhaled nitric oxide. The difference could be partly due to the limited accessibility to diagnostic tests. However, there have not been enough concrete data to support using these diagnostic criteria in ACO. Further large longitudinal data are required to validate these diagnostic criteria of ACO for an accurate diagnosis and proper treatment.

Keywords Asthma and COPD overlap · Diagnostic criteria · Prevalence of ACO

1 Introduction

Asthma and chronic obstructive pulmonary disease (COPD) are the most frequently encountered pulmonary diseases in clinical practice. Although both diseases are characterized by airflow limitation, the pathophysiology is quite different. Airway obstruction in asthma is mainly caused by type 2 eosinophilic

A. Koarai (✉)
Division of Respiratory Medicine, Sendai City Hospital, Sendai, Japan
e-mail: koarai-aki@hospital.city.sendai.jp

H. Nagase et al. (eds.), *Asthma-COPD Overlap*, Respiratory Disease Series: Diagnostic Tools and Disease Managements,
https://doi.org/10.1007/978-981-96-0217-9_13

inflammation, while the airflow limitation in COPD is due to neutrophilic type 1 inflammation induced by exposure to noxious particles or gases, mainly cigarette smoke [1]. On the other hand, COPD has been shown to be a heterogeneous disease as patients have diverse clinical characteristics [2]. A patient population of COPD with asthmatic features has been indicated, which shows higher numbers of eosinophils in sputum [3] and an increase in type 2 inflammation-related genes in the airways [4]. COPD patients with asthmatic features have been demonstrated to have greater respiratory symptoms, frequent exacerbations, and poor quality of life compared to patients with asthma or COPD alone [5–9]. Therefore, to identify these patients for proper treatment and to promote research for identifying the characteristics and underlying mechanisms, a new disease concept for "asthma and COPD overlap syndrome (ACOS)" was proposed by the Global Initiative for Asthma (GINA) and the Global Initiative for Chronic Obstructive Lung Disease (GOLD) in 2014 [10]. Afterwards, in 2017, GINA recommended the use of the term "ACO" rather than "ACOS," to avoid the misconception that this is a single disease entity [11]. Until now, various diagnostic algorithms of ACO have been proposed in different countries and committees around the world, but there is no single universally accepted definition for ACO. In this chapter, we describe the diagnostic criteria of ACO in the recent literature and compare them to clarify their differences.

2 Definition of ACO

In GINA 2021, ACO, which is also called asthma+COPD, was defined as "'Asthma-COPD overlap" and "asthma+COPD" are terms used to collectively describe patients who have persistent airflow limitation together with clinical features that are consistent with both asthma and COPD. This is not a definition of a single disease entity. Still, a descriptive term for clinical use that includes several different clinical phenotypes reflecting different underlying mechanisms" (Table 13.1) [12]. However, the GOLD committee declared that "they no longer refer to ACO. Still, instead they emphasized that asthma and COPD are different disorders, although they may share some common traits and clinical features (e.g., eosinophilia, some degree of reversibility)" since the revision of GOLD document in 2020 [1]. It is important to make a firm diagnosis of either asthma or COPD. Still, it is also obvious that there is little concrete evidence, including the epidemiology and pathophysiology of patients with ACO, for determining the optimal treatment strategies. Therefore, it remains necessary to define ACO and focus on this patient population.

Table 13.1 Current definition of asthma and COPD and clinical description of asthma-COPD overlap in GINA

Asthma
Asthma is a heterogeneous disease, usually characterized by chronic airway inflammation. It is defined by the history of respiratory symptoms such as wheeze, shortness of breath, chest tightness, and cough that vary over time and in intensity, together with variable expiratory airflow limitation. [GINA 2021] [12]
COPD
Chronic obstructive pulmonary disease (COPD) is a common, preventable, and treatable disease that is characterized by persistent respiratory symptoms and airflow limitation that is due to airway and/or alveolar abnormalities usually caused by significant exposure to noxious particles or gases and influenced by host factors including abnormal lung development. Significant comorbidities may have an impact on morbidity and mortality. [GOLD 2022] [1]
Asthma-COPD overlap, also called asthma+COPD
"Asthma-COPD overlap" and "asthma+COPD" are terms used to collectively describe patients who have persistent airflow limitation together with clinical features that are consistent with both asthma and COPD. This is not a definition of a single disease entity but a descriptive term for clinical use that includes several different clinical phenotypes reflecting different underlying mechanisms. [GINA 2021] [12]

Notes: Reproduced with permission from Global Initiative for Asthma. *GINA* Global initiative for asthma, *GOLD* Global Initiative for Chronic Obstructive Lung Disease

3 Comparison of Diagnostic Criteria of ACO

3.1 Diagnostic Criteria of GINA and GOLD Consensus

In the initial consensus for ACOS proposed by GINA and GOLD in 2014 [10], the diagnostic process was performed based on clinical feature-based criteria (Fig. 13.1). That approach consisted of two steps for the diagnosis of ACOS. The first step was to identify symptoms such as chronic or recurrent cough, sputum, or wheezing, suggesting chronic airway disease. In the second step, the features of either asthma or COPD that best described the patient, including age at onset, pattern of symptoms, lung function test results, and findings on chest radiographs, were identified and compared. When both features of asthma and COPD were detected, the patient was diagnosed with ACOS. Asthma is often allergic and begins in childhood with variable airflow limitation and intermittent wheezing, cough, sputum and dyspnea. In contrast, patients with COPD are usually current or former smokers and present with symptoms including chronic cough & sputum and exertional dyspnea. The diagnostic process is based on the typical clinical features of asthma or COPD, which could be easily understood by general physicians. However, there have been criticisms for not indicating how many clinical features are necessary for the diagnosis of ACOS and because the features are not sufficiently objective.

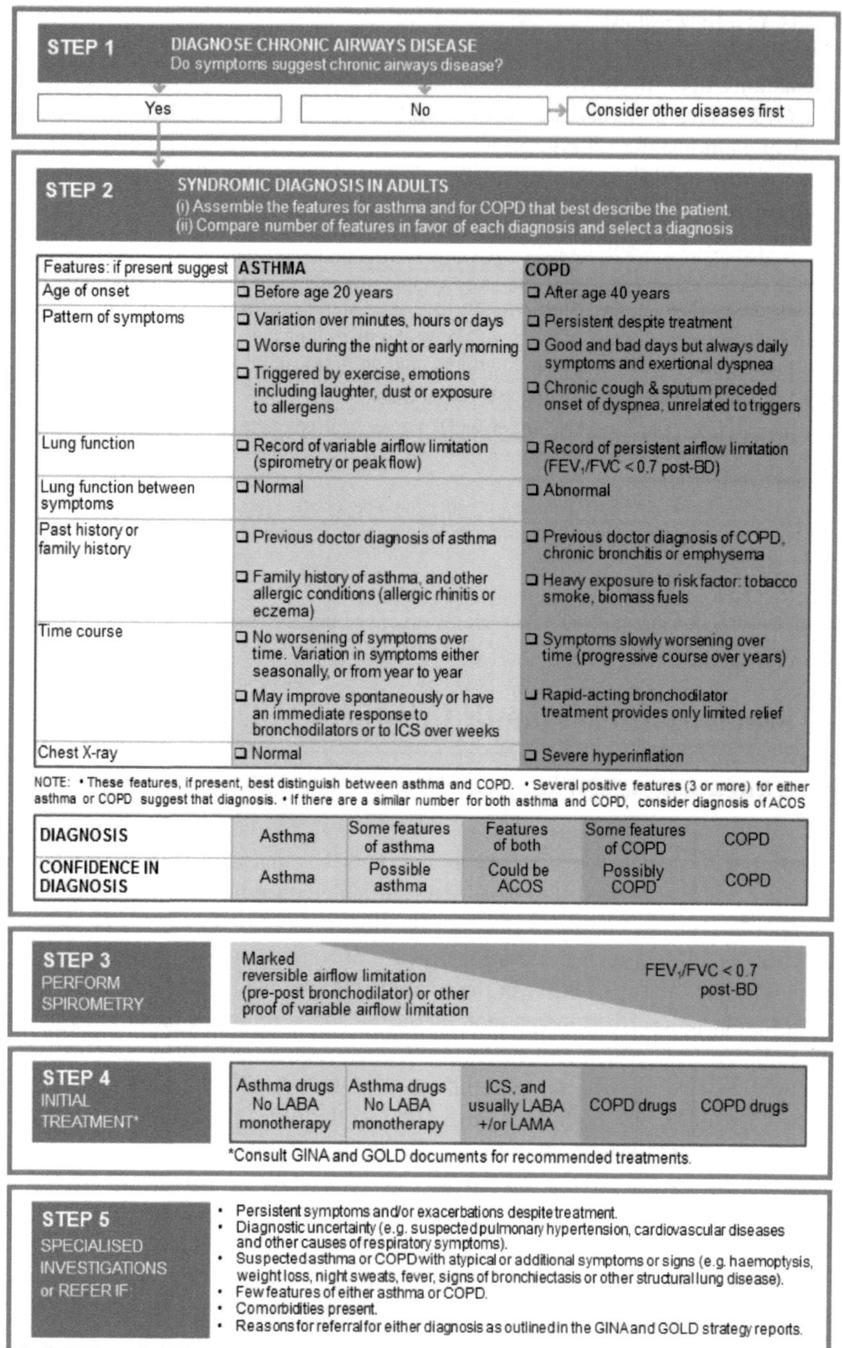

Fig. 13.1 Summary of syndromic approach to diseases of chronic airflow limitation. (Reproduced with permission from Ref. [10])

3.2 *Diagnostic Criteria of Global Expert Round Table Discussion*

In a global expert round table discussion held in 2015 for the purpose of defining ACOS more precisely, the committee proposed major and minor criteria for the diagnosis of ACOS (Table 13.2) [13]. They claimed that ACOS could be diagnosed when the patients meet all three major criteria of (1) persistent airflow limitation evaluated by spirometry in individuals 40 years of age or older, (2) a significant history of exposure to cigarette or air pollution, and (3) a history of asthma before 40 years of age or bronchodilator response of more than 400 ml in forced expiratory volume in 1 second (FEV1), and at least one minor criterion from among (1) documented history of atopy or allergic rhinitis, (2) bronchodilator response of 200 ml or more in FEV1 and 12% from baseline values on 2 or more visits, or (3) peripheral blood eosinophil count of 300 or more cells/μL. These diagnostic criteria employ a higher peripheral blood eosinophil count and greater bronchodilator response as

Table 13.2 Diagnostic criteria for ACO in different consensus and guidelines

Diagnostic criteria		
Global expert round table discussion [13]	ACOS is confirmed by the presence of all three major criteria and at least one minor criterion	
	Major criteria • Persistent airflow limitation [post-bronchodilator FEV1/FVC<0.70 or LLN] in individuals 40 years of age or older; LLN is preferred. • At least 10 pack-years of tobacco smoking OR equivalent indoor or outdoor air pollution exposure [e.g., biomass] • Documented history of asthma before 40 years of age OR BDR of >400 mL in FEV1	**Minor criteria** • Documented history of atopy or allergic rhinitis • BDR of FEV1 ≥200 mL and 12% from baseline values on 2 or more visits • Peripheral blood eosinophil count of ≥300 cells/μL.
Czech guideline [15]	ACO is confirmed by the presence of two major criteria or one major plus two minor criteria in patients with COPD	
	Major criteria • Strongly positive bronchodilator test (change FEV1 ≥15% and ≥400 ml) • History of bronchial asthma before 40 years established by physician • Presence of eosinophilia in peripheral blood (≥300 eosinophils/μl) • Sputum eosinophil count ≥3% • Positivity of metacholine bronchial challenge test • Increased FeNO (>45–50 ppb) in the stable phase of COPD	**Minor criteria** • Mild positivity of bronchodilator test (change FEV1 ≥12% and ≥200 ml) • History of atopy established by physician

(continued)

Table 13.2 (continued)

<table>
<tr><td rowspan="2">Finnish guideline [16]</td><td colspan="2">ACO is confirmed by the presence of two main criteria or one main criterion plus two additional criteria in patients with COPD</td></tr>
<tr><td>Main criteria
• Very positive BDT FEV_1 >15% and >400 mL
• Sputum eosinophilia or elevated FeNO (>50 ppb)
• Previous asthma symptoms (starting age at <40 years)</td><td>Additional criteria
• Elevated total IgE
• Atopy
• Repeated significant positive BDT (FEV_1 >12% and >200 mL)
• Peak expiratory flow follow-up typical of asthma</td></tr>
<tr><td rowspan="2">Spanish guideline [17]</td><td colspan="2">ACO is confirmed by the presence of three main criteria plus diagnosis of asthma or asthmatic criteria</td></tr>
<tr><td>Main criteria
• ≥35 years of age
• Smoker (or former smoker) ≥10 pack-years
• FEV1/FVC <0.70 post PBD <70%</td><td>Additional criteria
• Current diagnosis of asthma
• If not satisfied as asthma diagnosis:
→PBD ≥15% and 400 mL, and/or eosinophilia in blood ≥300 cells/μL</td></tr>
<tr><td rowspan="5">Belgian expert panel [19]</td><td colspan="2">A diagnosis of ACOS is accepted in both COPD and asthma patients when the two major criteria and at least one minor criterion are met.</td></tr>
<tr><td colspan="2">ACOS in a COPD patient</td></tr>
<tr><td>Main criteria
• High degree of variability in airway obstruction over time (PFTs): FEV1 variation ≥400 mL
• High degree of response to bronchodilators (PFTs): >200 mL and 12% predicted above baseline</td><td>Minor criteria
• Personal or family history of atopy and/or IgE sensitivity to one or more airborne allergens
• Elevated blood or sputum eosinophils or increased FeNO
• Diagnosed with asthma before the age of 40
• Symptom variability
• Age (in favor of asthma)</td></tr>
<tr><td colspan="2">ACOS in an asthma patient</td></tr>
<tr><td>Main criteria
• Persistence over time of airflow obstruction (persistence of FEV1/FVC ratio <0.7 or <lower normal limit)
• Exposure to noxious particles or gases, with ≥10 pack-years in case of smoking for (ex-)smokers</td><td>Minor criteria
• Lack of response on acute bronchodilator test
• Reduced lung diffusion capacity (on PFTs)
• Little variability in airway obstruction (PFTs)
• Age in favor of COPD (i.e., >40 years)
• Presence of emphysema on chest CT scan</td></tr>
</table>

Abbreviations: *ACO* Asthma–COPD overlap, *ACOS* Asthma–COPD overlap syndrome, *BDR* Bronchodilator respo+A1:E17nse using 400 μg of albuterol/ salbutamol [or equivalent], *BDT* Bronchodilator test, *CT* Computed tomography, *FEV1* Forced expiratory volume in 1 s, *FVC* Forced vital capacity, *FeNO* Fractioned exhaled nitric oxide, *IgE* Immunoglobulin E, *LLN* Lower limit of normal, *PBD* Post-bronchodilator, *PFTs* Pulmonary function tests objective criteria for the diagnosis of the asthmatic phenotype compared to those of the GINA and GOLD consensus. In the evaluation of ACO using various COPD cohorts, the diagnostic criteria proposed in this round table discussion such as bronchodilator response in FEV1, history of asthma, and history of atopy or allergic rhinitis have been used to detect asthmatic features [7, 14]. In the evaluation of ACOS in one of the large COPD cohort studies, the Evaluation of COPD Longitudinally to Identify Predictive Surrogate End-points (ECLIPSE), the presence of current asthma and wheeze was employed to detect asthmatic features for the diagnosis of ACOS in addition to a history of asthma, bronchodilator reversibility (change in FEV1 ≥12% and ≥200 mL) and history of atopy [7].

3.3 *Diagnostic Criteria of European Countries' Guidelines and Consensus*

At present, several committees in European countries have proposed criteria for the diagnosis of ACO (Table 13.2). In the Czech and Finnish guidelines for detecting ACO from COPD patients, the sets of criteria are similar to each other and include the evaluation of type 2 airway inflammation with sputum eosinophilia or an elevated fractioned exhaled nitric oxide (FeNO) in the major criteria instead of the peripheral blood eosinophil count. Therefore, the Czech and Finnish diagnostic criteria could more objectively diagnose the asthmatic phenotype in patients with COPD compared to those of the global expert round table discussion [15, 16].

On the other hand, the diagnostic criteria of the Spanish guidelines are more practical and similar to those of the global expert round table discussion. The first criterion for the diagnosis of COPD is based on Spanish guidelines, i.e. age >35 years with significant exposure to smoking and persistent respiratory symptoms and airflow limitation. After the diagnosis of COPD, co-existence of current asthma or an asthmatic feature is checked for the diagnosis of ACO, which is based on whether it fulfills the diagnostic criteria for asthma or shows a large bronchodilator response (≥400 mL and ≥15% in FEV1) and/or blood eosinophilia (≥300 cells/μL). Compared with the criteria of the global expert round table discussion, the age is younger (35 years or older vs 40 years or older) and a history of atopy or allergic rhinitis is excluded [17]. The Spanish guideline's criteria do not contain a type 2 airway inflammation biomarker such as FeNO and sputum eosinophilia for evaluation. In order to simplify the diagnostic criteria, the current diagnosis of asthma and high blood eosinophilia, which are both known as the best-documented factors associated with the response to ICS in COPD, are only included in the criteria [18].

In Belgium, an expert panel proposed criteria for diagnosing ACO in patients with asthma or COPD, respectively in 2017 [19]. In the diagnosis of patients with COPD, despite some variations, the diagnostic criteria are similar to those used in the Czech and Finnish diagnostic criteria. Concerning the diagnosis of patients with asthma, the committee first proposed criteria for the diagnosis of ACO, i.e., ACO could be diagnosed when the patients with asthma meet at least two major criteria: (1) persistent airflow obstruction over time (forced expiratory volume in 1 second/forced vital capacity ratio <0.7) and (2) exposure to noxious particles or gases, with 10 pack-years for (ex-) smokers, and at least one minor criteria such as (1) lack of response in an acute bronchodilator test, (2) reduced lung diffusion capacity, (3) little variability in airway obstruction, (4) age >40 years, or (5) emphysema on chest CT scan. This diagnostic approach employs lung diffusion capacity and chest CT scan as objective diagnostic tools for the emphysematous features of COPD.

3.4 Diagnostic Criteria of Japanese Respiratory Society

In Japan, the diagnostic criteria for ACO proposed by the Japanese Respiratory Society (JRS) in 2017 included each objective evaluation for the characteristics of COPD or asthma, the same as those in the Belgian consensus, i.e., a decreased level of DLCO and emphysematous changes in a chest CT scan for COPD or increased FeNO and sputum eosinophilia for asthma (Table 13.3) [20, 21]. This is because CT is widely used and measuring devices for FeNO are clinically available in more than 2000 facilities in Japan.

The diagnostic approach is as follows: first, in individuals with respiratory symptoms, such as cough, sputum and dyspnea, both criteria are essential, i.e., 40 years or older and chronic airflow obstruction (post-bronchodilator FEV1/FVC <0.70). At present, a differential diagnosis is recommended to be performed by taking a chest radiograph. Next, each feature of COPD and asthma is evaluated based on whether the individuals meet at least one criterion from (1) smoking history (>10 pack-years) or equivalent air pollution exposure, (2) presence of low attenuation area showing emphysematous changes on chest CT scan, or (3) impaired pulmonary diffusing capacity for the feature of COPD, and two features from (1) variable (daily, from day to day or seasonal) or paroxysmal respiratory symptom (cough, sputum and dyspnea), (2) history of asthma before 40 years of age, or (3) FeNO >35 ppb, or one of these three characteristics plus at least two characteristics from (4-1) history of perennial allergic rhinitis, (4-2) airway reversibility (post-bronchodilator response of FEV_1 >12% and >200 mL from baseline values), (4-3) peripheral blood eosinophil count of >5% or 300 cells/μL, or (4-4)) elevated level of IgE (total IgE or specific IgE to inhaled perennial antigens) for the feature of asthma. When both features of COPD and asthma are fulfilled, ACO is diagnosed.

Table 13.3 Diagnostic criteria for ACO in Japanese Respiratory Society

<table>
<tr><td colspan="5">Basic criteria</td></tr>
<tr><td colspan="5">Age ≥40 years and chronic airflow obstruction: post-bronchodilator FEV_1/FVC <70%</td></tr>
<tr><td colspan="2">[Characteristics of COPD]
One item from 1, 2, and 3</td><td colspan="3">[Characteristics of asthma]
Two items from 1, 2, and 3, or
One item out of 1, 2, and 3 and at least two items from 4</td></tr>
<tr><td>1.</td><td>Smoking history (10 pack-years or more) or career involving significant air pollution or biomass exposure</td><td>1.</td><td colspan="2">Variable (diurnally, daily, and seasonally) or paroxysmal respiratory symptoms (cough, sputum, and dyspnea)</td></tr>
<tr><td>2.</td><td>Presence of a low attenuation area on chest CT demonstrating emphysematous changes</td><td>2.</td><td colspan="2">History of asthma before age 40 years</td></tr>
<tr><td rowspan="5">3.</td><td rowspan="5">Impaired pulmonary diffusing capacity (%DLCO <80% or %DLCO/VA <80%)</td><td>3.</td><td colspan="2">FeNO >35 ppb</td></tr>
<tr><td rowspan="4">4.</td><td>(1)</td><td>Concomitant perennial allergic rhinitis</td></tr>
<tr><td>(2)</td><td>Airway reversibility (change in FEV1 >12% and >200 mL)</td></tr>
<tr><td>(3)</td><td>Peripheral blood eosinophils > 5% or 300 /μL</td></tr>
<tr><td>(4)</td><td>High IgE level (total IgE, or IgE specific to perennial inhalant antigens)</td></tr>
<tr><td>1.</td><td colspan="4">To be diagnosed as ACO, one item of the characteristics of COPD plus two items from 1, 2, and 3 or one item from 1, 2, and 3 and at least two items from criterion 4 of the characteristics of asthma are needed.</td></tr>
<tr><td>2.</td><td colspan="4">If the characteristics of COPD alone are present, it is diagnosed as COPD, and if the characteristics of asthma alone are present, it is diagnosed as asthma (with remodeling).</td></tr>
<tr><td>3.</td><td colspan="4">If the characteristics of asthma cannot be confirmed when diagnosing ACO, it is important to monitor for the presence of the characteristics of asthma over time.</td></tr>
<tr><td>4.</td><td colspan="4">Perennial inhalant antigens include house dust, mites, molds, scales from animals, and feathers, and seasonal inhalant antigens include pollen from trees, plants, and weeds.</td></tr>
</table>

Reprinted with permission from Ref. [20]

Note 1: Diseases of differential diagnosis (diffuse panbronchiolitis, congenital sinobronchial syndrome, obstructive panbronchiolitis, bronchiectasis, pulmonary tuberculosis, pneumoconiosis, lymphangioleiomyomatosis, congestive heart failure, interstitial lung disease, and lung cancer) should be ruled out by standard chest x-rays, etc.

Note 2: Respiratory symptoms such as cough, sputum, and dyspnea are variable (diurnally, daily, and seasonally) or paroxysmal in asthma and chronic and continuous in COPD

Abbreviations: *ACO* Asthma-COPD overlap, *COPD* Chronic obstructive pulmonary disease, *CT* Computed tomography, *DLCO* Diffusion capacity of carbon monoxide, *VA* Alveolar volume, *FeNO* Fraction of exhaled nitric oxide, *FEV1* Forced expiratory volume in 1 s, *IgE* Immunoglobulin E

4 What Is the Point of Difference?

In the above-mentioned definitions, there are differences mainly due to how many objective laboratory tests are included in the diagnostic criteria. For the global convenience and practical setting, the GINA/GOLD consensus provides a list of characteristics mainly based on symptoms of either asthma or COPD for the criteria [10]. In contrast, the global expert round table discussion consensus and the Spanish guideline only include universally available laboratory tests such as spirometry and peripheral blood eosinophil counts [13, 17]. On the other hand, the Czech and Finnish guidelines employ objective diagnostic evaluations for type 2 airway inflammation in asthmatic features with sputum eosinophil counts and FeNO instead of the peripheral blood eosinophil count [15, 16]. In addition to the type 2 airway inflammation evaluation tools, the Belgian expert panel proposal and Japanese guidelines include objective diagnostic tools for detecting emphysematous features of COPD, namely lung diffusion capacity and chest CT scan [19]. Compared to the Belgian expert panel proposal, the JRS diagnostic criteria for ACO do not require a diagnosis of asthma or COPD in advance because, in some patients with airflow limitation in spirometry, it is difficult to diagnose either asthma or COPD precisely [20, 21]. Overall, in Japan, the JRS diagnostic algorithm would be more precise for the diagnosis of ACO compared to those of other countries, as proposed by the global committee. Although the employment of these objective criteria would increase the certainty of the diagnosis of ACO, the accessibility to these diagnostic tools depends on the individual circumstances of each country and region, which causes differences in the diagnostic criteria among the countries and global committee. Also, there are differences in the cut off values of the laboratory tests for the evaluation of type 2 airway inflammation, including the blood or sputum eosinophil count, bronchodilator response in FEV1.

The differences in the criteria for the diagnosis of ACO could affect the prevalence [9, 22–24]. In primary care practices in the UK, the prevalence of ACO was reported to be 20%, which was determined mostly according to the diagnostic criteria of the global expert round table discussion [25]. In Czech, the prevalence of ACO in COPD was shown to be 3.9% based on the Czech guidelines compared to 11.4% evaluated by the Spanish guidelines [15]. However, in Spain, the prevalence was reported to be 27.4% [26]. In Japan, while the prevalence of ACO in COPD was reported to be 14.4% or 16.6% using a stepwise approach of the GINA/GOLD consensus [27, 28], the prevalence was recently demonstrated to be 30.6% or 25.5% by evaluation with the JRS diagnostic criteria [29, 30]. The variation from 3.9% to 30.6% in the prevalence of ACO could be due not only to the selected criteria, but also due to the populations included in the studies.

5 Conclusion

In this chapter, we described the diagnostic criteria of ACO in the Global consensus and several typical country's guidelines and showed the point of the difference. As with the individual circumstances of each country such as limited accessibility to diagnostic tools, there are variations in the diagnostic criteria based on only the symptoms of either asthma or COPD, or additionally employing several objective diagnostic tests. However, there have not been enough concrete data for supporting the use of these diagnostic criteria in ACO, such as the bronchodilator response threshold of 400 mL in FEV1, blood or sputum eosinophil count, serum IgE levels, and FeNO. Further large longitudinal data are required to validate these diagnostic criteria of ACO for an accurate diagnosis and proper treatment with better practical use. Also, additional studies to address differences in race and ethnicity and socio-economic status would also be needed to improve the diagnostic accuracy in ACO.

References

1. Global Initiative for Chronic Obstructive Lung Disease (GOLD) 2022 REPORT. Global strategy for the diagnosis, management, and prevention of chronic obstructive lung disease Update November 2021. Available from: http://www.goldcopd.org/.
2. Agusti A. The path to personalised medicine in COPD. Thorax. 2014;69:857–64.
3. Brightling CE, Monteiro W, Ward R, Parker D, Morgan MD, Wardlaw AJ, Pavord ID. Sputum eosinophilia and short-term response to prednisolone in chronic obstructive pulmonary disease: a randomised controlled trial. Lancet. 2000;356:1480–5.
4. Christenson SA, Steiling K, Van Den Berge M, Hijazi K, Hiemstra PS, Postma DS, Lenburg ME, Spira A, Woodruff PG. Asthma-COPD overlap. Clinical relevance of genomic signatures of type 2 inflammation in chronic obstructive pulmonary disease. Am J Respir Crit Care Med. 2015;191:758–66.
5. Gibson PG, Simpson JL. The overlap syndrome of asthma and COPD: what are its features and how important is it? Thorax. 2009;64:728–35.
6. Alshabanat A, Zafari Z, Albanyan O, Dairi M, Fitzgerald JM. Asthma and COPD overlap syndrome (ACOS): a systematic review and meta analysis. PLoS One. 2015;10:e0136065.
7. Wurst KE, Rheault TR, Edwards L, Tal-Singer R, Agusti A, Vestbo J. A comparison of COPD patients with and without ACOS in the ECLIPSE study. Eur Respir J. 2016;47:1559–62.
8. Kendzerska T, Sadatsafavi M, Aaron SD, To TM, Lougheed MD, Fitzgerald JM, Gershon AS, Canadian Respiratory Research N. Concurrent physician-diagnosed asthma and chronic obstructive pulmonary disease: a population study of prevalence, incidence and mortality. PLoS One. 2017;12:e0173830.
9. Barrecheguren M, Pinto L, Mostafavi-Pour-Manshadi SM, Tan WC, Li PZ, Aaron SD, Benedetti A, Chapman KR, Walker B, Fitzgerald JM, Hernandez P, Maltais F, Marciniuk DD, O'donnell DE, Sin DD, Bourbeau J. Identification and definition of asthma-COPD overlap: the CanCOLD study. Respirology. 2020;25:836–49.
10. Global Initiative for Asthma; Global Initiative for Chronic Obstructive Lung Disease. Diagnosis of diseases of chronic airflow limitation: Asthma, COPD, and Asthma-COPD Overlap Syndrome (ACOS). Updated 2015. http://goldcopd.org/asthma-copd-asthma-copd-overlap-synd.

11. Global Initiative for Asthma. Global strategy for asthma management and prevention. Updated 2017. http://ginasthma.org/2017-gina-report-globalstrategy-for-asthma-management-andprevention/.
12. Global Initiative for Asthma. Global strategy for asthma management and prevention. Updated 2021. https://ginasthma.org/gina-reports/.
13. Sin DD, Miravitlles M, Mannino DM, Soriano JB, Price D, Celli BR, Leung JM, Nakano Y, Park HY, Wark PA, Wechsler ME. What is asthma-COPD overlap syndrome? Towards a consensus definition from a round table discussion. Eur Respir J. 2016;48:664–73.
14. Cosentino J, Zhao H, Hardin M, Hersh CP, Crapo J, Kim V, Criner GJ. Analysis of asthma-chronic obstructive pulmonary disease overlap syndrome defined on the basis of bronchodilator response and degree of emphysema. Ann Am Thorac Soc. 2016;13:1483–9.
15. Zatloukal J, Brat K, Neumannova K, Volakova E, Hejduk K, Kocova E, Kudela O, Kopecky M, Plutinsky M, Koblizek V. Chronic obstructive pulmonary disease—diagnosis and management of stable disease; a personalized approach to care, using the treatable traits concept based on clinical phenotypes. Position paper of the Czech Pneumological and Phthisiological Society. Biomed Pap Med Fac Univ Palacky Olomouc Czech Repub. 2020;164:325–56.
16. Kankaanranta H, Harju T, Kilpeläinen M, Mazur W, Lehto JT, Katajisto M, Peisa T, Meinander T, Lehtimäki L. Diagnosis and pharmacotherapy of stable chronic obstructive pulmonary disease: the finnish guidelines. Basic Clin Pharmacol Toxicol. 2015;116:291–307.
17. Plaza V, Álvarez F, Calle M, Casanova C, Cosío BG, López-Viña A, Pérez De Llano L, Quirce S, Román-Rodríguez M, Soler-Cataluña JJ, Miravitlles M. Consensus on the asthma-COPD overlap syndrome (ACOS) between the Spanish COPD Guidelines (GesEPOC) and the Spanish Guidelines on the Management of Asthma (GEMA). Arch Bronconeumol. 2017;53:443–9.
18. Miravitlles M, Alvarez-Gutierrez FJ, Calle M, Casanova C, Cosio BG, López-Viña A, Pérez De Llano L, Quirce S, Roman-Rodríguez M, Soler-Cataluña JJ, Plaza V. Algorithm for identification of asthma-COPD overlap: consensus between the Spanish COPD and asthma guidelines. Eur Respir J. 2017;49:1700068.
19. Cataldo D, Corhay JL, Derom E, Louis R, Marchand E, Michils A, Ninane V, Peché R, Pilette C, Vincken W, Janssens W. A Belgian survey on the diagnosis of asthma-COPD overlap syndrome. Int J Chron Obstruct Pulmon Dis. 2017;12:601–13.
20. The Japanese Respiratory Society. The JRS guidelines for the management of ACO 2018. Tokyo: Medical Review; 2017. (In Japanese)
21. Yanagisawa S, Ichinose M. Definition and diagnosis of asthma-COPD overlap (ACO). Allergol Int. 2018;67:172–8.
22. Bonten TN, Kasteleyn MJ, De Mutsert R, Hiemstra PS, Rosendaal FR, Chavannes NH, Slats AM, Taube C. Defining asthma-COPD overlap syndrome: a population-based study. Eur Respir J. 2017;49:1602008.
23. Montes De Oca M, Victorina Lopez Varela M, Laucho-Contreras ME, Casas A, Schiavi E, Mora JC. Asthma-COPD overlap syndrome (ACOS) in primary care of four Latin America countries: the PUMA study. BMC Pulmon Med. 2017;17:69.
24. Barczyk A, Maskey-Warzęchowska M, Górska K, Barczyk M, Kuziemski K, Śliwiński P, Batura-Gabryel H, Mróz R, Kania A, Obojski A, Tażbirek M, Celejewska-Wójcik N, Guziejko K, Brajer-Luftmann B, Korzybski D, Damps-Kostańska I, Krenke R. Asthma-COPD overlap—a discordance between patient populations defined by different diagnostic criteria. J Allergy Clin Immunol Pract. 2019;7:2326–36.e5.
25. Krishnan JA, Nibber A, Chisholm A, Price D, Bateman ED, Bjermer L, Van Boven JFM, Brusselle G, Costello RW, Dandurand RJ, Diamant Z, Van Ganse E, Gouder C, Van Kampen SC, Kaplan A, Kocks J, Miravitlles M, Niimi A, Pizzichini E, Rhee CK, Soriano JB, Vogelmeier C, Roman-Rodriguez M, Carter V, D'urzo AD, Roche N. Prevalence and characteristics of asthma-chronic obstructive pulmonary disease overlap in routine primary care practices. Ann Am Thorac Soc. 2019;16:1143–50.
26. Toledo-Pons N, Van Boven JFM, Román-Rodríguez M, Pérez N, Valera Felices JL, Soriano JB, Cosío BG. ACO: time to move from the description of different phenotypes to the treatable traits. PLoS One. 2019;14:e0210915.

27. Kobayashi S, Hanagama M, Yamanda S, Ishida M, Yanai M. Inflammatory biomarkers in asthma-COPD overlap syndrome. Int J Chron Obstruct Pulmon Dis. 2016;11:2117–23.
28. Inoue H, Nagase T, Morita S, Yoshida A, Jinnai T, Ichinose M. Prevalence and characteristics of asthma-COPD overlap syndrome identified by a stepwise approach. Int J Chron Obstruct Pulmon Dis. 2017;12:1803–10.
29. Yamamura K, Hara J, Kobayashi T, Ohkura N, Abo M, Akasaki K, Nomura S, Yuasa M, Saeki K, Terada N, Matsuoka H, Tambo Y, Nishikawa S, Sone T, Kimura H, Kasahara K. The prevalence and clinical features of asthma-COPD overlap (ACO) definitively diagnosed according to the Japanese Respiratory Society Guidelines for the Management of ACO 2018. J Med Investig. 2019;66:157–64.
30. Hashimoto S, Sorimachi R, Jinnai T, Ichinose M. Asthma and chronic obstructive pulmonary disease overlap according to the Japanese respiratory society diagnostic criteria: the prospective, observational aco Japan cohort study. Adv Ther. 2021;38:1168–84.

Chapter 14
Role of FeNO: How Can FeNO Be Positioned in Practice?

Naoya Fujino

Abstract Chronic obstructive pulmonary disease (COPD) is a complex and heterogenous disease, which justifies the need for a precision medicine approach for the improvement of its assessment, treatment and outcomes. One of the treatable traits for airway diseases is "eosinophilic airway inflammation," which can be detected by elevated fractional exhaled nitric oxide (FeNO). NO is generated by inducible NO synthase, which is transcriptionally regulated by type 2 immunity-associated cytokines interleukin (IL)-4 and 13 in airway epithelial cells of asthmatics. Recent international guidelines have employed FeNO testing to support the diagnosis of asthma in combination with respiratory symptoms and pulmonary function tests. The FeNO testing can also be utilized to detect eosinophilic airway inflammation in patients with COPD, who can respond to inhaled corticosteroid therapy. Several studies attempted to provide diagnostic criteria including FeNO. This chapter describes why and how FeNO can be used to detect type 2 airway inflammation in the clinical practice setting, which is one of the characteristics of asthmatic components in asthma-COPD overlap.

Keywords Treatable traits · Eosinophilic airway inflammation · Fractional exhaled nitric oxide · Type 2 immunity

1 Introduction

Chronic obstructive pulmonary disease (COPD) is a complex and heterogeneous disease that consists of several components with nonlinear dynamic interactions. However, not all of these components are present in all subjects [1]. This multilevel

---

N. Fujino (✉)
Department of Respiratory Medicine, Tohoku University Graduate School of Medicine, Sendai, Japan
e-mail: nfujino@med.tohoku.ac.jp

H. Nagase et al. (eds.), *Asthma-COPD Overlap*, Respiratory Disease Series: Diagnostic Tools and Disease Managements,
https://doi.org/10.1007/978-981-96-0217-9_14

(i.e., clinical, functional, structural and biological) and dynamic (i.e., subjected to changes with time) heterogeneity of COPD justifies the need for a precision medicine approach for the improvement of its assessment, treatment and outcomes [2]. Precision medicine is defined as "treatments targeted to the needs of individual patients based on genetic, biomarker, phenotypic or psychosocial characteristics that distinguish a given patient from other patients with similar clinical presentations." Agusti et al. proposed that the identification of "treatable traits" can be applied to a precision medicine strategy for the management of patients with airway diseases such as COPD and asthma [3]. One of the well-characterized treatable traits for airway diseases is "eosinophilic airway inflammation" which can be diagnosed by increased eosinophil counts in blood and sputum and elevated fractional exhaled nitric oxide (FeNO) [4, 5]. Brightling et al. reported that airway obstruction with higher sputum eosinophil counts can be improved by inhaled corticosteroid (ICS) in patients with COPD [6]. They conducted a randomized, double-blind, crossover trial of placebo and mometasone furoate (800 μg/day) for 6 weeks with a 4-week washout period in subjects with COPD treated with bronchodilator therapy only. Although there were no significant improvements in forced expiratory volume in one second (FEV_1), symptoms and sputum characteristics overall, stratification into tertiles by baseline eosinophil counts in induced sputum revealed that the mean change in post-bronchodilator FEV_1 with mometasone compared with placebo in the highest tertile was 0.11 mL (95% confidence interval (CI) 0.03–0.19) [6]. Based on this successful research, much effort has been given to identify the ICS-responsive subset in subjects with COPD, because the improper use of ICS increases the risk of pulmonary infection such as bacterial pneumonia and tuberculosis for COPD patients. The rationale of this chapter is to describe how FeNO can be used to detect type 2 airway inflammation in the clinical practice setting, which is one of the characteristics of asthmatic components in asthma-COPD overlap (ACO).

2 Biology of Nitric Oxide in the Airway

Because the fundamental aspects of exhaled nitric oxide were well reviewed by Alving et al. [7], here I summarize the relevance of FeNO to clinical aspects from the point view of translational science. Originally, in the respiratory tract, NO was thought to be produced by a diverse range of cell types and generated through the oxidation of L-arginine that is catalyzed by three distinct NO synthase (NOS) isozymes: inducible NOS (iNOS), endothelial NOS (eNOS) and neuronal NOS (nNOS) [8]. However, among these NOS isozymes, several studies have supported the idea that iNOS is a main contributor to NO generation in the airway, which is predominantly released by epithelial cells. eNOS and nNOS are recognized as constitutive, calcium-dependent forms that produce femtomolar and picomolar concentrations of NO upon receptor stimulation by selective agonists such as acetylcholine. Meanwhile, NOS is regulated at a transcription level and produces larger quantities of NO at nanomolar concentrations, which may continue in a sustained manner [8].

In lower airways, iNOS appears to be predominantly expressed by epithelial cells in immunohistochemical analyses [9, 10]. This was further confirmed by a randomized, double-blind, placebo-controlled crossover trial using a selective iNOS inhibitor called SC-51, where SC-51 was administered in separate cohorts of healthy volunteers and patients with mild asthma [11]. This demonstrated a complete reduction of FeNO levels in both healthy subjects and asthmatic patients following oral and single administration of SC-51 compared to placebo controls. Taken together with the observational studies and interventional trial, exhaled NO is derived through iNOS from epithelial cells in human airways.

3 The Role of FeNO as an Indicator of Type 2 Inflammation in the Airway of Asthma

In 1993, Alving et al., for the first time, showed that the FeNO levels were increased two-to-three-fold in steroid-naïve asthmatics (range 21–31 parts per billion (ppb), $n = 8$) compared to healthy volunteers (range 5–16 ppb, $n = 12$) [12]. The increased levels of FeNO were warranted by the up-regulated expressions of iNOS mRNA and protein in the airways of asthmatic patients compared to healthy subjects [10, 13–15]. Hamid et al. observed that iNOS protein was more abundant in airway epithelial cells, especially in remaining basal cells after the detachment of columnar cells, representing the loss of epithelial integrity in asthma [13]. iNOS protein expression was also increased in inflammatory cells in induced sputum, and this was significantly correlated with FeNO in corticosteroid-naïve asthmatics ($n = 11$, $r = 0.74$, $P < 0.01$) [14]. Importantly, although iNOS protein expression was also increased in inflammatory cells in induced sputum from COPD patients, this was not correlated with FeNO levels [14]. This provides supportive evidence that FeNO can be used to detect asthma-associated inflammation in the airway and therefore may identify asthmatic components in subjects with COPD. Another question was whether this inflammation-inducible NOS was a target for regulation by corticosteroid treatment. Redington et al. showed that the proportion of iNOS-expressing epithelial cells in the airway was significantly higher in the steroid-naïve asthmatic subjects ($8.6 \pm 1.8\%$, $n = 7$) than either the steroid-treated asthmatics ($3.4 \pm 1.0\%$, $n = 8$, $P = 0.009$) or the non-asthmatic controls ($4.2 \pm 0.9\%$, $n = 10$, $P = 0.018$) [10]. Consistently, FeNO levels were significantly greater in asthmatic patients without corticosteroid treatment than in asthmatics with inhaled corticosteroid therapy [16].

The consequences of exhaled NO in the airway may not be functionally influential in asthma pathogenesis, such as airway obstruction. As discussed above, although the selective iNOS inhibitor completely suppressed FeNO levels, this compound did not change FEV_1 in patients with asthma [11]. However, FeNO is rather a simple, noninvasive and useful tool for the detection of type 2 inflammation in the airway. In fact, the levels of FeNO were significantly correlated with the eosinophil numbers in induced sputum [16], endobronchial biopsies [17] and bronchoalveolar lavage fluid [18] in patients with asthma. These clinical observations suggested that FeNO could be used as a diagnostic marker for eosinophilic airway inflammation. In accordance with these findings, a reduction in the FeNO levels by inhaled steroid administration for 8 weeks (beclomethasone 800 μg/day) in corticosteroid-naïve asthmatic patients was significantly correlated with the improvement of airway hyperresponsiveness (AHR) and FEV_1 [19].

The molecular mechanisms underlying these observations in asthma are now explained by the evidence that type 2 immunity-associated cytokines, interleukin (IL)-4 and IL-13 up-regulate the gene expression of *NOS2* encoding iNOS in airway epithelial cells. IL-4 and IL-13 are able to bind to a cell-surface receptor, IL-4 receptor α subunit, and activate their downstream transcription factor, signal transducer and activator of transcription (STAT)-6 [20]. This evidence firstly originated from in vitro culture assays using primary human airway epithelial cells, in which recombinant IL-4 was able to induce and maintain the iNOS mRNA expression in the presence of recombinant interferon-γ in the culture of human airway epithelial cells [21]. In addition, there are two reports demonstrating IL-13-driven iNOS expression in human airway epithelial cells. Suresh et al. measured gas phase NO concentrations in an air-liquid interface culture system of normal human bronchial epithelial cells with IL-13 for 48 h [22]. Remarkably IL-13 increased NO production by around 100 times from the baseline, which was almost completely suppressed by an iNOS inhibitor in this system [22]. Chibana et al. showed that iNOS mRNA and protein expressions were increased by IL-13 in bronchial epithelial cells derived from not only non-asthmatic subjects but also asthmatic patients [23]. The increased iNOS was functional in the air-liquid interface culture mimicking in vivo settings, because nitrate levels were accordantly elevated by IL-13 treatment [23]. The role of the IL-4- and IL-13-triggered signaling pathways in the elevation of NO production in the airway was confirmed by the IL-4/IL-13 signaling blockade in three independent clinical trials. First, in a double-blind, placebo-controlled trial of nebulized altrakincept (soluble recombinant human IL-4 receptor), 25 patients with moderate atopic asthma were assigned to a single nebulized dose of IL-4R 1500 μg, IL-4R 500 μg or placebo after discontinuation of inhaled corticosteroids [24]. FeNO increased in both the placebo and the low dose of IL-4R groups, but the high-dose group reduced FeNO levels with significant improvements of FEV_1, asthma symptom scores and exacerbations [24]. Second, in a double-blind, placebo-controlled group trial of pitrakinra (an IL-4 variant which has the ability to inhibit the binding of both IL-14 and IL-13 to IL-4Rα complexes), patients with atopic asthma were challenged with inhaled allergens before and after 4 weeks of the treatment [25]. Resting (pre-allergen challenge) FeNO was significantly lower after 4 weeks of inhaled pitrakinra than placebo (34.9 ppb vs 63.1 ppb, treatment difference 23.3 ppb, 95% CI 9.4–47.2, $P = 0.005$). In accordance with the anti-inflammatory effect of inhaled pitrakinra, there was a 4.4% decrease in FEV_1 in the pitrakinra group, whereas the decrease was 15.9% in the placebo group (3.7 times [95% CI 2.08–6.25] lower in the pitrakinra group, $P = 0.0001$) [25]. Third, dupilumab (a fully human monoclonal antibody to the alpha subunit of the IL-4 receptor) for patients with moderate-to-severe asthma reduced FeNO levels in both phase 2 and phase 3 trials [26, 27]. These translational research and clinical trials indicate that exhaled NO is increased by type 2 immunity-associated cytokines IL-4 and IL-13, and FeNO could be a biomarker for detecting eosinophilic or type 2 inflammation in the airway.

4 The Utility of FeNO Testing for the Diagnosis and Management of Asthma

Based on the basic and translational research that shed light on the fundamental role of FeNO in the detection of type 2 airway inflammation, great efforts have been made to apply FeNO testing to the diagnosis of asthma in the setting of clinical practice. Four studies reported the sensitivity and specificity of FeNO in detecting 3% or more eosinophils in induced sputum, which indicates a hallmark of eosinophilic airway inflammation (Table 14.1). However, because these studies included heterogeneous patients, especially those receiving ICS (even high doses) that reduced FeNO values [28–31], the sensitivity and specificity were around 60–70%. In 2011, Matsunaga et al. reported optimal FeNO cut-off values to support the diagnosis of asthma [32]. In this study, FeNO values were measured in 142 corticosteroid-naïve patients with asthma and 224 non-asthmatic subjects, where asthma was diagnosed by the presence of airway reversibility or airway hyperresponsiveness. The receiver operating characteristics curves indicated that 22 ppb of FeNO was the optimal cut-off value with the highest combination of 90.8% sensitivity and 83.9% specificity with 0.896 of the area under the curve. In addition, the normal upper limit for healthy individuals, 37 ppb, had a 52% sensitivity and 99% specificity for the diagnosis of asthma [32, 33]. Based on these multicenter observational studies for Japanese subjects, if patients who have symptoms suggestive of asthma without receiving ICS have FeNO values of 22 ppb or more, asthma diagnosis is likely. If the FeNO value is more than 35 ppb, it is almost certain that the diagnosis of asthma can be made [34]. In addition, the comorbidity of allergic rhinitis and the smoking history affected the FeNO values: patients with rhinitis showed higher levels of FeNO compared with subjects without rhinitis, and the FeNO values were lower for current smokers than for non-smokers in both controls and asthmatics.

Recent guidelines in the US (the National Asthma Education and Prevention Program Coordinating Committee (NAEPPCC) in 2020 [35]), the UK (National Institute for Health and Care Excellence (NICE) guideline [36]) and Japan (Japanese Respiratory Society (JRS) guideline [34]) have addressed key questions regarding the utility of FeNO for asthma diagnosis, management and prognosis (Table 14.2). The NAEPPCC guideline recommends the addition of FeNO measurement as an adjunct to the evaluation process in individuals aged 5 years and older for whom the diagnosis of asthma is uncertain using history, clinical findings, clinical course and spirometry, including bronchodilator responsiveness testing, or in whom spirometry cannot be performed. The expert panel has also stated that FeNO test results should

Table 14.1 Clinical studies reporting FeNO values to detect 3% or more eosinophils in induced sputum

References	Patient characteristics	Asthma diagnosis/severity	Device (an exhalation flow late)	Cut-off values to detect >3% sputum eosinophils
Berry et al. [28]	Total number, 556 Female, 57% Smokers, 31% ICS user, 56% Atopy, 51% FEV_1%pred 85%	Airway hyperresponsiveness and/or airflow variability. Stable with symptoms	LR2000 (250 mL/s)	8.3 ppb (sensitivity 71%, specificity 72%, AUC 0.77 [95% CI 0.73–0.82] in non-smokers
Schleich et al. [29]	Total number, 295 Female, 56% Smokers, 20% ICS user, 76% Atopy, 71% FEV_1%pred 86%	Symptoms Airway hyperresponsiveness and/or airflow variability.	NIOX (50 mL/s)	41 ppb (sensitivity 65%, specificity 79%, AUC 0.78)
Hastie et al. [30]	Total number, 238	Mild-to-severe asthma, nonsmoking subjects (<5 pack years) who met American Thoracic Society criteria for the diagnosis of asthma	N.D.	30 ppb (sensitivity 65%, specificity 64%, AUC 0.71)
Westerhof, et al. [31]	Total number, 336 Female, 16% Smokers, 16% Atopy, 10% FEV_1%pred 97%	Adult-onset asthma. Patients aged >18 years were eligible if they had a confirmed diagnosis of asthma based on international guidelines (history of variable respiratory symptoms and documented variable expiratory airflow limitation)	NIOX (50 mL/s)	12.2 ppb (sensitivity 96%, specificity 28%), 64.5 ppb (sensitivity 39%, specificity 95%), AUC 0.82

ICS Inhaled corticosteroids, *FEV_1%pred* Forced expiratory volume in 1 second % predicted, *N.D.* Not described

not be used alone to diagnose asthma and that FeNO measurements can serve as an adjunct test that may aid in diagnosing asthma in the appropriate setting. In this guideline, the interpretation of FeNO test results for asthma diagnosis in nonsmoking individuals not receiving corticosteroids is applied from the official American Thoracic Society guideline [37] (Table 14.2). In the NICE guideline, the FeNO test is recommended to adults (aged 17 and over) if a diagnosis of asthma is being considered, where 40 ppb of a FeNO level is regarded as a positive test [36]. Compared to the NAEPPCC guideline, the NICE guideline interprets FeNO results for asthma diagnosis in combination with other clinical tests indicating bronchodilator reversibility or bronchial hyperreactivity.

Table 14.2 Summary of the interpretations of FeNO test results for the diagnosis of asthma in clinical practice

Guidelines	Ranges of FeNO levels supporting asthma diagnosis	Interpretations
NAEPPCC [35] (according to the ATS guideline [37])	>50 ppb (>35 in children aged 5–12 years)	• Eosinophilic airway inflammation likely • Phenotype more likely to respond to ICS • Allergic asthma • Eosinophilic bronchitis
NICE [36]	• Positive reversible airflow obstruction & >40 ppb (adults aged 17 and over) • Positive variability in peak flow readings & >40 ppb (adults aged 17 and over)	Asthma diagnosis
JRS [34]	1. >22 ppb in ICS-naïve cases showing symptoms suggestive of asthma 2. >35 ppb in ICS-naïve patients showing symptoms suggestive of asthma.	1. Asthma diagnosis is likely 2. Asthma diagnosis is almost certain

NAEPPCC The National Asthma Education and Prevention Program Coordinating Committee, *ATS* American Thoracic Society, *ppb* parts per billion, *ICS* Inhaled corticosteroids, *NICE* National Institute for Health and Care Excellence, *JRS* Japanese Respiratory Society

As discussed above, although it has been widely recognized that FeNO is a useful test to support the diagnosis of asthma, recent studies have shown that FeNO may be used to predict FEV_1 decline and a treatment response in asthmatics. A three-year prospective study that examined the changes in FEV_1 and FeNO in 140 patients with mild-to-moderate, controlled asthma demonstrated that a FeNO level >40.3 ppb yielded 43% sensitivity and 86% specificity for identifying patients with a rapid decline in FEV_1 (42.7 ± 37.5 mL (FeNO >40 ppb) vs 16.7 ± 31.5 mL (FeNO <40 ppb), mean ± standard deviation) [38]. A prospective 5-year follow-up study in 200 adults with newly diagnosed asthma demonstrated that a FeNO level ≥57 ppb was independently associated with a decline in FEV_1 (a change in FEV_1 of −37.8 mL per year) [39]. In addition to the prediction of lung function decline, FeNO can be a marker to identify a subset of asthmatic patients who have a better response to anti-inflammatory therapies, including biologics. Clinical trials indicated that the effects of omalizumab [40] and dupilumab [27] on a decrease in exacerbations were more evident in patients with high FeNO values. A meta-analysis including seven adult clinical studies was conducted to evaluate the efficacy of tailoring asthma interventions based on FeNO in comparison to clinical symptoms-based management [41]. In this meta-analysis, there was a significant difference in exacerbations between the groups, favoring the FeNO group (odds ratio 0.60, 95% CI 0.43–0.84).

5 The Aspect of ICS in the Context of Airway Infection of Patients with COPD

It has been widely recognized that patients with COPD have a higher risk of pulmonary infection compared to non-COPD subjects. A case-control study performed in Spain, including 859,033 subjects, showed a significant relationship between COPD and community-acquired pneumonia, which was independent of other clinical factors such as cigarette smoking, sudden temperature changes at work, contact with children, civil status, previous hospitalization, history of upper respiratory tract infection, chronic bronchitis, asthma, epilepsy, oxygen therapy and use of inhaler with or without plastic pear-spacers (OR 1.84 [95% CI, 1.32–2.59]) [42]. A prospective case-control study with more than 170,000 COPD subjects conducted in Canada also demonstrated that current use of ICS increased the risk of hospitalization for pneumonia (rate ratio (RR) 1.70 [95% CI, 1.63–1.77]) and pneumonia followed by death within 30 days (RR 1.53 [95% CI, 1.30–1.80]) [43]. The risk of hospitalization for pneumonia was highest in a group with high doses of ICS equivalent to fluticasone at 1000 μg/day or more (RR 2.25 [95% CI, 2.07–2.44]). Among ICS users in COPD subjects, a subset who had both less than 100 cells/μL of blood eosinophils and chronic bronchial infection by potentially pathogenic microorganisms (PPM) was at higher risk of pneumonia (OR 3.238 [95% CI, 1.426–7.231]), where the following bacteria were considered as PPM: *Haemophilus influenzae, Streptococcus pneumoniae, Moraxella catarrhalis, Haemophilus parainfluenzae, Staphylococcus aureus, Pseudomonas aeruginosa, Klebsiella pneumoniae, and other gram-negative rods* [44]. The current use of ICS in subjects even without oral corticosteroid also increased the risk of tuberculosis (TB) in a low-prevalence country (RR 1.33 [95% CI, 1.04–1.71]) [45] as well as in an intermediate-burden setting (OR 1.20 [95% CI 1.08–1.34]) [46]. In addition, the increased risk of TB infection was significantly associated with higher doses of ICS (RR 1.97 [95% CI 1.18–3.30] [45]; OR 2.14 [95% CI 1.71–2.66] [46]). These studies highlighted the importance of the risk of pulmonary infection in COPD patients who are treated with ICS (especially high doses) and therefore treatment with ICS may not be recommended to all COPD patients. This provides the clinically relevant question to address which subset of COPD subjects would benefit from ICS therapy.

6 The Role of FeNO to Detect ICS-Responsive Phenotypes in COPD

In 1998 and 1999, it was recognized that FeNO levels could be increased in at least a subset in COPD patients [47, 48]. This subset was later reported to have the reversibility of airflow limitation to salbutamol and therefore exhibited asthma-like features in patients with COPD [49]. This discovery addressed how the differential diagnosis of patients aged 40 or over with respiratory symptoms should be made. This was because COPD was becoming more common in older adults and distinguishing between asthma with persistent airflow obstruction and COPD was problematic [50, 51]. From 2007 onward, asthmatic components were widely known to possibly exist in patients with COPD. In 2007, *Canadian Thoracic Society recommendations for management of chronic obstructive pulmonary disease—2007 update* first provided a description of "combined COPD and asthma" to support the idea that ICS could be used to COPD patients if the COPD patients had evident features of asthma [52]. In 2009, Gibson and Simpson described "the overlap syndrome of asthma and COPD" and noted that, since these patients had been largely excluded from clinical trials for both asthma and COPD, their diagnosis and treatment were poorly defined and lacking evidence [53].

Because retrospective studies consistently suggested that patients with both asthma and COPD had worse respiratory symptoms [54], higher frequency of exacerbations [54, 55] and more rapid decline in FEV_1 [56], there have been researches to ask whether FeNO can be used to identify asthma-related components representing favorable ICS responses for COPD patients. Five clinical studies demonstrated that FeNO levels at baseline were significantly correlated with the improvement of airway obstruction after ICS treatment [57–61] (Table 14.3). Importantly this correlation was observed in ex-smokers but not in current smokers, indicating that clinicians should pay attention to the interpretation of FeNO values in smoking COPD patients. Although these studies supported the utility of FeNO testing in clinical practice to discriminate ACO from COPD without asthmatic components, a FeNO cut-off value to identify an ICS-responsive subset of COPD patients has been still unclear [62]. Recent clinical studies confirmed the high accuracy of FeNO testing for the diagnosis to discriminate ACO from COPD without asthmatic features [63–67] (Table 14.4).

7 Application of FeNO Measurement to Diagnostic Criteria for ACO

To maximize the benefits of ICS, which include its anti-inflammatory effects for COPD patients, while avoiding pulmonary infection related to its inappropriate use, a combination of several biomarkers may be promising for precisely defining an ICS-responsive subset in COPD. Based on this concept, Akamatsu et al. sought to determine whether the combination of FeNO and serum IgE discriminated ICS-responsive ACO from COPD without asthmatic features. All of the patients who had both FeNO >35 ppb and a positive result for specific IgE (atopy+) showed reversibility of airway obstruction to 12-week inhalation therapy of fluticasone propionate (FP)/Salmeterol (SAL) [60]. In addition, no patients with both less than 35 ppb of FeNO and a negative result of specific IgE responded to FP/SAL. Tamada et al.

Table 14.3 Studies showing an association of increased FeNO levels with the improvement of airway obstruction by inhaled corticosteroids in patients with COPD

References	Subject numbers	Lung function/ severity	Doses and duration of inhaled corticosteroids	Results
Zietkowski et al. [57]	COPD 47 (current smoker 28, ex-smoker 19) Healthy control 40 (current smoker 17, non-smoker 23)	Post-bronchodilator FEV_1 47.07 ± 14.55% (smoking COPD), 48.9 ± 15.3% (ex-smoking COPD) FEV_1 95.47 ± 6.1% (smoking control), 108.71 ± 10.78% (non-smoking control)	Budesoide 800 μg/day, 8 weeks	A statistically significant correlation between initial FeNO levels and postbronchodilator FEV_1 (% predicted) was observed in the group of ex-smokers COPD patients ($r = 0{:}47$; $P = 0{:}04$), but not in currently smoking COPD patients ($r = 0{:}27$; $P = 0{:}15$)
Kunisaki et al. [58]	COPD 60 (all ex-smokers)	Pre-bronchodilator FEV_1 35.6 ± 10.6%	Fluticasone propionate 500 μg + Salmeterol 50 μg, twice daily, 4 weeks	ICS responders (increase in FEV_1 >200 mL after 4 weeks ICS) have higher baseline FeNO (46.5 ppb vs 25.0 ppb)
Lehtimaki et al. [59]	COPD 40 (current smoker 29, ex-smoker 11)	Post-bronchodilator FEV_1 64.6 ± 2.7% (smoking COPD), 53.3 ± 4.8% (ex-smoking COPD)	Fluticasone propionate 500 μg/day, 4 weeks	Baseline FeNO was positively correlated with changes in FEV_1/FVC ($r = 0.334$, $P = 0.038$): ex-smokers ($r = 0.621$, $P = 0.042$), current smokers ($r = 0.152$, $P = 0.432$).
Akamatsu et al. [60]	COPD 14 (all ex-smokers)	Post-bronchodilator FEV_1 57.6 ± 4.4%	Fluticasone propionate 250 μg + Salmeterol 50 μg, twice daily, 12 weeks	FeNO >35 ppb and IgE positive was correlated with airway obstruction improvement evaluated by FEV_1 (>200 mL).
Yamaji et al. [61]	COPD 44 (all ex-smokers)	FEV_1 1.80 ± 0.40 (L), GOLD stage 1/2/3/4, n = 0/34/9/0	Ciclesonide 400 μg/day, 12 weeks	Baseline FeNO was positively correlated with changes in FEV_1 and correlated with the improvement of COPD assessment test score.

FEV_1 Forced expiratory volume in one second, *FeNO* Fractional exhaled nitric oxide, *ICS* Inhaled corticosteroids

further reported that the prevalence of expected high ICS responders (i.e. FeNO >35 ppb and atopy+) was 7.8% of Japanese COPD subjects, whereas that of patients who were not likely given the benefits of ICS (i.e. FeNO ≤35 ppb and atopy−) was 54.8% [68]. These clinical proof-of-concept studies may explain that a combination of biomarkers related to type 2 inflammation could be useful for a more precise

Table 14.4 Studies reporting FeNO cut-off values to diagnose ACO

Reference	ACO patient numbers	Definition of asthmatic features	FeNO values
Alcazar-Navarrete B, et al. [63]	$N = 22$ ICS 72.7% Current smoke 22.7%	One of the major criteria or two of the minor criteria Major criteria • Previous history of asthma/wheezing outside chest infections • A documented very positive bronchodilator test (>14% and >400 mL) Minor criteria • Blood eosinophil count >3% • IgE levels >100 UI/L • 2 documented positive bronchodilator tests with >12% or 200 mL gain in FEV1 • Atopy or previous history of sensibilization to allergens demonstrated by positive skin prick test or specific IgE to allergens	19 ppb Sensitivity 0.68 Specificity 0.75 AUC 0.79
Goto, et al. [64]	$N = 48$ ICS 5% Current smoke 48%	One of the major criteria or two of the minor criteria Major criteria • History of asthma • Bronchodilator response of >15% and 400 mL Minor criteria • History of hay fever • Bronchodilator responses to salbutamol of >12% and 200 mL • Blood eosinophils >5%	AUC 0.63
Chen, et al. [65]	$N = 57$ Smoking history 40.4%	Positive bronchodilator test with >12% and 200 mL gain in FEV_1, and presence of clinical characteristics of asthma (previous history of asthma/wheezing).	22.5 ppb Sensitivity 0.70 Specificity 0.75 AUC 0.78
Takayama, et al. [66]	$N = 56$ ICS 41.1% Current smoke 21.4%	According to syndromic and spirometric features of the ACO from the GINA/GOLD joint document [70]	25.0 ppb Sensitivity 0.61 Specificity 0.88 AUC 0.73 for corticosteroid-naïve patients
Guo, et al. [67]	$N = 53$	Two primary criteria or one primary and two secondary criteria Primary criteria • Strong positive bronchial dilation test (BDT) in patients with COPD (FEV_1 improved >400 mL, improvement rate >15%) • Increased sputum eosinophilia Secondary criteria • Elevated total serum IgE • History of allergies • Positive BDTs (FEV1 improved >200 mL, improvement rate >12%) on ≥2 occasions	25.5 ppb Sensitivity 0.74 Specificity 0.77 AUC 0.815

definition of ACO. Given this concept, in 2018 the Japanese Respiratory Society (JRS) issued guidelines for new definitions and diagnostic criteria of ACO [69]. It is noteworthy that these two biomarkers (FeNO and IgE) were included in the criteria to identify the features of asthma among COPD subjects.

References

1. Faner R, Agustí Á. Multilevel, dynamic chronic obstructive pulmonary disease heterogeneity. A challenge for personalized medicine. Ann Am Thorac Soc. 2016;13:S466–70.
2. Agustí A, Antó JM, Auffray C, et al. Personalized respiratory medicine: exploring the horizon, addressing the issues. Summary of a BRN-AJRCCM Workshop Held in Barcelona on June 12, 2014. Am J Respir Crit Care Med. 2015;191:391–401.
3. Agusti A, Bel E, Thomas M, et al. Treatable traits: toward precision medicine of chronic airway diseases. Eur Respir J. 2016;47:410–9.
4. Zhang X-Y, Simpson JL, Powell H, et al. Full blood count parameters for the detection of asthma inflammatory phenotypes. Clin Exp Allergy. 2014;44:1137–45.
5. Wagener AH, de Nijs SB, Lutter R, Sousa AR, Weersink EJM, Bel EH, Sterk PJ. External validation of blood eosinophils, FENO and serum periostin as surrogates for sputum eosinophils in asthma. Thorax. 2015;70:115.
6. Brightling CE, McKenna S, Hargadon B, et al. Sputum eosinophilia and the short term response to inhaled mometasone in chronic obstructive pulmonary disease. Thorax. 2005;60:193–8.
7. Alving K, Malinovschi A. Basic aspects of exhaled nitric oxide; 2010. p. 1–31.
8. Ricciardolo FLM, Sterk PJ, Gaston B, Folkerts G. Nitric oxide in health and disease of the respiratory system. Physiol Rev. 2004;84:731–65.
9. Guo FH, Raeve HRD, Rice TW, Stuehr DJ, Thunnissen FB, Erzurum SC. Continuous nitric oxide synthesis by inducible nitric oxide synthase in normal human airway epithelium in vivo. Proc Natl Acad Sci U S A. 1995;92:7809–13.
10. Redington AE, Meng QH, Springall DR, Evans TJ, Créminon C, Maclouf J, Holgate ST, Howarth PH, Polak JM. Increased expression of inducible nitric oxide synthase and cyclo-oxygenase-2 in the airway epithelium of asthmatic subjects and regulation by corticosteroid treatment. Thorax. 2001;56:351–7.
11. Hansel TT, Kharitonov SA, Donnelly LE, Erin EM, Currie MG, Moore WM, Manning PT, Recker DP, Barnes PJ. A selective inhibitor of inducible nitric oxide synthase inhibits exhaled breath nitric oxide in healthy volunteers and asthmatics. FASEB J. 2003;17:1298–300.
12. Alving K, Weitzberg E, Lundberg JM. Increased amount of nitric oxide in exhaled air of asthmatics. Eur Respir J. 1993;6:1368–70.
13. Hamid Q, Springall DR, Polak J, Riveros-Moreno V, Chanez P, Bousquet J, Godard P, Holgate S, Howarth P, Redington A. Induction of nitric oxide synthase in asthma. Lancet. 1993;342:1510–3.
14. Ichinose M, Sugiura H, Yamagata S, Koarai A, Shirato K. Increase in reactive nitrogen species production in chronic obstructive pulmonary disease airways. Am J Respir Crit Care Med. 2000;162:701–6.
15. Guo FH, Comhair SAA, Zheng S, Dweik RA, Eissa NT, Thomassen MJ, Calhoun W, Erzurum SC. Molecular mechanisms of increased nitric oxide (NO) In asthma: evidence for transcriptional and post-translational regulation of NO synthesis. J Immunol. 2000;164:5970–80.
16. Berlyne GS, Parameswaran K, Kamada D, Efthimiadis A, Hargreave FE. A comparison of exhaled nitric oxide and induced sputum as markers of airway inflammation. J Allergy Clin Immunol. 2000;106:638–44.

17. Payne DN, Adcock IM, Wilson NM, Oates T, Scallan M, Bush A. Relationship between exhaled nitric oxide and mucosal eosinophilic inflammation in children with difficult asthma, after treatment with oral prednisolone. Am J Respir Crit Care Med. 2001;164:1376–81.
18. Warke TJ, Fitch PS, Brown V, Taylor R, Lyons JDM, Ennis M, Shields MD. Exhaled nitric oxide correlates with airway eosinophils in childhood asthma. Thorax. 2002;57:383–7.
19. Ichinose M, Takahashi T, Sugiura H, Endoh N, Miura M, Mashito Y, Shirato K. Baseline airway hyperresponsiveness and its reversible component: role of airway inflammation and airway calibre. Eur Respir J. 2000;15:248–53.
20. Hershey GKK. IL-13 receptors and signaling pathways: an evolving web. J Allergy Clin Immunol. 2003;111:677–90.
21. Guo FH, Uetani K, Haque SJ, Williams BR, Dweik RA, Thunnissen FB, Calhoun W, Erzurum SC. Interferon gamma and interleukin 4 stimulate prolonged expression of inducible nitric oxide synthase in human airway epithelium through synthesis of soluble mediators. J Clin Invest. 1997;100:829–38.
22. Suresh V, Mih JD, George SC. Measurement of IL-13–induced iNOS-derived gas phase nitric oxide in human bronchial epithelial cells. Am J Respir Cell Mol Biol. 2007;37:97–104.
23. Chibana K, Trudeau JB, Mustovich AT, Mustovitch AT, Hu H, Zhao J, Balzar S, Chu HW, Wenzel SE. IL-13 induced increases in nitrite levels are primarily driven by increases in inducible nitric oxide synthase as compared with effects on arginases in human primary bronchial epithelial cells. Clin Exp Allergy. 2008;38:936–46.
24. Borish LC, Nelson HS, Lanz MJ, Claussen L, Whitmore JB, Agosti JM, Garrison L. Interleukin-4 receptor in moderate atopic asthma. Am J Respir Crit Care Med. 1999;160:1816–23.
25. Wenzel S, Wilbraham D, Fuller R, Getz EB, Longphre M. Effect of an interleukin-4 variant on late phase asthmatic response to allergen challenge in asthmatic patients: results of two phase 2a studies. Lancet. 2007;370:1422–31.
26. Wenzel S, Ford L, Pearlman D, et al. Dupilumab in persistent asthma with elevated eosinophil levels. N Engl J Med. 2013;368:2455–66.
27. Castro M, Corren J, Pavord ID, et al. Dupilumab efficacy and safety in moderate-to-severe uncontrolled asthma. N Engl J Med. 2018;378:2486–96.
28. Berry MA, Shaw DE, Green RH, Brightling CE, Wardlaw AJ, Pavord ID. The use of exhaled nitric oxide concentration to identify eosinophilic airway inflammation: an observational study in adults with asthma. Clin Exp Allergy. 2005;35:1175–9.
29. Schleich FN, Seidel L, Sele J, Manise M, Quaedvlieg V, Michils A, Louis R. Exhaled nitric oxide thresholds associated with a sputum eosinophil count ≥3% in a cohort of unselected patients with asthma. Thorax. 2010;65:1039.
30. Hastie AT, Moore WC, Li H, Rector BM, Ortega VE, Pascual RM, Peters SP, Meyers DA, Bleecker ER, Program NH Lung, and Blood Institute's Severe Asthma Research. Biomarker surrogates do not accurately predict sputum eosinophil and neutrophil percentages in asthmatic subjects. J Allergy Clin Immunol. 2013;132:72–80.e12.
31. Westerhof GA, Korevaar DA, Amelink M, de Nijs SB, de Groot JC, Wang J, Weersink EJ, ten Brinke A, Bossuyt PM, Bel EH. Biomarkers to identify sputum eosinophilia in different adult asthma phenotypes. Eur Respir J. 2015;46:688–96.
32. Matsunaga K, Hirano T, Akamatsu K, Koarai A, Sugiura H, Minakata Y, Ichinose M. Exhaled nitric oxide cutoff values for asthma diagnosis according to rhinitis and smoking status in Japanese subjects. Allergol Int. 2011;60:331–6.
33. Matsunaga K, Hirano T, Kawayama T, Tsuburai T, Nagase H, Aizawa H, Akiyama K, Ohta K, Ichinose M. Reference ranges for exhaled nitric oxide fraction in healthy Japanese adult population. Allergol Int. 2010;59:363–7.
34. Matsunaga K, Kuwahira I, Hanaoka M, Saito J, Tsuburai T, Fukunaga K, Matsumoto H, Sugiura H, Ichinose M, Physiology JRSA on P. An official JRS statement: the principles of fractional exhaled nitric oxide (FeNO) measurement and interpretation of the results in clinical practice. Respir Investig. 2021;59:34–52.

35. (NAEPPCC) EPWG of the NH Lung, and Blood Institute (NHLBI) administered and coordinated National Asthma Education and Prevention Program Coordinating Committee, Cloutier MM, Baptist AP, et al. 2020 Focused updates to the asthma management guidelines: a report from the National Asthma Education and Prevention Program Coordinating Committee Expert Panel Working Group. J Allergy Clin Immunol. 2020;146:1217–70.
36. Asthma: diagnosis, monitoring and chronic asthma management. https://www.nice.org.uk/guidance/ng245
37. Dweik RA, Boggs PB, Erzurum SC, Irvin CG, Leigh MW, Lundberg JO, Olin A-C, Plummer AL, Taylor DR, Applications on behalf of the ATSC on I of ENOL (FeNO) for C. An official ATS clinical practice guideline: interpretation of exhaled nitric oxide levels (FeNO) for clinical applications. Am J Respir Crit Care Med. 2011;184:602–15.
38. Matsunaga K, Hirano T, Oka A, Ito K, Edakuni N. Persistently high exhaled nitric oxide and loss of lung function in controlled asthma. Allergol Int. 2016;65:266–71.
39. Coumou H, Westerhof GA, de Nijs SB, Zwinderman AH, Bel EH. Predictors of accelerated decline in lung function in adult-onset asthma. Eur Respir J. 2018;51:1701785.
40. Hanania NA, Wenzel S, Rosén K, Hsieh H-J, Mosesova S, Choy DF, Lal P, Arron JR, Harris JM, Busse W. Exploring the effects of omalizumab in allergic asthma. Am J Respir Crit Care Med. 2013;187:804–11.
41. Petsky HL, Kew KM, Turner C, Chang AB. Exhaled nitric oxide levels to guide treatment for adults with asthma. Cochrane Database Syst Rev. 2016;2016:CD011440.
42. Almirall J, Bolíbar I, Serra-Prat M, et al. New evidence of risk factors for community-acquired pneumonia: a population-based study. Eur Respir J. 2008;31:1274–84.
43. Ernst P, Gonzalez AV, Brassard P, Suissa S. Inhaled corticosteroid use in chronic obstructive pulmonary disease and the risk of hospitalization for pneumonia. Am J Respir Crit Care Med. 2007;176:162–6.
44. Martinez-Garcia MA, Faner R, Oscullo G, de la Rosa D, Soler-Cataluña J-J, Ballester M, Agusti A. Inhaled steroids, circulating eosinophils, chronic airway infection, and pneumonia risk in chronic obstructive pulmonary disease. a network analysis. Am J Respir Crit Care Med. 2020;201:1078–85.
45. Brassard P, Suissa S, Kezouh A, Ernst P. Inhaled corticosteroids and risk of tuberculosis in patients with respiratory diseases. Am J Respir Crit Care Med. 2012;183:675–8.
46. Lee C-H, Kim K, Hyun MK, Jang EJ, Lee NR, Yim J-J. Use of inhaled corticosteroids and the risk of tuberculosis. Thorax. 2013;68:1105.
47. Maziak W, Loukides S, Culpitt S, Sullivan P, Kharitonov SA, Barnes PJ. Exhaled nitric oxide in chronic obstructive pulmonary disease. Am J Respir Crit Care Med. 1998;157:998–1002.
48. Corradi M, Majori M, Cacciani GC, Consigli GF, de'Munari E, Pesci A. Increased exhaled nitric oxide in patients with stable chronic obstructive pulmonary disease. Thorax. 1999;54:572.
49. Papi A, Romagnoli M, Baraldo S, Braccioni F, Guzzinati I, Saetta M, Ciaccia A, Fabbri LM. Partial reversibility of airflow limitation and increased exhaled NO and sputum eosinophilia in chronic obstructive pulmonary disease. Am J Respir Crit Care Med. 2000;162:1773–7.
50. van Schayck CP, Levy ML, Chen JC, Isonaka S, Halbert RJ. Coordinated diagnostic approach for adult obstructive lung disease in primary care. Prim Care Respir J. 2004;13:218–21.
51. Guerra S, Sherrill DL, Kurzius-Spencer M, Venker C, Halonen M, Quan SF, Martinez FD. The course of persistent airflow limitation in subjects with and without asthma. Respir Med. 2008;102:1473–82.
52. Denis EO, Shawn A, Jean B, et al. Canadian thoracic society recommendations for management of chronic obstructive pulmonary disease—2007 update. Can Respir J. 2007;14:5B–32B.
53. Gibson PG, Simpson JL. The overlap syndrome of asthma and COPD: what are its features and how important is it? Thorax. 2009;64:728.
54. Miravitlles M, Soriano JB, Ancochea J, Muñoz L, Duran-Tauleria E, Sánchez G, Sobradillo V, García-Río F. Characterisation of the overlap COPD–asthma phenotype. Focus on physical activity and health status. Respir Med. 2013;107:1053–60.

55. Menezes AMB, de Oca MM, Pérez-Padilla R, et al. Increased risk of exacerbation and hospitalization in subjects with an overlap phenotype COPD-asthma. Chest. 2014;145:297–304.
56. Silva GE, Sherrill DL, Guerra S, Barbee RA. Asthma as a risk factor for COPD in a longitudinal study. Chest. 2004;126:59–65.
57. Zietkowski Z, Kucharewicz I, Bodzenta-Lukaszyk A. The influence of inhaled corticosteroids on exhaled nitric oxide in stable chronic obstructive pulmonary disease. Respir Med. 2005;99:816–24.
58. Kunisaki KM, Rice KL, Janoff EN, Rector TS, Niewoehner DE. Exhaled nitric oxide, systemic inflammation, and the spirometric response to inhaled fluticasone propionate in severe chronic obstructive pulmonary disease: a prospective study. Ther Adv Respir Dis. 2008;2:55–64.
59. Lehtimaki L, Kankaanranta H, Saarelainen S, Annila I, Aine T, Nieminen R, Moilanen E. Bronchial nitric oxide is related to symptom relief during fluticasone treatment in COPD. Eur Respir J. 2009;35:72–8.
60. Akamatsu K, Matsunaga K, Sugiura H, Koarai A, Hirano T, Minakata Y, Ichinose M. Improvement of airflow limitation by fluticasone propionate/salmeterol in chronic obstructive pulmonary disease: what is the specific marker? Front Pharmacol. 2011;2:36.
61. Yamaji Y, Oishi K, Hamada K, et al. Detection of type2 biomarkers for response in COPD. J Breath Res. 2020;14:026007.
62. Mostafavi-Pour-Manshadi S-M-Y, Naderi N, Barrecheguren M, Dehghan A, Bourbeau J. Investigating fractional exhaled nitric oxide in chronic obstructive pulmonary disease (COPD) and asthma-COPD overlap (ACO): a scoping review. COPD. 2018;15:1–15.
63. Alcázar-Navarrete B, Romero-Palacios PJ, Ruiz-Sancho A, Ruiz-Rodriguez O. Diagnostic performance of the measurement of nitric oxide in exhaled air in the diagnosis of COPD phenotypes. Nitric Oxide. 2016;54:67–72.
64. Goto T, Camargo CA, Hasegawa K. Fractional exhaled nitric oxide levels in asthma–COPD overlap syndrome: analysis of the National Health and Nutrition Examination Survey, 2007–2012. Int J Chron Obstruct Pulmon Dis. 2016;11:2149–55.
65. Chen F, Huang X, Liu Y, Lin G, Xie C. Importance of fractional exhaled nitric oxide in the differentiation of asthma–COPD overlap syndrome, asthma, and COPD. Int J Chron Obstruct Pulmon Dis. 2016;11:2385–90.
66. Takayama Y, Ohnishi H, Ogasawara F, Oyama K, Kubota T, Yokoyama A. Clinical utility of fractional exhaled nitric oxide and blood eosinophils counts in the diagnosis of asthma-COPD overlap. Int J Chron Obstruct Pulmon Dis. 2018;13:2525–32.
67. Guo Y, Hong C, Liu Y, Chen H, Huang X, Hong M. Diagnostic value of fractional exhaled nitric oxide for asthma-chronic obstructive pulmonary disease overlap syndrome. Medicine. 2018;97:e10857.
68. Tamada T, Sugiura H, Takahashi T, Matsunaga K, Kimura K, Katsumata U, Takekoshi D, Kikuchi T, Ohta K, Ichinose M. Biomarker-based detection of asthma–COPD overlap syndrome in COPD populations. Int J Chron Obstruct Pulmon Dis. 2015;10:2169–76.
69. Yanagisawa S, Ichinose M. Definition and diagnosis of asthma–COPD overlap (ACO). Allergol Int. 2018;67(2):172–8.
70. 2015 Asthma COPD and Asthma—COPD Overlap Syndrome (ACOS). https://goldcopd.org/wpcontent/uploads/2016/04/GOLD_ACOS_2015.pdf

Chapter 15
Role of IgE and Eosinophils: The Use of Type 2 Biomarkers in Practice

Hiroyuki Nagase and Hikaru Toyota

Abstract Most patients with asthma and some patients with chronic obstructive pulmonary disease (COPD) demonstrate the features of type 2 inflammation. The association between eosinophils and pathophysiology is less clear in COPD than in asthma, but eosinophil testing in COPD is important to determine patients with response to steroids, and a blood eosinophil count of 300/μl is listed as an item in the guidelines for asthma–COPD overlap (ACO).

Allergic sensitization is related to increased symptoms and risk of exacerbations in COPD, and some guidelines for ACO have introduced immunoglobulin E (IgE) into the diagnostic criteria. We comprehensively compared the positivity of specific IgE between ACO and non-ACO COPD, and only the positivity for house dust and *Dermatophagoides pteronyssinus* was significantly higher in ACO, indicating the specifically important role of mite-specific IgE in diagnosing ACO among COPD.

This chapter discusses the role of eosinophils and IgE in the diagnosis and treatment of ACO.

Keywords Asthma–COPD overlap · *Dermatophagoides pteronyssinus*
Eosinophils · IgE

1 Introduction

The concept of asthma–chronic obstructive pulmonary disease (COPD) overlap (ACO) was introduced in the early 2010s, and various diagnostic criteria have been proposed [1]. However, the recognition of treatable traits in chronic airway diseases has been emphasized [2], and ACO was not defined according to the latest GOLD document [3].

H. Nagase (✉) · H. Toyota
Division of Respiratory Medicine and Allergology, Department of Medicine, Teikyo University School of Medicine, Tokyo, Japan
e-mail: nagaseh@med.teikyo-u.ac.jp

H. Nagase et al. (eds.), *Asthma-COPD Overlap*, Respiratory Disease Series: Diagnostic Tools and Disease Managements,
https://doi.org/10.1007/978-981-96-0217-9_15

However, cluster analysis based on transcription factors characterizing the subset of helper T cells identified the ACO phenotype with elevated IgE and blood eosinophils, indicating the existence of ACO endotypes [4]. Most patients with asthma demonstrate type 2 inflammation, which comprises Th2 and type 2 innate lymphoid cells (ILC2) and cytokines, including interleukin (IL)-4, IL-5, and IL-13 derived from these cells. The representative biomarkers for type 2 inflammation are the blood eosinophil count, exhaled nitric oxide (FeNO) fraction, and immunoglobulin E (IgE) level. Some patients with COPD demonstrated the characteristics of type 2 inflammation, and the relationship between type 2 inflammation and steroid responsiveness has been reported. Thus, eosinophilic or IgE-mediated inflammation is potentially a treatable trait for these diseases. This chapter discusses the role of eosinophils and IgE in the diagnosis and treatment of ACO.

2 Role of Eosinophils

Blood eosinophil count and sputum eosinophil ratio are related to clinical features or steroid responsiveness, as in both asthma and COPD, and the analysis concerning the relationship is widely investigated. This chapter reviews the relationship between eosinophil counts and the clinical index or treatment response in COPD and asthma (Table 15.1) and discusses the role of eosinophil testing.

Table 15.1 Clinical features and use of the sputum eosinophil ratio and blood eosinophil count

	Sputum eosinophil ratio	Blood eosinophil count (ratio)
Asthma	• Upper Normal Limit: 2.2%	• 210–415/μl correspond to 2% sputum eosinophil • Decrease in smoking in patients with asthma
	Correlated with • FEV1, severity • Basement membrane thickness • Tissue eosinophilia • Airway hyperresponsiveness • ICS responsiveness • Exacerbation after the withdrawal of ICS	Correlated with • Diagnosis of asthma • Symptom • FEV1, exacerbation • Cut-off value for the prediction of exacerbation: 400/μl
COPD	• Above 3% 4.5%: predicts better responsiveness to ICS	• 162–300/μl correspond to sputum eosinophil 3% • Cut-off value for the prediction of exacerbation: 340/μl or 3.3% • Above 150/μl or 2%: predicts better responsiveness to ICS

2.1 Eosinophils in COPD

The existence of Th2 and ILC2 have been reported in the lung tissue of patients with COPD, [5, 6] as well as the local expression of cytokines that induce eosinophilic or type 2 inflammation, including IL-5 [7], GM-CSF [8], CCL5 [8], thymic stromal lymphopoietin (TSLP) [9], and IL-33 [10]. Elevated expressions of genes observed in asthma with type 2 inflammation have been reported in some patients with COPD, and the expression was related to airway reversibility or steroid responsiveness but not to the history of asthma [11]. This finding indicates that among patients with COPD without a history of asthma, a subgroup of patients possessed the feature of type 2 inflammation.

However, the association between the sputum eosinophil ratio or blood eosinophil count and pathophysiology is less clear in COPD than in asthma [12–14]. Eosinophils in the lung tissue of patients with COPD are not as degranulate as those with asthma [15], and gene expression associated with blood eosinophilia has minimal similarities between patients with COPD and those with asthma, indicating the different mechanisms of eosinophilic inflammation in these diseases [16]. Additionally, the presence of tissue eosinophils involved in homeostasis (resident eosinophils) has been indicated [17, 18]. Thus, numerical differences in tissue eosinophils may not be directly related to the pathogenesis of COPD, warranting further investigation into the involvement of local eosinophils in the pathogenesis.

2.1.1 Sputum Eosinophils in COPD

The sputum eosinophil ratio is significantly higher in patients with COPD than in healthy individuals [19], with 25%~44% of patients having a ratio of >3% [12, 20]. However, the association between the sputum eosinophil ratio and symptoms [12–14] or airway reversibility [12] is inconsistent.

Conversely, the sputum eosinophil ratio is useful for predicting steroid responsiveness, and the higher efficacy of oral corticosteroids [13, 21] and inhaled corticosteroids (ICS) [14] has been reported when the ratio exceeds 3%~4.5%. Patients with preexisting asthma were excluded in all but one of these trials, and sputum eosinophils were studied in the absence of ICS. A sputum eosinophil ratio of ≥3% has been associated with more exacerbations after ICS discontinuation [22]. These results reveal the use of sputum eosinophils to predict steroid responsiveness in COPD.

2.1.2 Blood Eosinophils in Patients with COPD

The mean blood eosinophil count in COPD is not significantly different from that in the non-COPD population [23, 24], but 57%~75% of patients with COPD have a blood eosinophil ratio of >2%, and 37.3% of patients with multiple tests always demonstrated >2% [25].

The correlation between blood eosinophil counts and lung tissue eosinophilia is inconsistent [24, 26], but a certain correlation with the sputum eosinophil ratio has been observed [14]. The blood eosinophil count was superior in predicting sputum eosinophil ratio compared with FeNO and serum IgE levels. A blood eosinophil count of 300/μl is considered the best threshold for a corresponding sputum eosinophil ratio of ≥3% [27]. The optimal cut-off is 162/μl or 2.6% and 215/μl or 2.3% if ICS is used [28]. The use of blood eosinophil count to predict COPD exacerbation is inconsistent [24], but eosinophil count is a better indicator than eosinophil ratio [23, 29] and 340/μl or 3.3% [23] was reported to be associated with exacerbations.

Conversely, some studies have reported that patients with consistent blood eosinophil ratios of >2% have better FEV1, better symptoms and quality of life, and less emphysema progression [25], and patients with blood eosinophil ratios of >150/μl have a better prognosis for survival [24]. Thus, the association between blood eosinophil counts and clinical indicators in COPD is not always as consistent as in asthma.

In contrast, many reports have revealed an association between blood eosinophil count and steroid responsiveness (Table 15.2). A post hoc analysis of a large clinical trial comparing the efficacy of ICS/long-acting β2-agonist (LABA) and LABA revealed that patients with a blood eosinophil count of >2% [30] or 279.8/μl [31] demonstrated a better response to ICS. Both the IMPACT [32] and ETHOS [33] studies revealed that a blood eosinophil count of ≥150/μl was associated with a superior response to the LABA/long-acting muscarinic antagonist (LAMA) combination in preventing exacerbations regarding the triple combination ICS/LABA/LAMA therapy. The TRIBUTE study revealed that the triple combination was significantly more effective in preventing exacerbations than the LABA/LAMA combination in peripheral blood eosinophils of ≥2% [34].

Based on these findings, the significance of eosinophil testing in COPD lies in identifying patients with response to steroids.

Table 15.2 Relationships between blood eosinophil count and response to inhaled corticosteroids in patients with COPD

Trial Year	Drugs	*N*	Cut-off value of blood eosinophil count	Endpoint	Reference
2015	FF/VI vs VI	3177	2%, 150/μl	Exacerbation	[30]
FORWARD 2015	BDP/FOR vs FOR	1186	279.8/μl	Exacerbation FEV1, SGRQ	[31]
IMPACT 2018	FF/VI/UMEC vs VI/UMEC	10,355	150/μl	Exacerbation	[32]
ETHOS 2020	BUD/FOR/GLY FOR/GLY	8509	150/μl	Exacerbation	[33]
TRIBUTE 2018	BDP/FOR/GLY IND/GLY	1532	2%	Exacerbation	[34]

BDP Beclomethasone, *BUD* Budesonide, *FF* Fluticasone furoate, *FOR* Formoterol, *GLY* Glycopyrronium, *IND* Indacaterol, *SGRQ* St. George Respiratory Questionnaire, *UMEC* Umeclidinium, *VI* Vilanterol

2.2 *Eosinophils in Asthma*

2.2.1 Significance of Sputum Eosinophils in Asthma

Eosinophils have cytotoxic granules and are believed to play a crucial role in airway inflammation in asthma [35]. Many studies have reported a relationship between sputum eosinophils and asthma pathogenesis. The sputum eosinophil ratio correlates with tissue eosinophil count [36], basement membrane thickening [37], decreased FEV1 [38], airway hyperresponsiveness [38], and asthma severity [39] (Table 15.1). It correlates better with asthma control status than the sputum neutrophil ratio [39]. Furthermore, the sputum eosinophil ratio is useful in predicting ICS responsiveness [40] and exacerbations after ICS discontinuation [41]. The sputum eosinophil ratio is more accurate than symptoms in controlling exacerbations for adjusting the ICS dose in long-term management [42, 43]. The method of sputum eosinophil quantification is recommended by the eosinophil ratio [44], and the upper limit in healthy individuals is 2.2% [45, 46].

Sputum eosinophils are an excellent indicator for asthma control. However, their role in clinical practice is limited because not all patients can expectorate the sputum, inhalation of a beta2-stimulant inhalation is required to prevent airway constriction caused by hypertonic saline inhalation, and processing is required after collection [44].

2.2.2 Significance of Blood Eosinophils in Asthma

Blood eosinophil count has been correlated with asthma diagnosis, symptoms, and pulmonary function, with a cut-off value of 400/μL for exacerbation prediction [47, 48]. However, the degree of correlation with clinical indicators is lower than the sputum eosinophil ratio [49].

The blood eosinophil count corresponding to a 2% sputum eosinophil ratio was 220/μl [50] or 210–415/μl in patients with asthma without ICS treatment [51]. Absolute numbers, not ratios, are recommended for laboratory values for blood eosinophils [44].

2.3 *Eosinophils in the ACO*

2.3.1 Eosinophils as Biomarkers in ACO

ACO consists of two groups: COPD with eosinophilic or type 2 inflammation and asthma with a smoking history, which have different inflammatory backgrounds [52, 53]. The sputum eosinophil ratio [54–56] and blood eosinophil counts are significantly higher in ACO compared with pure COPD [54, 56, 57]. In contrast, blood eosinophil counts in asthma are lower in patients who are smoking [52, 58]; thus, a significant difference in eosinophil count between asthma and the whole ACO population has not been observed [56].

Significant differences were found in FeNO and serum IgE levels when the entire group of patients with fixed airflow obstruction was classified into two groups based on blood eosinophil counts [52]. Therefore, considering increased blood eosinophil counts as a treatable trait is more useful, and the question of defining ACO as a single disease group has been raised [59].

However, monitoring blood eosinophil count may be useful in determining the ICS responding ACO among patients with COPD. A blood eosinophil count of 300/μl or higher is listed as an auxiliary item in the international consensus criteria [60] or Spanish guidelines [61]. The diagnostic criteria for ACO in the Japanese Respiratory Society guideline published in 2018 describe a blood eosinophil count of 5% or 300/μl as one of the characteristics of ACO among patients with COPD [62]. A threshold of 150–280/μl or 2% of blood eosinophils in COPD has been effective in preventing exacerbations with ICS (Table 15.2). A blood eosinophil count of 300/μl in ACO guidelines is set higher than these thresholds; thus, the specificity of the additional effect of ICS in COPD is assumed to be high.

2.3.2 Eosinophils as a Treatable Trait for ACO

IL-5 is a representative activation factor for eosinophils; however, local lung eosinophil counts during COPD exacerbations do not correlate with IL-5 levels [63]. The effect of anti-IL-5 therapy in COPD is not consistent, even in subgroups with increased eosinophil counts [64–66].

Conversely, the efficacy of anti-IL-5 therapy in asthma with eosinophilia has been consistently revealed [67–69], indicating the prominent contribution of IL-5 in the pathogenesis of eosinophilic asthma. A similar real-world effectiveness of mepolizumab for ACO has been shown in patients with asthma with a history of smoking, as in non-smokers [70, 71]. These findings reveal that anti-IL-5 therapy is effective in ACO with a history of asthma and smoking history but with no clear efficacy in pure COPD with eosinophilia.

3 Role of IgE

3.1 IgE in COPD

Allergic sensitization is an established feature of asthma, and assessment of the sensitization status is highly recommended for patients with asthma [35]. In contrast, allergic sensitization may not be routinely assessed in patients with COPD, and the Global Initiative for Chronic Obstructive Lung Disease guideline does not recommend the diagnosis of allergy [3]. The positivity of *Dermatophagoides pteronyssinus* and house dust-specific IgE was lower in patients with COPD than in those with asthma [72, 73]. However, allergic sensitization is related to increased respiratory symptoms and the risk of exacerbations in patients with COPD [74] and may be a treatable trait for allergen avoidance or anti-IgE treatment [2].

Allergic sensitization in patients with COPD has not been extensively investigated, and the positivity of only 5–6 allergen-specific IgE has been analyzed [74, 75]. The relationship between allergen-specific IgE and patient characteristics was not fully elucidated.

We comprehensively analyzed the positivity of various allergen-specific IgE in COPD [76] (Fig. 15.1). The positivity for moth (31.5%), *Candida* (23.7%), *D. pteronyssinus* (22.4%), and house dust (22.4%) regarding the perennial aeroallergens was >20% (Fig. 15.1). The positivity for Japanese cedar (35.5%) and Japanese cypress (22.2%) regarding pollen allergens exceeded 20% in Japanese patients with COPD.

Moreover, we compared the characteristics of patients who were positive with those who were negative for specific IgE. Residual volume (RV) was significantly higher (136.7% vs. 110.2%) and FEV_1 tended to be lower (69.5% vs 78.7%) in patients with positive IgE for cockroaches than in those with negative IgE [76]. The positivity for cockroach-specific IgE in COPD is higher than in the control group and comparable with asthma [73, 77]. Cockroach extract induces various cytokine secretions [78, 79], and the allergen component of cockroach, per a 10, is a serine protease that induces the generation of IL-6, IL-8, and GM-CSF from airway epithelial cells by activating protease-activated receptor 2 [80, 81]. A high exposure level to cockroaches has been reported to increase the risk of asthma development [82] and its severity [83]. These proinflammatory natures of the cockroach allergen may harm the airway structure of COPD, which warrants further investigation.

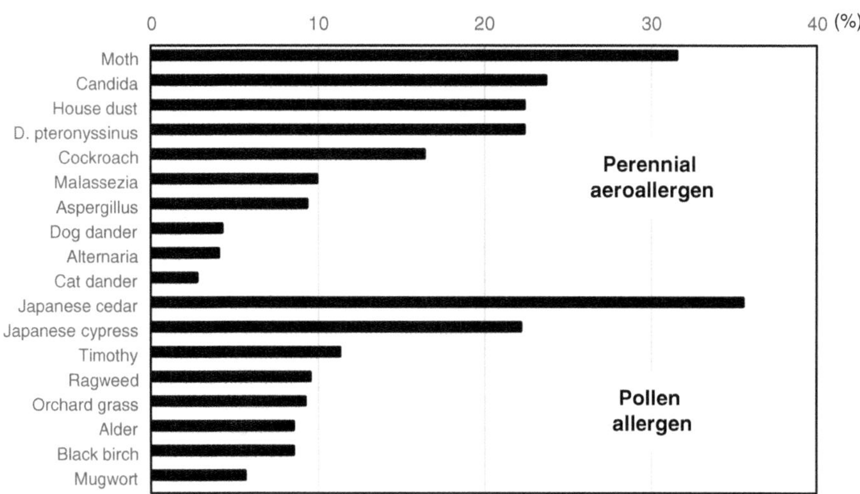

Fig. 15.1 Positivity of specific immunoglobulin E (IgE) in chronic obstructive pulmonary disease. Specific IgE levels were judged as positive when the class was ≥1. (Modified from Reference [76])

3.2 *IgE in Asthma–COPD Overlap*

3.2.1 Significance of Mite-Specific IgE in Diagnosing ACO

Allergic sensitization results in type 2 inflammation, a prominent feature of asthma that may be an important component of ACO diagnosis. The diagnostic criteria of ACO did not always include IgE categories, but some recent guidelines, including the Japanese guideline, introduced IgE into the diagnostic criteria [60, 62, 84].

Some studies compared the total and several allergen-specific IgE levels between ACO and pure COPD and revealed higher total IgE [75] or *Dermatophagoides*-specific IgE levels [1, 75] in ACO. However, the number of tested allergens was limited, and which allergen-specific IgE is important for ACO diagnosis remained unclear. Additionally, the guidelines stated no cut-off level of IgE and types of allergen-specific IgE to be measured [62].

We comprehensively compared the positivity of specific IgE between ACO and non-ACO COPD [76] and revealed that only the positivity for house dust and *D. pteronyssinus* was significantly higher in ACO among various aeroallergens (Table 15.3). The positivity for moth, *Candida*, and *Malassezia* appeared higher in

Table 15.3 Comparison of positivity in specific IgE between ACO and non-ACO COPD

	ACO	Non-ACO COPD	Total	*P*-value
Perennial aeroallergen				
Moth	38.7	26.2	31.5	0.26
Candida	29.4	19.1	23.7	0.29
House dust	35.3	11.9	22.4	0.015**
D. pteronyssinus	35.3	11.9	22.4	0.015**
Cockroach	19.4	14.3	16.4	0.56
Malassezia	13.3	7.3	9.9	0.40
Aspergillus	12.1	7.1	9.3	0.46
Dog dander	3.3	4.8	4.2	0.76
Alternaria	6.1	2.4	4.0	0.42
Cat dander	6.1	0.0	2.7	0.11
Pollen allergen				
Japanese cedar	44.1	28.6	35.5	0.16
Japanese cypress	19.4	24.4	22.2	0.61
Orchard grass	14.7	9.5	11.8	0.49
Timothy	13.3	9.8	11.3	0.64
Ragweed	11.8	7.1	9.2	0.49
Alder	3.3	12.2	8.5	0.18
Black birch	3.3	12.2	8.5	0.18
Mugwort	3.3	7.3	5.6	0.47

Modified from reference [76]. $P < 0.01$** between ACO and non-ACO COPD groups ($n = 76$). Specific IgE was judged as positive when the class was ≥1. *ACO* asthma-COPD overlap, *COPD* chronic obstructive pulmonary disease, *D. pteronyssinus Dermatophagoides pteronyssinus*

ACO for other perennial aeroallergens. Regarding pollen, the positivity for Japanese cedar tended to be higher in ACO.

Moreover, we analyzed the relationship between the value of the IgE class and the proportion of patients diagnosed with ACO (Fig. 15.2) [76]. Only house dust- and *D. pteronyssinus*-specific IgE demonstrated a significant relationship between the class of specific IgE and ACO diagnosis. Multivariate analysis revealed a significant contribution of total IgE, house dust, and *D. pteronyssinus*-specific IgE to ACO diagnosis [76].

Mites have been identified as a major antigenic substance in house dust [85]; thus, these results indicate the specifically important role of sensitization in mite allergens in the pathology or diagnosis of ACO among COPD.

3.2.2 Comparison of IgE and Other Type 2 Biomarkers for Diagnosing ACO

The diagnostic criteria for ACO included FeNO and blood eosinophil count, in addition to IgE levels [62]. Thus, we compared the use of these biomarkers in ACO diagnosis. Weak or no significant relationships were found between these biomarkers, but the area under the curve for ACO diagnosis was comparable among them (Fig. 15.3) [76]. The best cut-off value for diagnosis was 234 count/μl for blood eosinophils, 158 IU/mL for serum total IgE, and 31.0 ppb for FeNO. Regarding IgE factors, all the following criteria significantly contributed to ACO diagnosis: total IgE of >100 IU/mL, positive house dust-specific IgE, and positive *D. pteronyssinus*-specific IgE. In summary, by analyzing a panel of specific IgE in COPD, we revealed the important role of mite-specific IgE in diagnosing ACO.

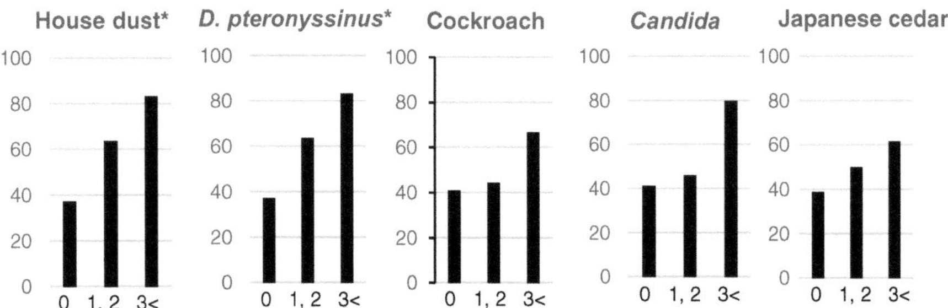

Fig. 15.2 The relationship between the value of the immunoglobulin E (IgE) class and the proportion of patients diagnosed with asthma–COPD overlap. $P < 0.05$* indicates a significant difference between groups. *D. pteronyssinus, Dermatophagoides pteronyssinus.* (Modified from Reference [76])

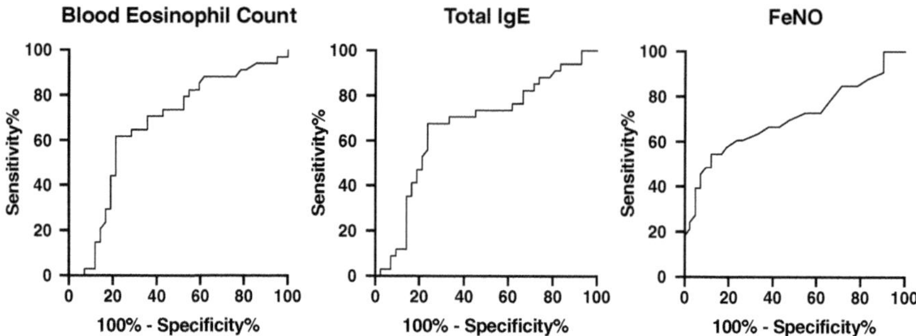

Fig. 15.3 Receiver operating characteristic analysis of biomarkers to detect the diagnosis of asthma–COPD overlap. The area under the curve was 0.666 for blood eosinophil count, 0.665 for total immunoglobulin E (IgE), and 0.703 for the fraction of exhaled nitric oxide (FeNO). The best cut-off value was 234 count/μl for blood eosinophils (sensitivity of 0.618 and specificity of 0.786), 158 IU/mL for serum total IgE (sensitivity of 0.677 and specificity of 0.662), and 31.0 ppb for FeNO (sensitivity of 0.546 and specificity of 0.881). (Modified from Reference [76])

3.3 IgE in Patients with Asthma with Smoking History

Serum IgE levels consistently decreased with increasing age in never-smoker asthmatics [86]. However, IgE levels were higher in current smokers, followed by ex-smokers and never-smokers in the elderly group. Additionally, the total and specific IgE levels against mites, cedar pollen, and *Candida* were higher in current smokers with asthma than in never-smokers [87]. Tobacco smoke exposure induces eosinophilia and type 2 inflammation in murine models of allergy. One possible mechanism underlying persistent type 2 inflammation in smokers is increased TSLP expression, which promotes type 2 skewed immune responses. Sputum TSLP levels in current smokers and ex-smokers were significantly higher than those in never-smokers [86]. These results indicate the importance of IgE as a treatable trait in ACO with asthma history.

3.4 IgE as a Treatable Trait for ACO

The importance of sensitized allergen avoidance has been stressed for asthma [2], and the effect of the anti-IgE antibody omalizumab is expected in ACO. A small retrospective analysis of omalizumab revealed an improvement in the symptoms of patients with severe asthma who had a smoking history and fixed airway obstruction [88]. However, studies on ACO are limited [89, 90], and another exploratory study of omalizumab in patients with COPD with elevated IgE levels was terminated because of difficulty in recruiting eligible patients (NCT00851370).

Our analysis revealed that patients diagnosed with ACO demonstrated lower FEV_1 compared with non-ACO COPD, and patients with cockroach-specific IgE exhibited higher RV than nonsensitized patients. Hence, future studies should establish the efficacy of anti-IgE treatment for ACO with COPD.

4 Conclusion

This chapter discussed the role of eosinophils and IgE in the diagnosis and treatment of ACO. The significance of diagnosing ACO by these biomarkers was more prominent in COPD than in asthma because the initial treatment for COPD excludes ICS, and finding steroid responders from COPD is an important issue. Further research is required to establish the significance of eosinophils and IgE as treatable traits in patients with ACO.

References

1. Yanagisawa S, Ichinose M. Definition and diagnosis of asthma-COPD overlap (ACO). Allergol Int. 2018;67(2):172–8.
2. Sterk PJ. Chronic diseases like asthma and COPD: do they truly exist? Eur Respir J. 2016;47(2):359–61.
3. Global strategy for the diagnosis, management, and prevention of chronic obstructive pulmonary disease (2023 Report); 2023.
4. Hirai K, Shirai T, Suzuki M, Akamatsu T, Suzuki T, Hayashi I, et al. A clustering approach to identify and characterize the asthma and chronic obstructive pulmonary disease overlap phenotype. Clin Exp Allergy. 2017;47(11):1374–82.
5. De Grove KC, Provoost S, Verhamme FM, Bracke KR, Joos GF, Maes T, Brusselle GG. Characterization and quantification of innate lymphoid cell subsets in human lung. PLoS One. 2016;11(1):e0145961.
6. Barczyk A, Pierzchala W, Kon OM, Cosio B, Adcock IM, Barnes PJ. Cytokine production by bronchoalveolar lavage T lymphocytes in chronic obstructive pulmonary disease. J Allergy Clin Immunol. 2006;117(6):1484–92.
7. Bafadhel M, Saha S, Siva R, McCormick M, Monteiro W, Rugman P, et al. Sputum IL-5 concentration is associated with a sputum eosinophilia and attenuated by corticosteroid therapy in COPD. Respiration. 2009;78(3):256–62.
8. Costa C, Rufino R, Traves SL, Lapa ESJR, Barnes PJ, Donnelly LE. CXCR3 and CCR5 chemokines in induced sputum from patients with COPD. Chest. 2008;133(1):26–33.
9. Ying S, O'Connor B, Ratoff J, Meng Q, Fang C, Cousins D, et al. Expression and cellular provenance of thymic stromal lymphopoietin and chemokines in patients with severe asthma and chronic obstructive pulmonary disease. J Immunol. 2008;181(4):2790–8.
10. Tworek D, Majewski S, Szewczyk K, Kiszalkiewicz J, Kurmanowska Z, Gorski P, et al. The association between airway eosinophilic inflammation and IL-33 in stable non-atopic COPD. Respir Res. 2018;19(1):108.
11. Christenson SA, Steiling K, van den Berge M, Hijazi K, Hiemstra PS, Postma DS, et al. Asthma-COPD overlap. Clinical relevance of genomic signatures of type 2 inflammation in chronic obstructive pulmonary disease. Am J Respir Crit Care Med. 2015;191(7):758–66.

12. Leigh R, Pizzichini MM, Morris MM, Maltais F, Hargreave FE, Pizzichini E. Stable COPD: predicting benefit from high-dose inhaled corticosteroid treatment. Eur Respir J. 2006;27(5):964–71.
13. Brightling CE, Monteiro W, Ward R, Parker D, Morgan MD, Wardlaw AJ, Pavord ID. Sputum eosinophilia and short-term response to prednisolone in chronic obstructive pulmonary disease: a randomised controlled trial. Lancet (London, England). 2000;356(9240):1480–5.
14. Brightling CE, McKenna S, Hargadon B, Birring S, Green R, Siva R, et al. Sputum eosinophilia and the short term response to inhaled mometasone in chronic obstructive pulmonary disease. Thorax. 2005;60(3):193–8.
15. Louis RE, Cataldo D, Buckley MG, Sele J, Henket M, Lau LC, et al. Evidence of mast-cell activation in a subset of patients with eosinophilic chronic obstructive pulmonary disease. Eur Respir J. 2002;20(2):325–31.
16. George L, Taylor AR, Esteve-Codina A, Soler Artigas M, Thun GA, Bates S, et al. Blood eosinophil count and airway epithelial transcriptome relationships in COPD versus asthma. Allergy. 2020;75(2):370–80.
17. Mesnil C, Raulier S, Paulissen G, Xiao X, Birrell MA, Pirottin D, et al. Lung-resident eosinophils represent a distinct regulatory eosinophil subset. J Clin Invest. 2016;126(9):3279–95.
18. Weller PF, Spencer LA. Functions of tissue-resident eosinophils. Nat Rev Immunol. 2017;17(12):746–60.
19. Rutgers SR, Timens W, Kaufmann HF, van der Mark TW, Koëter GH, Postma DS. Comparison of induced sputum with bronchial wash, bronchoalveolar lavage and bronchial biopsies in COPD. Eur Respir J. 2000;15(1):109–15.
20. Eltboli O, Bafadhel M, Hollins F, Wright A, Hargadon B, Kulkarni N, Brightling C. COPD exacerbation severity and frequency is associated with impaired macrophage efferocytosis of eosinophils. BMC Pulm Med. 2014;14:112.
21. Pizzichini E, Pizzichini MM, Gibson P, Parameswaran K, Gleich GJ, Berman L, et al. Sputum eosinophilia predicts benefit from prednisone in smokers with chronic obstructive bronchitis. Am J Respir Crit Care Med. 1998;158(5 Pt 1):1511–7.
22. Liesker JJ, Bathoorn E, Postma DS, Vonk JM, Timens W, Kerstjens HA. Sputum inflammation predicts exacerbations after cessation of inhaled corticosteroids in COPD. Respir Med. 2011;105(12):1853–60.
23. Vedel-Krogh S, Nielsen SF, Lange P, Vestbo J, Nordestgaard BG. Blood eosinophils and exacerbations in chronic obstructive pulmonary disease. The copenhagen general population study. Am J Respir Crit Care Med. 2016;193(9):965–74.
24. Turato G, Semenzato U, Bazzan E, Biondini D, Tinè M, Torrecilla N, et al. Blood eosinophilia neither reflects tissue eosinophils nor worsens clinical outcomes in chronic obstructive pulmonary disease. Am J Respir Crit Care Med. 2018;197(9):1216–9.
25. Singh D, Kolsum U, Brightling CE, Locantore N, Agusti A, Tal-Singer R. Eosinophilic inflammation in COPD: prevalence and clinical characteristics. Eur Respir J. 2014;44(6):1697–700.
26. Eltboli O, Mistry V, Barker B, Brightling CE. Relationship between blood and bronchial submucosal eosinophilia and reticular basement membrane thickening in chronic obstructive pulmonary disease. Respirology. 2015;20(4):667–70.
27. Negewo NA, McDonald VM, Baines KJ, Wark PA, Simpson JL, Jones PW, Gibson PG. Peripheral blood eosinophils: a surrogate marker for airway eosinophilia in stable COPD. Int J Chron Obstruct Pulmon Dis. 2016;11:1495–504.
28. Schleich F, Corhay JL, Louis R. Blood eosinophil count to predict bronchial eosinophilic inflammation in COPD. Eur Respir J. 2016;47(5):1562–4.
29. Wedzicha JA. Eosinophils as biomarkers of chronic obstructive pulmonary disease exacerbation risk. Maybe just for some? Am J Respir Crit Care Med. 2016;193(9):937–8.
30. Pascoe S, Locantore N, Dransfield MT, Barnes NC, Pavord ID. Blood eosinophil counts, exacerbations, and response to the addition of inhaled fluticasone furoate to vilanterol in patients with chronic obstructive pulmonary disease: a secondary analysis of data from two parallel randomised controlled trials. Lancet Respir Med. 2015;3(6):435–42.

31. Siddiqui SH, Guasconi A, Vestbo J, Jones P. Blood eosinophils: a biomarker of response to extrafine beclomethasone/Formoterol in chronic obstructive pulmonary disease. Am J Respir Crit Care Med. 2015;192:523–5.
32. Lipson DA, Barnhart F, Brealey N, Brooks J, Criner GJ, Day NC, et al. Once-daily single-inhaler triple versus dual therapy in patients with COPD. N Engl J Med. 2018;378(18):1671–80.
33. Rabe KF, Martinez FJ, Ferguson GT, Wang C, Singh D, Wedzicha JA, et al. Triple inhaled therapy at two glucocorticoid doses in moderate-to-very-severe COPD. N Engl J Med. 2020;383(1):35–48.
34. Papi A, Vestbo J, Fabbri L, Corradi M, Prunier H, Cohuet G, et al. Extrafine inhaled triple therapy versus dual bronchodilator therapy in chronic obstructive pulmonary disease (TRIBUTE): a double-blind, parallel group, randomised controlled trial. Lancet. 2018;391(10125):1076–84.
35. Nakamura Y, Tamaoki J, Nagase H, Yamaguchi M, Horiguchi T, Hozawa S, et al. Japanese guidelines for adult asthma 2020. Allergol Int. 2020;69(4):519–48.
36. Grootendorst DC, Sont JK, Willems LNA, Kluin-Nelemans JC, Van Krieken JHJM, Veselic-Charvat M, Sterk PJ. Comparison of inflammatory cell counts in asthma: induced sputum vs bronchoalveolar lavage and bronchial biopsies. Clin Exp Allergy. 1997;27(7):769–79.
37. Berry M, Morgan A, Shaw DE, Parker D, Green R, Brightling C, et al. Pathological features and inhaled corticosteroid response of eosinophilic and non-eosinophilic asthma. Thorax. 2007;62(12):1043–9.
38. Woodruff PG, Khashayar R, Lazarus SC, Janson S, Avila P, Boushey HA, et al. Relationship between airway inflammation, hyperresponsiveness, and obstruction in asthma. J Allergy Clin Immunol. 2001;108(5):753–8.
39. Louis R, Lau LC, Bron AO, Roldaan AC, Radermecker M, Djukanović R. The relationship between airways inflammation and asthma severity. Am J Respir Crit Care Med. 2000;161(1):9–16.
40. Pavord ID, Brightling CE, Woltmann G, Wardlaw AJ. Non-eosinophilic corticosteroid unresponsive asthma. Lancet (London, England). 1999;353(9171):2213–4.
41. Deykin A, Lazarus SC, Fahy JV, Wechsler ME, Boushey HA, Chinchilli VM, et al. Sputum eosinophil counts predict asthma control after discontinuation of inhaled corticosteroids. J Allergy Clin Immunol. 2005;115(4):720–7.
42. Jayaram L, Pizzichini MM, Cook RJ, Boulet LP, Lemiere C, Pizzichini E, et al. Determining asthma treatment by monitoring sputum cell counts: effect on exacerbations. Eur Respir J. 2006;27(3):483–94.
43. Green RH, Brightling CE, McKenna S, Hargadon B, Parker D, Bradding P, et al. Asthma exacerbations and sputum eosinophil counts: a randomised controlled trial. Lancet (London, England). 2002;360(9347):1715–21.
44. Szefler SJ, Wenzel S, Brown R, Erzurum SC, Fahy JV, Hamilton RG, et al. Asthma outcomes: biomarkers. J Allergy Clin Immunol. 2012;129(3 Suppl):S9–23.
45. Belda J, Leigh R, Parameswaran K, O'Byrne PM, Sears MR, Hargreave FE. Induced sputum cell counts in healthy adults. Am J Respir Crit Care Med. 2000;161(2 Pt 1):475–8.
46. Spanevello A, Confalonieri M, Sulotto F, Romano F, Balzano G, Migliori GB, et al. Induced sputum cellularity. Reference values and distribution in normal volunteers. Am J Respir Crit Care Med. 2000;162(3 Pt 1):1172–4.
47. Price DB, Rigazio A, Campbell JD, Bleecker ER, Corrigan CJ, Thomas M, et al. Blood eosinophil count and prospective annual asthma disease burden: a UK cohort study. Lancet Respir Med. 2015;3(11):849–58.
48. Zeiger RS, Schatz M, Li Q, Chen W, Khatry DB, Gossage D, Tran TN. High blood eosinophil count is a risk factor for future asthma exacerbations in adult persistent asthma. J Allergy Clin Immunol Pract. 2014;2(6):741–50.
49. Pizzichini E, Pizzichini MM, Efthimiadis A, Dolovich J, Hargreave FE. Measuring airway inflammation in asthma: eosinophils and eosinophilic cationic protein in induced sputum compared with peripheral blood. J Allergy Clin Immunol. 1997;99(4):539–44.

50. McGrath KW, Icitovic N, Boushey HA, Lazarus SC, Sutherland ER, Chinchilli VM, et al. A large subgroup of mild-to-moderate asthma is persistently noneosinophilic. Am J Respir Crit Care Med. 2012;185(6):612–9.
51. Korevaar DA, Westerhof GA, Wang J, Cohen JF, Spijker R, Sterk PJ, et al. Diagnostic accuracy of minimally invasive markers for detection of airway eosinophilia in asthma: a systematic review and meta-analysis. Lancet Respir Med. 2015;3(4):290–300.
52. Cosio BG, Perez de Llano L, Lopez Vina A, Torrego A, Lopez-Campos JL, Soriano JB, et al. Th-2 signature in chronic airway diseases: towards the extinction of asthma-COPD overlap syndrome? Eur Respir J. 2017;49(5):1602397.
53. Toledo-Pons N, van Boven JFM, Roman-Rodriguez M, Perez N, Valera Felices JL, Soriano JB, Cosio BG. ACO: time to move from the description of different phenotypes to the treatable traits. PLoS One. 2019;14(1):e0210915.
54. Kitaguchi Y, Komatsu Y, Fujimoto K, Hanaoka M, Kubo K. Sputum eosinophilia can predict responsiveness to inhaled corticosteroid treatment in patients with overlap syndrome of COPD and asthma. Int J Chron Obstruct Pulmon Dis. 2012;7:283–9.
55. Iwamoto H, Gao J, Koskela J, Kinnula V, Kobayashi H, Laitinen T, Mazur W. Differences in plasma and sputum biomarkers between COPD and COPD-asthma overlap. Eur Respir J. 2014;43(2):421–9.
56. Peng J, Wang M, Wu Y, Shen Y, Chen L. Clinical indicators for asthma-COPD overlap: a systematic review and meta-analysis. Int J Chron Obstruct Pulmon Dis. 2022;17:2567–75.
57. Cosio BG, Soriano JB, Lopez-Campos JL, Calle-Rubio M, Soler-Cataluna JJ, de-Torres JP, et al. Defining the asthma-COPD overlap syndrome in a COPD cohort. Chest. 2016;149(1):45–52.
58. Sunyer J, Springer G, Jamieson B, Conover C, Detels R, Rinaldo C, et al. Effects of asthma on cell components in peripheral blood among smokers and non-smokers. Clin Exp Allergy. 2003;33(11):1500–5.
59. Papi A. Asthma COPD overlap PRO-CON Debate. ACO: the mistaken term. COPD. 2020;17(5):474–6.
60. Sin DD, Miravitlles M, Mannino DM, Soriano JB, Price D, Celli BR, et al. What is asthma-COPD overlap syndrome? Towards a consensus definition from a round table discussion. Eur Respir J. 2016;48(3):664–73.
61. Plaza V, Alvarez F, Calle M, Casanova C, Cosio BG, Lopez-Vina A, et al. Consensus on the asthma-COPD overlap syndrome (ACOS) between the Spanish COPD guidelines (GesEPOC) and the Spanish guidelines on the management of asthma (GEMA). Arch Bronconeumol. 2017;53(8):443–9.
62. Hashimoto S, Sorimachi R, Jinnai T, Ichinose M. Asthma and chronic obstructive pulmonary disease overlap according to the Japanese respiratory society diagnostic criteria: the prospective, observational aco Japan cohort study. Adv Ther. 2020;38(2):1168–84.
63. Saetta M, Di Stefano A, Maestrelli P, Turato G, Mapp CE, Pieno M, et al. Airway eosinophilia and expression of interleukin-5 protein in asthma and in exacerbations of chronic bronchitis. Clin Exp Allergy. 1996;26(7):766–74.
64. Pavord ID, Chanez P, Criner GJ, Kerstjens HAM, Korn S, Lugogo N, et al. Mepolizumab for eosinophilic chronic obstructive pulmonary disease. N Engl J Med. 2017;377(17):1613–29.
65. Pavord ID, Chapman KR, Bafadhel M, Sciurba FC, Bradford ES, Schweiker Harris S, et al. Mepolizumab for eosinophil-associated COPD: analysis of METREX and METREO. Int J Chron Obstruct Pulmon Dis. 2021;16:1755–70.
66. Brightling CE, Bleecker ER, Panettieri RA Jr, Bafadhel M, She D, Ward CK, et al. Benralizumab for chronic obstructive pulmonary disease and sputum eosinophilia: a randomised, double-blind, placebo-controlled, phase 2a study. Lancet Respir Med. 2014;2(11):891–901.
67. Ortega HG, Liu MC, Pavord ID, Brusselle GG, FitzGerald JM, Chetta A, et al. Mepolizumab treatment in patients with severe eosinophilic asthma. N Engl J Med. 2014;371(13):1198–207.

68. Bleecker ER, FitzGerald JM, Chanez P, Papi A, Weinstein SF, Barker P, et al. Efficacy and safety of benralizumab for patients with severe asthma uncontrolled with high-dosage inhaled corticosteroids and long-acting β(2)-agonists (SIROCCO): a randomised, multicentre, placebo-controlled phase 3 trial. Lancet (London, England). 2016;388(10056):2115–27.
69. FitzGerald JM, Bleecker ER, Nair P, Korn S, Ohta K, Lommatzsch M, et al. Benralizumab, an anti-interleukin-5 receptor α monoclonal antibody, as add-on treatment for patients with severe, uncontrolled, eosinophilic asthma (CALIMA): a randomised, double-blind, placebo-controlled phase 3 trial. Lancet. 2016;388(10056):2128–41.
70. Isoyama S, Ishikawa N, Hamai K, Matsumura M, Kobayashi H, Nomura A, et al. Efficacy of mepolizumab in elderly patients with severe asthma and overlapping COPD in real-world settings: a retrospective observational study. Respir Investig. 2021;59(4):478–86.
71. Nagase H, Tamaoki J, Suzuki T, Nezu Y, Akiyama S, Cole AL, et al. Reduction in asthma exacerbation rate after mepolizumab treatment initiation in patients with severe asthma: a real-world database study in Japan. Pulm Pharmacol Ther. 2022;75:102130.
72. Adachi M, Ohta K, Morikawa A, Nishima S. [Asthma insights & reality in Japan 2005]. Arerugi 2006;55(10):1340–3.
73. Bozek A, Rogala B. IgE-dependent sensitization in patients with COPD. Ann Agric Environ Med. 2018;25(3):417–20.
74. Jamieson DB, Matsui EC, Belli A, McCormack MC, Peng E, Pierre-Louis S, et al. Effects of allergic phenotype on respiratory symptoms and exacerbations in patients with chronic obstructive pulmonary disease. Am J Respir Crit Care Med. 2013;188(2):187–92.
75. Hersh CP, Zacharia S, Prakash Arivu Chelvan R, Hayden LP, Mirtar A, Zarei S, et al. Immunoglobulin E as a biomarker for the overlap of atopic asthma and chronic obstructive pulmonary disease. COPD. 2020;7(1):1–12.
76. Toyota H, Sugimoto N, Kobayashi K, Suzuki Y, Takeshita Y, Ito A, et al. Comprehensive analysis of allergen-specific IgE in COPD: mite-specific IgE specifically related to the diagnosis of asthma-COPD overlap. Allergy Asthma Clin Immunol. 2021;17(1):13.
77. Minami T, Fukutomi Y, Inada R, Tsuda M, Sekiya K, Miyazaki M, et al. Regional differences in the prevalence of sensitization to environmental allergens: analysis on IgE antibody testing conducted at major clinical testing laboratories throughout Japan from 2002 to 2011. Allergol Int. 2019;68(4):440–9.
78. Page K, Hughes VS, Odoms KK, Dunsmore KE, Hershenson MB. German cockroach proteases regulate interleukin-8 expression via nuclear factor for interleukin-6 in human bronchial epithelial cells. Am J Respir Cell Mol Biol. 2005;32(3):225–31.
79. Pomes A, Mueller GA, Randall TA, Chapman MD, Arruda LK. New insights into cockroach allergens. Curr Allergy Asthma Rep. 2017;17(4):25.
80. Hong JH, Lee SI, Kim KE, Yong TS, Seo JT, Sohn MH, Shin DM. German cockroach extract activates protease-activated receptor 2 in human airway epithelial cells. J Allergy Clin Immunol. 2004;113(2):315–9.
81. Kale SL, Arora N. Per a 10 activates human derived epithelial cell line in a protease dependent manner via PAR-2. Immunobiology. 2015;220(4):525–32.
82. Litonjua AA, Carey VJ, Burge HA, Weiss ST, Gold DR. Exposure to cockroach allergen in the home is associated with incident doctor-diagnosed asthma and recurrent wheezing. J Allergy Clin Immunol. 2001;107(1):41–7.
83. Do DC, Zhao Y, Gao P. Cockroach allergen exposure and risk of asthma. Allergy. 2016;71(4):463–74.
84. Soler-Cataluña JJ, Cosío B, Izquierdo JL, López-Campos JL, Marín JM, Agüero R, et al. Consensus document on the overlap phenotype COPD–asthma in COPD. Arch Bronconeumol (Engl Ed). 2012;48(9):331–7.
85. Miyamoto T, Oshima S, Ishizaki T, Sato SH. Allergenic identity between the common floor mite (Dermatophagoides farinae Hughes, 1961) and house dust as a causative antigen in bronchial asthma. J Allergy. 1968;42(1):14–28.

86. Nagasaki T, Matsumoto H, Nakaji H, Niimi A, Ito I, Oguma T, et al. Smoking attenuates the age-related decrease in IgE levels and maintains eosinophilic inflammation. Clin Exp Allergy. 2013;43(6):608–15.
87. Tsukioka K, Toyabe S, Akazawa K. [Total and specific IgE levels in adolescents and adults with bronchial asthma]. Nihon Kokyuki Gakkai Zasshi. 2010;48(6):409–18.
88. Maltby S, Gibson PG, Powell H, McDonald VM. Omalizumab treatment response in a population with severe allergic asthma and overlapping COPD. Chest. 2017;151(1):78–89.
89. Tat TS, Cilli A. Evaluation of long-term safety and efficacy of omalizumab in elderly patients with uncontrolled allergic asthma. Ann Allergy Asthma Immunol. 2016;117(5):546–9.
90. Yalcin AD, Celik B, Yalcin AN. Omalizumab (anti-IgE) therapy in the asthma-COPD overlap syndrome (ACOS) and its effects on circulating cytokine levels. Immunopharmacol Immunotoxicol. 2016;38(3):253–6.

Chapter 16
Rhinosinusitis in ACO: What Is the Implication of Nasal Comorbidity?

Satoshi Hamada

Abstract The airway is subdivided into the upper and lower airway, but similar anatomical and morphological features and the immunological relationship between the two have led to the concept of "united airway disease" (UAD). Allergic rhinitis and asthma are the classic UAD, although there is considerable evidence that UAD may involve other clinical phenotypes of sinonasal disease (e.g., chronic rhinosinusitis [CRS]) and lower-airway disease (e.g., chronic obstructive pulmonary disease [COPD] and asthma-COPD overlap [ACO]). The data relating to the association between ACO and CRS is limited, and the present paper aims to review the concept of UAD in the context of ACO and CRS, providing a comprehensive description of the state of the literature and highlighting avenues for future research.

Keywords Asthma · Asthma-chronic obstructive pulmonary disease overlap · Chronic rhinosinusitis · Chronic obstructive pulmonary disease · United airway disease

Abbreviations

ACO	Asthma- chronic obstructive pulmonary disease overlap
AR	Allergic rhinitis
COPD	Chronic obstructive pulmonary disease
CRS	Chronic rhinosinusitis
CRSsNP	Chronic rhinosinusitis without nasal polyps
CRSwNP	Chronic rhinosinusitis with nasal polyps
CT	Computed tomography

S. Hamada (✉)
Department of Advanced Medicine for Respiratory Failure, Graduate School of Medicine, Kyoto University, Kyoto, Japan
e-mail: sh1124@kuhp.kyoto-u.ac.jp

H. Nagase et al. (eds.), *Asthma-COPD Overlap*, Respiratory Disease Series: Diagnostic Tools and Disease Managements,
https://doi.org/10.1007/978-981-96-0217-9_16

FEV_1	Forced expiratory volume in 1 s
FeNO	Fractional exhaled nitric oxide level
ICS	Inhaled corticosteroid
IL	Interleukin
LMS	Lund-Mackay score
MRI	Magnetic resonance imaging
Th2	T helper cell type 2
UAD	United airway disease

1 Introduction

In recent years, the upper and lower airways have been found to share elements of pathogenesis, which has led to the belief that they represent a unified morphological and functional unit. This has led to the concept of "united airway disease" (UAD), arising from the idea that these airways form a single organ [1]. The concept of UAD is based on anatomical features, histological similarities, and immunological relationships between the upper and lower airways. Anatomically, the location of the upper-airway facilitates maintenance of the homeostasis of the lower airway by functioning as a heat exchanger, humidifier for inhaled air, and physical filter to inflammatory and other irritants [2]. With regards to histology, the upper and lower airways share features such as a pseudostratified columnar ciliated epithelium with a continuous basement membrane, although they differ in that the lower airway has smooth muscle and the upper airway has prominent glands within the submucosa [3]. In terms of immunology, inflammatory cells of the upper airway propagate into the lower airway via postnasal drip and systemic circulation. Furthermore, inflammatory mediators of both airways mutually propagate via systemic circulation [3, 4].

Allergic rhinitis (AR) and asthma is the classic example of UAD [5]. The Allergic Rhinitis and its Impact on Asthma report reported that up to 40% of patients with AR have asthma, while almost all patients with asthma have AR [6]. In addition, the risk of developing asthma later in life is about threefold higher for patients with AR [7]. Numerous reports have suggested that UAD is not restricted to the relationship between AR and asthma but can involve other clinical phenotypes of sinonasal disease (e.g., chronic rhinosinusitis [CRS]) and lower-airway disease (e.g., chronic obstructive pulmonary disease [COPD], asthma-COPD overlap (ACO), and bronchiectasis) [8].

The clinical indications of CRS are inflammation of the nose and paranasal sinuses, and the condition is defined by the presence of symptoms and objective findings of nasal endoscopy and/or sinus computed tomography (CT) [9]. The symptomatic criteria are the presence of two or more of the following: nasal discharge (rhinorrhea or postnasal drip), nasal obstruction or congestion, hyposmia, and facial pressure or pain [9]. Nasal endoscopic criteria are the presence of polyps in one or both nasal cavities and/or mucopurulent discharge and/or edema or mucosal obstruction primarily in the middle nasal cavity [9]. Radiological criteria are mucosal changes within the ostiomeatal complex or sinuses [9]. Generally, CRS is divided into the two clinical phenotypes: CRS without nasal polyps (CRSsNP) or CRS with nasal polyps (CRSwNP). Tokunaga et al. classified intractable CRSwNP as eosinophilic CRS (ECRS) in the recent Japanese Epidemiological Survey of Refractory Eosinophilic Chronic Rhinosinusitis Study [10]. Both CRSwNP and ECRS are mainly caused by a type 2 immune response with infiltration of eosinophil-dominant inflammatory cells. In contrast, CRSsNP is mainly caused by a type 1 immune response with infiltration of neutrophil-dominant inflammatory cells. Epidemiological studies have shown the prevalence of CRSwNP and CRSsNP to be higher among patients with asthma compared with those without asthma [11–13]. Øie et al. reported that CRSsNP was present in 51% of patients with COPD [14]. Our previous studies have highlighted the association of abnormal sinus CT findings with COPD and ACO [15]. Thus, the concept of UAD might apply to CRS and conditions other than asthma, such as COPD and ACO. Published data on the association between ACO and CRS is limited, and so the present paper aims to present a review of the current status of the literature relating to UAD in the context of ACO and CRS.

2 Prevalence of CRS in Patients with Lower-Airway Disease

2.1 Prevalence of CRS in Patients with Asthma

The association between CRS and asthma has been extensively evaluated. The Global Allergy and Asthma Network of Excellence conducted a postal questionnaire in 12 countries of Europe, which revealed a strong association between asthma and CRS (adjusted odds ratio: 3.47; 95% confidence interval: 3.20–3.76) for all ages [12]. Another questionnaire-based epidemiological survey conducted in China showed the prevalence of CRS to be 23% among asthmatic patients, compared with 7% in participants without asthma [13]. Bresciani et al. reported that 70% of patients with mild-to-moderate asthma and 74% of patients with severe asthma had symptoms of ~~rhinositis~~ rhinosinusitis [16]. They also reported that 100% of patients with steroid-dependent asthma and 88% of patients with mild-to-moderate asthma had abnormal sinus CT findings [16]. Abnormal sinus CT findings have been detected in 94.9% of asthma patients who had a forced expiratory volume ratio in 1 s (FEV_1) to forced vital capacity of less than 70% [15]. The Lund-Mackay score (LMS) system is the standard method of determining radiological severity of CRS from sinus CT findings [17], and LMS score has been shown to increase with increasing severity of asthma [16, 18, 19]. The presence of nasal polyps is common in the context of asthma, with 26.5% of patients with mild-to-moderate asthma and 53.8% of patients with severe asthma found to exhibit this symptom [20], and the prevalence of CRSwNP reported to be higher in patients with asthma (7%) than the general population (4%) [21]. Together, the evidence suggests that CRS, particularly CRSwNP, is a common complication among patients with asthma.

2.2 *Prevalence of CRS Among Patients with COPD*

Despite being considered a lower-airway disease, there is increasing evidence to suggest that COPD as well as asthma frequently occurs with concomitant involvement of upper-airway diseases ~~such as asthma~~ [8]. An early questionnaire-based epidemiological study conducted in southern Sweden reported that 40.1% of patients with self-reported chronic bronchiolitis or emphysema had nasal symptoms, compared with 32.7% of the total study population [22]. A more recent epidemiological survey, conducted in China and obtained using questionnaires, reported patients with COPD to be about twice as likely to develop CRS than participants without COPD [13]. Imaging studies of sinonasal inflammation using sinus CT [23], magnetic resonance imaging (MRI) [24], and endoscopy [14] identified abnormal sinus CT findings in about 60% of patients with COPD, particularly those with more severe obstructive pulmonary function [15, 23]. Hansen et al. reported that the prevalence of paranasal sinus opacification—as evaluated by MRI—was six times higher among patients with COPD than healthy participants [24]. Furthermore, endoscopic investigations have revealed ~~CRSnNP~~ CRSsNP to be present in 51% of patients with COPD [14]. Therefore, CRS—particularly CRSsNP—is a common complication of COPD.

2.3 *Prevalence of CRS Among Patients with Asthma-COPD Overlap*

The association between CRS and asthma and COPD leads to the speculation that patients with ACO will frequently exhibit CRS such as CRSwNP, ECRS, or CRSsNP. Sinonasal inflammation—evaluated using sinus CT—has been found to be present in 72.2% of patients with ACO [15], and patients with ACO are more than twice as likely to develop AR than those with COPD according to the Nord-Trøndelag Health Study, a large-population study [25]. However, there is a paucity of evidence relating to the association between CRS and ACO.

3 Effects of CRS on Control of Lower-Airway Disease

3.1 *Effects of CRS on Lower-Airway Function in Patients Without Asthma and COPD*

There ~~is~~ are clinical evidences of the influence of CRS, including CRSsNP, CRSwNP, and ECRS, on lower-airway function, regardless of the existence of asthma and/or COPD. Williamson et al. reported that 30% of patients with CRSwNP and without asthma had marked elevation of fractional exhaled nitric oxide (FeNO), increased eosinophilic airway inflammation, and asymptomatic bronchial hyperactivity [26]. It has also been shown that patients with CRSwNP and CRSsNP exhibit changes in latent obstructive lung function, which are correlated with levels of interleukin (IL)-5—a T helper cell type 2 (Th2)-related cytokine—in nasal secretions [27, 28]. In addition, patients with ECRS and without asthma were found to have higher FeNO levels and increased peripheral airway obstruction compared with those without ECRS or asthma [29, 30]. The mechanism underlying the association between upper- and lower-airway dysfunction is currently considered to be as follows: Obstruction of the upper airway leads to favoring mouth breathing, increased exposure of the lower airways to allergens, and increased inflammation of the lower airways [31]. Next, absorption of inflammatory mediators such as IL-5 and eotaxin from the upper airway releases eosinophils, basophils, and their progenitor cells from the bone marrow. The systemic allergic response then facilitates the migration of inflammatory cells into the lower airway [32]. However, the precise mechanism is complex and studies to clarify specific details are ongoing [32, 33]. Recent studies into the nasal microbiome have begun to unravel the role of upper-airway inflammation in lower-airway dysfunction [33].

3.2 Effects of CRS on Asthma Control

It is thought that asthma might be more difficult to control and more prone to exacerbation when comorbid with CRSwNP [11, 34, 35], supported by the increase in asthma severity with increased radiological severity of CRS [16, 19, 36, 37]. Markers of systemic and lower-airway eosinophilic inflammation, such as eosinophil levels of sputum and blood and FeNO levels, have also been shown to increase according to radiological CRS severity in patients with asthma, particularly in the case of severe asthma [37]. These associations are markedly increased in patients with asthma and CRSwNP [20, 38, 39]. Furthermore, the upregulation of Th2-related cytokine activity induced by type-2 innate lymphoid cells might contribute to uncontrolled asthma status in patients with asthma comorbid with CRS [33, 40].

3.3 Effects of CRS on Control of COPD and Asthma-COPD Overlap

The presence of CRS, particularly CRSsNP, is associated with impaired health-related quality of life in patients with COPD, according to the findings of the St. Georges Respiratory Questionnaire and COPD Assessment Test [41–43]. Furthermore, nasal symptoms have been shown to be associated with more frequent exacerbation [44] and treatment failure of acute exacerbation in patients with

COPD [45]. Furthermore, the impact of CRS on lower-airway function and exacerbation of lower-airway disease suggest that CRS might influence the control of ACO. However, this possibility has ~~net~~ not been examined to date.

4 Treatment with Lower-Airway Disease Comorbid with CRS

4.1 Inhaled Therapy

Antibiotics, topical steroids, short-course systemic steroids, and endoscopic sinus surgery are all effective treatments for CRS [46]. Inhaled therapeutics, including corticosteroids (ICSs) and bronchodilators such as long-acting β_2 agonists and long-acting muscarinic antagonists are the first-line asthma treatments [47]. Previous studies have paid little attention to exhaled particles; however, we previously identified the presence of ICS particles in the nasally and orally exhaled breath using a particle image velocimetry laser [48] and high-performance liquid chromatography analysis [49]. This led us to propose a technique involving nasal exhalation of ICSs to simultaneously manage asthma comorbid with CRSwNP and ECRS [48–50]. A blinded, placebo-controlled study showed that nasal exhalation of ICSs resulted in decreased FeNO levels and blood eosinophil counts, as well as improved nasal polyp scores and sinus CT findings in patients with asthma and ECRS [51]. Therefore, nasally exhaling ICSs may be beneficial for patients with ACO if there is a comorbidity of CRSwNP and ECRS.

4.2 Biologics

Biologics that target Th2-related cytokines such as IL-4, IL-5, IL-13, and immunoglobulin E (IgE) have been developed to treat severe asthma [52]. Currently available biologics include monoclonal antibodies such as omalizumab (anti-IgE), mepolizumab, reslizumab and benralizumab (anti-IL-5 pathways) and dupilumab (anti-IL-4/IL-13) [52], which may reduce exacerbation of asthma, support maintenance systemic steroids, and improve pulmonary function (FEV_1) [53]. If single-biologic therapy does not sufficiently control symptoms, recent studies have suggested that switching to another biologic and implementing dual- or cycling-biologic therapy using a combination of omalizumab or dupilumab with mepolizumab, benralizumab, reslizumab, or dupilumab, may be beneficial approaches [54–57]. Omalizumab and dupilumab are currently approved by the U.S. Food and Drug Administration for the treatment of CRSwNP [58]. Mepolizumab has also been reported to decrease nasal polyp size and improve symptoms of nasal obstruction and sinus CT findings [59, 60]. Thus, patients with asthma, COPD, and ACO may benefit from the administration of biologics such as omalizumab, dupilumab, and mepolizumab with the view to continuously treat UAD, if CRSwNP and ECRS are suspected.

Conflict of Interest Satoshi Hamada reports grants from Teijin Pharma, outside the submitted work.

Financial Conflicts The Department of Advanced Medicine for Respiratory Failure is a Department of Collaborative Research Laboratory funded by Teijin Pharma.

References

1. Passalacqua G, Ciprandi G, Canonica GW. United airways disease: therapeutic aspects. Thorax. 2000;55(Suppl 2):S26–7. https://doi.org/10.1136/thorax.55.suppl_2.s26.
2. Hens G, Hellings PW. The nose: gatekeeper and trigger of bronchial disease. Rhinology. 2006;44(3):179–87.
3. Bergeron C, Hamid Q. Relationship between asthma and rhinitis: epidemiologic, pathophysiologic, and therapeutic aspects. Allergy Asthma Clin Immunol. 2005;1(2):81–7. https://doi.org/10.1186/1710-1492-1-2-81.
4. Braunstahl GJ. The unified immune system: respiratory tract-nasobronchial interaction mechanisms in allergic airway disease. J Allergy Clin Immunol. 2005;115(1):142–8. https://doi.org/10.1016/j.jaci.2004.10.041.
5. Grossman J. One airway, one disease. Chest. 1997;111:11S–6S. https://doi.org/10.1378/chest.111.2_supplement.11s.
6. Bousquet J, Khaltaev N, Cruz AA, Denburg J, Fokkens WJ, Togias A, Zuberbier T, Baena-Cagnani CE, Canonica GW, van Weel C, Agache I, Aït-Khaled N, Bachert C, Blaiss MS, Bonini S, Boulet LP, Bousquet PJ, Camargos P, Carlsen KH, Chen Y, Custovic A, Dahl R, Demoly P, Douagui H, Durham SR, van Wijk RG, Kalayci O, Kaliner MA, Kim YY, Kowalski ML, Kuna P, Le LT LC, Li J, Lockey RF, Mavale-Manuel S, Meltzer EO, Mohammad Y, Mullol J, Naclerio R, O'Hehir RE, Ohta K, Ouedraogo S, Palkonen S, Papadopoulos N, Passalacqua G, Pawankar R, Popov TA, Rabe KF, Rosado-Pinto J, Scadding GK, Simons FE, Toskala E, Valovirta E, van Cauwenberge P, Wang DY, Wickman M, Yawn BP, Yorgancioglu A, Yusuf OM, Zar H, Annesi-Maesano I, Bateman ED, Ben Kheder A, Boakye DA, Bouchard J, Burney P, Busse WW, Chan-Yeung M, Chavannes NH, Chuchalin A, Dolen WK, Emuzyte R, Grouse L, Humbert M, Jackson C, Johnston SL, Keith PK, Kemp JP, Klossek JM, Larenas-Linnemann D, Lipworth B, Malo JL, Marshall GD, Naspitz C, Nekam K, Niggemann B, Nizankowska-Mogilnicka E, Okamoto Y, Orru MP, Potter P, Price D, Stoloff SW, Vandenplas O, Viegi G, Williams D, World Health Organization; GA(2)LEN; AllerGen. Allergic Rhinitis and its Impact on Asthma (ARIA) 2008 update (in collaboration with the World Health Organization, GA(2)LEN and AllerGen). Allergy. 2008;63 Suppl 86:8–160. https://doi.org/10.1111/j.1398-9995.2007.01620.x.
7. Guerra S, Sherrill DL, Martinez FD, Barbee RA. Rhinitis as an independent risk factor for adult-onset asthma. J Allergy Clin Immunol. 2002;109(3):419–25. https://doi.org/10.1067/mai.2002.121701.
8. Yii ACA, Tay TR, Choo XN, Koh MSY, Tee AKH, Wang DY. Precision medicine in united airways disease: a "treatable traits" approach. Allergy. 2018;73(10):1964–78. https://doi.org/10.1111/all.13496.

9. Orlandi RR, Kingdom TT, Smith TL, Bleier B, DeConde A, Luong AU, Poetker DM, Soler Z, Welch KC, Wise SK, Adappa N, Alt JA, Anselmo-Lima WT, Bachert C, Baroody FM, Batra PS, Bernal-Sprekelsen M, Beswick D, Bhattacharyya N, Chandra RK, Chang EH, Chiu A, Chowdhury N, Citardi MJ, Cohen NA, Conley DB, DelGaudio J, Desrosiers M, Douglas R, Eloy JA, Fokkens WJ, Gray ST, Gudis DA, Hamilos DL, Han JK, Harvey R, Hellings P, Holbrook EH, Hopkins C, Hwang P, Javer AR, Jiang RS, Kennedy D, Kern R, Laidlaw T, Lal D, Lane A, Lee HM, Lee JT, Levy JM, Lin SY, Lund V, McMains KC, Metson R, Mullol J, Naclerio R, Oakley G, Otori N, Palmer JN, Parikh SR, Passali D, Patel Z, Peters A, Philpott C, Psaltis AJ, Ramakrishnan VR, Ramanathan M Jr, Roh HJ, Rudmik L, Sacks R, Schlosser RJ, Sedaghat AR, Senior BA, Sindwani R, Smith K, Snidvongs K, Stewart M, Suh JD, Tan BK, Turner JH, van Drunen CM, Voegels R, Wang Y, Woodworth BA, Wormald PJ, Wright ED, Yan C, Zhang L, Zhou B. International consensus statement on allergy and rhinology: rhinosinusitis 2021. Int Forum Allergy Rhinol. 2021;11(3):213–739. https://doi.org/10.1002/alr.22741.
10. Tokunaga T, Sakashita M, Haruna T, Asaka D, Takeno S, Ikeda H, Nakayama T, Seki N, Ito S, Murata J, Sakuma Y, Yoshida N, Terada T, Morikura I, Sakaida H, Kondo K, Teraguchi K, Okano M, Otori N, Yoshikawa M, Hirakawa K, Haruna S, Himi T, Ikeda K, Ishitoya J, Iino Y, Kawata R, Kawauchi H, Kobayashi M, Yamasoba T, Miwa T, Urashima M, Tamari M, Noguchi E, Ninomiya T, Imoto Y, Morikawa T, Tomita K, Takabayashi T, Fujieda S. Novel scoring system and algorithm for classifying chronic rhinosinusitis: the JESREC Study. Allergy. 2015;70(8):995–1003. https://doi.org/10.1111/all.12644.
11. Laidlaw TM, Mullol J, Woessner KM, Amin N, Mannent LP. Chronic rhinosinusitis with nasal polyps and asthma. J Allergy Clin Immunol Prac. 2021;9(3):1133–41. https://doi.org/10.1016/j.jaip.2020.09.063.
12. Jarvis D, Newson R, Lotvall J, Hastan D, Tomassen P, Keil T, Gjomarkaj M, Forsberg B, Gunnbjornsdottir M, Minov J, Brozek G, Dahlen SE, Toskala E, Kowalski ML, Olze H, Howarth P, Krämer U, Baelum J, Loureiro C, Kasper L, Bousquet PJ, Bousquet J, Bachert C, Fokkens W, Burney P. Asthma in adults and its association with chronic rhinosinusitis: the GA2LEN survey in Europe. Allergy. 2012;67(1):91–8. https://doi.org/10.1111/j.1398-9995.2011.02709.x.
13. Shi JB, Fu QL, Zhang H, Cheng L, Wang YJ, Zhu DD, Lv W, Liu SX, Li PZ, Ou CQ, Xu G. Epidemiology of chronic rhinosinusitis: results from a cross-sectional survey in seven Chinese cities. Allergy. 2015;70(5):533–9. https://doi.org/10.1111/all.12577.
14. Øie MR, Dahlslett SB, Sue-Chu M, Helvik AS, Steinsvåg SK, Thorstensen WM. Rhinosinusitis without nasal polyps in COPD. ERJ Open Res. 2020;6(2):00015–2020. https://doi.org/10.1183/23120541.00015-2020.
15. Hamada S, Tatsumi S, Kobayashi Y, Matsumoto H, Yasuba H. Radiographic evidence of sinonasal inflammation in asthma-chronic obstructive pulmonary disease overlap syndrome: an underrecognized association. J Allergy Clin Immunol Pract. 2017;5(6):1657–62. https://doi.org/10.1016/j.jaip.2017.03.031.
16. Bresciani M, Paradis L, Des Roches A, Vernhet H, Vachier I, Godard P, Bousquet J, Chanez P. Rhinosinusitis in severe asthma. J Allergy Clin Immunol. 2001;107(1):73–80. https://doi.org/10.1067/mai.2001.111593.
17. Lund VJ, Mackay IS. Staging in rhinosinusitis. Rhinology. 1993;31(4):183–4.
18. Pearlman AN, Chandra RK, Chang D, Conley DB, Tripathi-Peters A, Grammer LC, Schleimer RT, Kern RC. Relationships between severity of chronic rhinosinusitis and nasal polyposis, asthma, and atopy. Am J Rhinol Allergy. 2009;23(2):145–8. https://doi.org/10.2500/ajra.2009.23.3284.
19. Lin DC, Chandra RK, Tan BK, Zirkle W, Conley DB, Grammer LC, Kern RC, Schleimer RP, Peters AT. Association between severity of asthma and degree of chronic rhinosinusitis. Am J Rhinol Allergy. 2011;25(4):205–8. https://doi.org/10.2500/ajra.2011.25.3613.
20. Amelink M, de Groot JC, de Nijs SB, Lutter R, Zwinderman AH, Sterk PJ, ten Brinke A, Bel EH. Severe adult-onset asthma: a distinct phenotype. J Allergy Clin Immunol. 2013;132(2):336–41. https://doi.org/10.1016/j.jaci.2013.04.052.

21. Settipane GA, Chafee FH. Nasal polyps in asthma and rhinitis. A review of 6,037 patients. J Allergy Clin Immunol. 1977;59(1):17–21. https://doi.org/10.1016/0091-6749(77)90171-3.
22. Montnémery P, Svensson C, Adelroth E, Löfdahl CG, Andersson M, Greiff L, Persson CG. Prevalence of nasal symptoms and their relation to self-reported asthma and chronic bronchitis/emphysema. Eur Respir J. 2001;17(4):596–603. https://doi.org/10.1183/09031936.01.17405960.
23. Kelemence A, Abadoglu O, Gumus C, Berk S, Epozturk K, Akkurt I. The frequency of chronic rhinosinusitis/nasal polyp in COPD and its effect on the severity of COPD. COPD. 2011;8(1):8–12. https://doi.org/10.3109/15412555.2010.540272.
24. Hansen AG, Helvik AS, Thorstensen WM, Nordgård S, Langhammer A, Bugten V, Stovner LJ, Eggesbø HB. Paranasal sinus opacification at MRI in lower airway disease (the HUNT study-MRI). Eur Arch Otorhinolaryngol. 2016;273(7):1761–8. https://doi.org/10.1007/s00405-015-3790-7.
25. Henriksen AH, Langhammer A, Steinshamn S, Mai XM, Brumpton BM. The prevalence and symptom profile of asthma-COPD overlap: the HUNT study. COPD. 2018;15(1):27–35. https://doi.org/10.1080/15412555.2017.1408580.
26. Williamson PA, Vaidyanathan S, Clearie K, Barnes M, Lipworth BJ. Airway dysfunction in nasal polyposis: a spectrum of asthmatic disease? Clin Exp Allergy. 2011;41(10):1379–85. https://doi.org/10.1111/j.1365-2222.2011.03793.x.
27. Kariya S, Okano M, Oto T, Higaki T, Makihara S, Haruna T, Nishizaki K. Pulmonary function in patients with chronic rhinosinusitis and allergic rhinitis. J Laryngol Otol. 2014;128(3):255–62. https://doi.org/10.1017/S0022215114000450.
28. Lee SY, Yoon SH, Song WJ, Lee SH, Kang HR, Kim SS, Cho SH. Influence of chronic sinusitis and nasal polyp on the lower airway of subjects without lower airway diseases. Allergy Asthma Immunol Res. 2014;6(4):310–5. https://doi.org/10.4168/aair.2014.6.4.310.
29. Kambara R, Minami T, Akazawa H, Tsuji F, Sasaki T, Inohara H, Horii A. Lower airway inflammation in eosinophilic chronic rhinosinusitis as determined by exhaled nitric oxide. Int Arch Allergy Immunol. 2017;173(4):225–32. https://doi.org/10.1159/000479387.
30. Uraguchi K, Kariya S, Makihara S, Okano M, Haruna T, Oka A, Fujiwara R, Noda Y, Nishizaki K. Pulmonary function in patients with eosinophilic chronic rhinosinusitis. Auris Nasus Larynx. 2018;45(3):476–81. https://doi.org/10.1016/j.anl.2017.07.020.
31. Izuhara Y, Matsumoto H, Nagasaki T, Kanemitsu Y, Murase K, Ito I, Oguma T, Muro S, Asai K, Tabara Y, Takahashi K, Bessho K, Sekine A, Kosugi S, Yamada R, Nakayama T, Matsuda F, Niimi A, Chin K, Mishima M, Nagahama Study Group. Mouth breathing, another risk factor for asthma: the Nagahama Study. Allergy. 2016;71(7):1031–6. https://doi.org/10.1111/all.12885.
32. Lee TJ, Fu CH, Wang CH, Huang CC, Huang CC, Chang PH, Chen YW, Wu CC, Wu CL, Kuo HP. Impact of chronic rhinosinusitis on severe asthma patients. PLoS One. 2017;12(2):e0171047. https://doi.org/10.1371/journal.pone.0171047.
33. Yang HJ, LoSavio PS, Engen PA, Naqib A, Mehta A, Kota R, Khan RJ, Tobin MC, Green SJ, Schleimer RP, Keshavarzian A, Batra PS, Mahdavinia M. Association of nasal microbiome and asthma control in patients with chronic rhinosinusitis. Clin Exp Allergy. 2018;48(12):1744–7. https://doi.org/10.1111/cea.13255.
34. Stevens WW, Peters AT, Hirsch AG, Nordberg CM, Schwartz BS, Mercer DG, Mahdavinia M, Grammer LC, Hulse KE, Kern RC, Avila P, Schleimer RP. Clinical characteristics of patients with chronic rhinosinusitis with nasal polyps, asthma, and aspirin-exacerbated respiratory disease. J Alergy Clin Immunol Pract. 2017;5(4):1061–1070.e3. https://doi.org/10.1016/j.jaip.2016.12.027.
35. Klossek JM, Neukirch F, Pribil C, Jankowski R, Serrano E, Chanal I, El Hasnaoui A. Prevalence of nasal polyposis in France: a cross-sectional, case-control study. Allergy. 2005;60(2):233–7. https://doi.org/10.1111/j.1398-9995.2005.00688.x.

36. Kimura H, Konno S, Nakamaru Y, Makita H, Taniguchi N, Shimizu K, Suzuki M, Ono J, Ohta S, Izuhara K, Nishimura M, Hokkaido-based Investigative Cohort Analysis for Refractory Asthma Investigators. Sinus computed tomographic findings in adult smokers and non-smokers with asthma. Analysis of clinical indices and biomarkers. Ann Am Thorac Soc. 2017;14(3):332–41. https://doi.org/10.1513/AnnalsATS.201606-463OC.
37. ten Brinke A, Grootendorst DC, Schmidt JT, De Bruïne FT, van Buchem MA, Sterk PJ, Rabe KF, Bel EH. Chronic sinusitis in severe asthma is related to sputum eosinophilia. J Allergy Clin Immunol. 2002;109(4):621–6. https://doi.org/10.1067/mai.2002.122458.
38. Bilodeau L, Boulay ME, Prince P, Boisvert P, Boulet LP. Comparative clinical and airway inflammatory features of asthmatics with or without polyps. Rhinology. 2010;48(4):420–5. https://doi.org/10.4193/Rhino09.095.
39. Novelli F, Bacci E, Latorre M, Seccia V, Bartoli ML, Cianchetti S, Dente FL, Franco AD, Celi A, Paggiaro P. Comorbidities are associated with different features of severe asthma. Clin Mol Allergy. 2018;16:25. https://doi.org/10.1186/s12948-018-0103-x.
40. Håkansson K, Bachert C, Konge L, Thomsen SF, Pedersen AE, Poulsen SS, Martin-Bertelsen T, Winther O, Backer V, von Buchwald C. Airway inflammation in chronic rhinosinusitis with nasal polyps and asthma: the united airways concept further supported. PLoS One. 2015;10(7):e0127228. https://doi.org/10.1371/journal.pone.0127228.
41. Hurst JR, Wilkinson TM, Donaldson GC, Wedzicha JA. Upper airway symptoms and quality of life in chronic obstructive pulmonary disease (COPD). Respir Med. 2004;98(8):767–70. https://doi.org/10.1016/j.rmed.2004.01.010.
42. Arndal E, Sørensen AL, Lapperre TS, Said N, Trampedach C, Aanæs K, Alanin MC, Christensen KB, Backer V, von Buchwald C. Chronic rhinosinusitis in COPD: a prevalent but unrecognized comorbidity impacting health related quality of life. Respir Med. 2020;171:106092. https://doi.org/10.1016/j.rmed.2020.106092.
43. Øie MR, Sue-Chu M, Helvik AS, Steinsvåg SK, Steinsbekk S, Thorstensen WM. Rhinosinusitis without nasal polyps is associated with poorer health-related quality of life in COPD. Respir Med. 2021;189:106661. https://doi.org/10.1016/j.rmed.2021.106661.
44. Huerta A, Donaldson GC, Singh R, Mackay AJ, Allinson JP, Brill SE, Kowlessar B, Torres A, Wedzicha JA. Upper respiratory symptoms worsen over time and relate to clinical phenotype in chronic obstructive pulmonary disease. Ann Am Thorac Soc. 2015;12(7):997–1004. https://doi.org/10.1513/AnnalsATS.201408-359OC.
45. Dewan NA, Rafique S, Kanwar B, Satpathy H, Ryschon K, Tillotson GS, Niederman MS. Acute exacerbation of COPD: factors associated with poor treatment outcome. Chest. 2000;117(3):662–71. https://doi.org/10.1378/chest.117.3.662.
46. Fokkens WJ, Lund VJ, Hopkins C, Hellings PW, Kern R, Reitsma S, Toppila-Salmi S, Bernal-Sprekelsen M, Mullol J, Alobid I, Terezinha Anselmo-Lima W, Bachert C, Baroody F, von Buchwald C, Cervin A, Cohen N, Constantinidis J, De Gabory L, Desrosiers M, Diamant Z, Douglas RG, Gevaert PH, Hafner A, Harvey RJ, Joos GF, Kalogjera L, Knill A, Kocks JH, Landis BN, Limpens J, Lebeer S, Lourenco O, Meco C, Matricardi PM, O'Mahony L, Philpott CM, Ryan D, Schlosser R, Senior B, Smith TL, Teeling T, Tomazic PV, Wang DY, Wang D, Zhang L, Agius AM, Ahlstrom-Emanuelsson C, Alabri R, Albu S, Alhabash S, Aleksic A, Aloulah M, Al-Qudah M, Alsaleh S, Baban MA, Baudoin T, Balvers T, Battaglia P, Bedoya JD, Beule A, Bofares KM, Braverman I, Brozek-Madry E, Richard B, Callejas C, Carrie S, Caulley L, Chussi D, de Corso E, Coste A, El Hadi U, Elfarouk A, Eloy PH, Farrokhi S, Felisati G, Ferrari MD, Fishchuk R, Grayson W, Goncalves PM, Grdinic B, Grgic V, Hamizan AW, Heinichen JV, Husain S, Ping TI, Ivaska J, Jakimovska F, Jovancevic L, Kakande E, Kamel R, Karpischenko S, Kariyawasam HH, Kawauchi H, Kjeldsen A, Klimek L, Krzeski A, Kopacheva Barsova G, Kim SW, Lal D, Letort JJ, Lopatin A, Mahdjoubi A, Mesbahi A, Netkovski J, Nyenbue Tshipukane D, Obando-Valverde A, Okano M, Onerci M, Ong YK, Orlandi R, Otori N, Ouennoughy K, Ozkan M, Peric A, Plzak J, Prokopakis E, Prepageran N, Psaltis A, Pugin B, Raftopulos M, Rombaux P, Riechelmann H, Sahtout S, Sarafoleanu CC, Searyoh K, Rhee CS, Shi J, Shkoukani M, Shukuryan AK, Sicak M, Smyth D, Sindvongs K, Soklic Kosak T, Stjarne P, Sutikno B, Steinsvag S, Tantilipikorn P, Thanaviratananich S,

Tran T, Urbancic J, Valiulius A, Vasquez de Aparicio C, Vicheva D, Virkkula PM, Vicente G, Voegels R, Wagenmann MM, Wardani RS, Welge-Lussen A, Witterick I, Wright E, Zabolotniy D, Zsolt B, Zwetsloot CP. European position paper on rhinosinusitis and nasal polyps 2020. Rhinology. 2020;58(Suppl S29):1–464. https://doi.org/10.4193/Rhin20.600.

47. Dekhuijzen PN, Bjermer L, Lavorini F, Ninane V, Molimard M, Haughney J. Guidance on handheld inhalers in asthma and COPD guidelines. Respir Med. 2014;108(5):694–700. https://doi.org/10.1016/j.rmed.2014.02.013.
48. Hamada S, Matsumoto H, Kobayashi Y, Asako M, Yasuba H. Nasal exhalation of inhaled beclomethasone hydrofluoroalkane-134a to treat chronic rhinosinusitis. J Allergy Clin Immunol Pract. 2016;4(4):751–2. https://doi.org/10.1016/j.jaip.2015.11.018.
49. Hamada S, Hira D, Kobayashi Y, Yasuba H. Effect of nasally exhaling budesonide/formoterol dry powder inhaled at “fast” inspiratory flow on eosinophilic chronic rhinosinusitis. Int J Clin Pharmacol Ther. 2018;56(11):539–43. https://doi.org/10.5414/CP203272.
50. Kobayashi Y, Asako M, Kanda A, Tomoda K, Yasuba H. A novel therapeutic use of HFA-BDP metereddose inhaler for asthmatic patients with rhinosinusitis: case series. Int J Clin Pharmacol Ther. 2014;52(10):914–9. https://doi.org/10.5414/CP202100.
51. Kobayashi Y, Yasuba H, Asako M, Yamamoto T, Takano H, Tomoda K, Kanda A, Iwai H. HFA-BDP metered-dose inhaler exhaled through the nose improves eosinophilic chronic rhinosinusitis with bronchial asthma: a blinded, placebo-controlled study. Front Immunol. 2018;9:2192. https://doi.org/10.3389/fimmu.2018.02192.
52. Busse WW. Biological treatments for severe asthma: a major advance in asthma care. Allergol Int. 2019;68(2):158–66. https://doi.org/10.1016/j.alit.2019.01.004.
53. Busse WW, Kraft M, Rabe KF, Deniz Y, Rowe PJ, Ruddy M, Castro M. Understanding the key issues in the treatment of uncontrolled persistent asthma with type 2 inflammation. Eur Respir J. 2021;58(2):2003393. https://doi.org/10.1183/13993003.03393-2020.
54. Hamada S, Ogino E, Yasuba H. Cycling therapy with benralizumab and dupilumab for severe eosinophilic asthma with eosinophilic chronic rhinosinusitis and eosinophilic otitis media. Allergol Int. 2021;70(3):389–91. https://doi.org/10.1016/j.alit.2021.02.002.
55. Hamada S, Ogino E, Yasuba H. Cycling biologic therapy for severe asthma. Pulmonology. 2022;28(1):65–7. https://doi.org/10.1016/j.pulmoe.2021.07.009.
56. Ortega G, Tongchinsub P, Carr T. Combination biologic therapy for severe persistent asthma. Ann Allergy Asthma Immunol. 2019;123(3):309–11. https://doi.org/10.1016/j.anai.2019.06.013.
57. Menzies-Gow AN, McBrien C, Unni B, Porsbjerg CM, Al-Ahmad M, Ambrose CS, Dahl Assing K, von Bülow A, Busby J, Cosio BG, FitzGerald JM, Garcia Gil E, Hansen S, Heaney LG, Hew M, Jackson DJ, Kallieri M, Loukides S, Lugogo NL, Papaioannou AI, Larenas-Linnemann D, Moore WC, Perez-de-Llano LA, Rasmussen LM, Schmid JM, Siddiqui S, Alacqua M, Tran TN, Suppli Ulrik C, Upham JW, Wang E, Bulathsinhala L, Carter VA, Chaudhry I, Eleangovan N, Murray RB, Price CA, Price DB. Real world biologic use and switch patterns in severe asthma: data from the international severe asthma registry and the US CHRONICLE study. J Asthma Allergy. 2022;15:63–78. https://doi.org/10.2147/JAA.S328653.
58. Morse CJ, Miller C, Senior B. Management of chronic rhinosinusitis with nasal polyposis in the era of biologics. J Asthma Allergy. 2021;14:873–82. https://doi.org/10.2147/JAA.S258438.
59. Bachert C, Sousa AR, Lund VJ, Scadding GK, Gevaert P, Nasser S, Durham SR, Cornet ME, Kariyawasam HH, Gilbert J, Austin D, Maxwell AC, Marshall RP, Fokkens WJ. Reduced need for surgery in severe nasal polyposis with mepolizumab: randomized trial. J Allergy Clin Immunol. 2017;140(4):1024–1031.414. https://doi.org/10.1016/j.jaci.2017.05.044.
60. Han JK, Bachert C, Fokkens W, Desrosiers M, Wagenmann M, Lee SE, Smith SG, Martin N, Mayer B, Yancey SW, Sousa AR, Chan R, Hopkins C, SYNAPSE Study Investigators. Mepolizumab for chronic rhinosinusitis with nasal polyps (SYNAPSE): a randomised, double-blind, placebo-controlled, phase 3 trial. Lancet Respir Med. 2021;9(10):1141–53. https://doi.org/10.1016/S2213-2600(21)00097-7.

Part V
Treatment

Chapter 17
Current Evidence of Treatment for Asthma-COPD Overlap (ACO): Is There Emerging Evidence of Optimal Therapy?—In Asthma COPD Overlap: Updated Concept, Pathophysiology, Diagnosis and Treatment

Yoshihisa Ishiura, Shosaku Nomura, Takeshi Tamaki, Toshiki Shimizu, Naoyuki Miyashita, and Tomoki Ito

Abstract Asthma-COPD overlap (ACO), a phenotype involving asthma and COPD, is an important disease entity because patients with ACO have significantly worse outcomes, conferring greater economic and social burdens. Some guidelines for ACO recommend add-on therapy of long-acting muscarinic antagonists (LAMAs) to inhaled corticosteroids (ICS) and long-acting β_2 agonists (LABAs). However, this approach is based on extrapolation from patients with asthma or COPD alone. Therefore, there is still no consensus on the treatment strategy for ACO based on sufficient evidence.

When ACO is diagnosed for the first time, the severity of asthma and COPD is determined. The more severe severity of each is used as a reference. The following treatment is recommended: ICS+LABA, ICS+LABA, and ICS+LABA+LAMA starting from the mildest disease, followed by theophylline, leukotriene receptor antagonist, anti-IgE antibody, anti-IL5 antibody, oral steroids, and in cases of high sputum production, macrolides, and expectorants, etc., are added sequentially when sputum production is increased.

The degree of exacerbation of ACO is classified into three categories: mild, moderate, and severe. Mild disease presents with mild dyspnea and wheezing attacks, and inhalation of a short-acting β_2 agonist (SABA) is recommended for asthma and

Y. Ishiura (✉) · S. Nomura · T. Tamaki · T. Shimizu · N. Miyashita · T. Ito
First Department of Internal Medicine, Kansai Medical University, Osaka, Japan
e-mail: ishiuray@takii.kmu.ac.jp

H. Nagase et al. (eds.), *Asthma-COPD Overlap*, Respiratory Disease Series: Diagnostic Tools and Disease Managements,
https://doi.org/10.1007/978-981-96-0217-9_17

COPD, as is the case for ACO. If the patient has been treated with budesonide/formoterol in the stable phase, this drug can also treat attacks. If SABA inhalation or additional budesonide/formoterol inhalation fails to improve, i.e., moderate or severe exacerbations, systemic administration of steroids has to be indicated.

Keywords Asthma-COPD overlap · Triple therapy · Treatable traits

1 Goals of Treatment and Management

There is still no consensus on the treatment strategy for ACO based on sufficient evidence. This is because clinical trials in asthma patients have excluded patients with a smoking history and elderly patients. At the same time, clinical trials in COPD patients have also excluded patients with asthma complications, and only a few prospective clinical studies have been conducted in ACO patients [1–4]. Therefore, the current treatment strategy for ACO is based on the treatment strategy for asthma and COPD, with recommendations for treatment as deemed appropriate.

Since ACO patients have characteristics of both asthma and COPD, Table 17.1 is determined by the Japanese Respiratory Society; considering the management goals of both diseases to achieve the management goals of ACO, the following items should be considered.

1.1 Pathological Evaluation

The disease type and severity are evaluated in terms of asthma and COPD by referring to various biomarkers, physiological indices, imaging findings, and quality of life questionnaires in ACO patients, and the disease progression and response to treatment are carefully monitored.

Table 17.1 Management objectives of ACO

1. Improvement of symptoms and quality of life
2. Improvement of respiratory dysfunction and airway hyperresponsiveness
3. Improvement and maintenance of exercise tolerance and physical activity
4. suppression of disease progression and airway remodeling
5. Prevention of exacerbations
6. Prevention and treatment of complications and dependence
7. Improvement of life expectancy
8. Avoidance of adverse effects of therapeutic drugs

1.2 Avoidance of Risk Factors

Avoid exposure to allergens, tobacco smoke, air pollutants, and infectious agents such as viruses and bacteria, and consider reducing risk factors by cleaning rooms and installing air purifiers. Drugs, stress, and overwork should also be avoided.

1.3 Long-Term Management During the Stable Period

Appropriate long-term management of both asthma and COPD is essential during the stable period. Therefore, ACO should provide pharmacotherapy according to the disease state and comprehensive management through environmental conditioning, patient education, respiratory rehabilitation, influenza and pneumococcal vaccination, nutritional therapy, oxygen therapy, ventilatory support therapy, etc. In COPD, the combination of influenza and pneumococcal vaccine is recommended to be combined with the influenza vaccine alone. In COPD, combining influenza and pneumococcal vaccines reduces the frequency of COPD exacerbations caused by infectious diseases compared to influenza vaccination alone, so both vaccines should be administered in ACO. Currently, two types of pneumococcal vaccines are available: 23-valent pneumococcal polysaccharide vaccine (Pneumovax NP) and 13-valent pneumococcal conjugate vaccine (Prevenar 13).

2 Basic Concept of Treatment

The basic approach to the treatment of ACO is to "treat both asthma and COPD" because patients with ACO have a higher frequency of imaging [5–7], higher medical costs [8], lower quality of life [9], and a faster decline in respiratory function [10] than patients with asthma or COPD alone. Low quality of life [9] and rapid decline in respiratory function [10], more extensive and intensive treatment should be considered in ACO. The basic ACO treatment strategy and evaluation are as follows.

2.1 Inhaled Steroids and Bronchodilators

Initial treatment should be initiated as soon as ACO is diagnosed. If an inhaled steroid (ICS) is not being administered at diagnosis, the patient should be started on an ICS. At the same time, long-acting β_2 agonists (LABAs) and long-acting muscarinic antagonists (LAMAs) are added as bronchodilators [1–4]. It is important to note that LABAs and LAMAs should not be used alone because of the presence of asthma and must be combined with ICS [11].

There is no established standardized evaluation of the benefit of ICS/LABA or ICS+LAMA for ACOs; LAMA has been reported to be a more severe exacerbation inhibitor than LABA in COPD [12], but comparative studies in ACOs are needed. Several studies have recommended ICS/LAMA/LABA as treatable traits for ACO, which can be used as a reference for future treatment [2–4].

There is no standardized dosage of ICS for the treatment of ACO. In general, smokers are less responsive to ICS [13]. In addition, because of the high degree of airway inflammation caused by smoking, it has been reported that patients with ACO require more intensive ICS to overcome the higher degree of airway inflammation compared to pure asthmatics [2–4]. At present, it is reasonable to use ICS in combination with long-acting bronchodilators from the beginning of treatment, and the dose of ICS should be determined according to the severity of the disease.

2.2 *Other Drugs*

Macrolide antimicrobial agents may reduce ACO exacerbations. Macrolides have effects such as inhibiting neutrophil activation and antiviral activity, improving airway clearance, and reducing the risk of acute exacerbations in patients with COPD [14]. Macrolide administration to asthma patients with repeated exacerbations also significantly reduced the frequency of asthma exacerbations in a subanalysis of non-neutrophilic severe asthma patients with peripheral blood eosinophils below 200/μL [15], suggesting that macrolides may be helpful in patients with neutrophilic inflammation.

Anti-IgE and anti-IL5 antibody drugs suppress eosinophilic inflammation and may help treat the asthmatic component of the ACO condition. Other asthma medications include leukotriene receptor antagonists, but there is no evidence of their efficacy in COPD, and the pros and cons of their aggressive administration in ACO are unknown.

Expectorants such as carbocisteine have been reported to be effective in treating ACOs. These agents suppress airway mucus secretion and improve airway clearance impairment, thereby preventing exacerbation of the disease.

3 Treatment Practice

The first pattern of ACO treatment is that untreated patients are diagnosed with ACO for the first time. Second, patients who have been treated for asthma are diagnosed with ACO. Third, COPD patients are diagnosed with ACO. These three cases are assumed. The actual treatment in each case is described below.

3.1 When ACO Is Diagnosed for the First Time

First, the severity of asthma and COPD is determined. The more severe severity of each is used as a reference, and the following treatment is recommended: ICS+LABA, ICS+LABA, and ICS+LABA+LAMA starting from the mildest disease, followed by theophylline, leukotriene receptor antagonist, anti-IgE antibody, anti-IL5 antibody, oral steroids, and in cases of high sputum production, macrolides, and expectorants. Macrolides, expectorants, etc., are added sequentially when sputum production is increased.

3.2 When a Patient with Asthma Is Diagnosed with ACO

When ACO is suspected in patients treated for asthma (smoking history, insufficient reversibility of respiratory function tests, emphysematous changes, chronic and progressive shortness of breath, etc.), the addition of LAMA to the treatment for asthma (ICS or ICS/LABA ± leukotriene receptor antagonist) may improve symptoms. Even if the airflow obstruction is fixed, ICS should be continued, and if there is a solid atopic predisposition.

Leukotriene receptor antagonists may also be helpful if the patient has a strong predisposition to atopy [16].

3.3 When a COPD Patient Is Diagnosed with ACO

Suppose ACO is suspected in a COPD patient (paroxysmal dyspnea/wheezing, airway reversibility, atopic predisposition, high exhaled nitric oxide (FeNO) levels, etc.). In that case, ICS should be promptly added to COPD medications (LAMA, LABA, LAMA/LABA), depending on symptoms. ICS should be reduced after 3–6 months of good control. Leukotriene receptor antagonists should be continued for 2–4 weeks after initiation before evaluation.

4 Determination of Treatment Response

Objective measures used to determine treatment response include the Asthma Control Test (ACT), Asthma Control Questionnaire (ACQ), COPD Assessment Test (CAT), mMRC shortness of breath scale, modified Borg scale, Visual Analogue Scale (VAS), forced expiratory volume in one second (FEV1), forced vital capacity (FVC), FEV1/FVC and Visual Analogue Scale (VAS). Spirometry should be measured at the first visit and repeated 1–3 months after treatment and at least once a year after that. Mostographs, sputum eosinophil ratio and FeNO, peripheral blood eosinophil count, exacerbation frequency, arterial blood gas analysis, transcutaneous arterial blood oxygen saturation (SPO2) measurement, and 6-min walk test should also be performed as necessary.

5 Treatment of Exacerbations

There are no clear guidelines for treating ACO exacerbations, and existing guidelines for asthma and COPD should be consulted. An exacerbation of ACO is defined as "an increase in dyspnea, wheezing, coughing or sputum production compared with the stable phase, which requires a change in treatment during the stable phase, such as the administration of systemic steroids or antibacterial agents." It is defined as "a condition in which there is an increase in dyspnea, wheezing, cough, and sputum compared to the stable phase, and a need for a change in treatment during the stable phase, such as the administration of systemic steroids or antimicrobials."

The degree of exacerbation of ACO is classified into three categories according to the degree of exacerbation of COPD: mild (when only short-acting bronchodilators are needed), moderate (when antibacterial agents or systemic steroids are needed in addition to short-acting bronchodilators), and severe (when emergency department visits or hospitalization are required). Mild disease presents with mild dyspnea and wheezing attacks, and inhalation of a short-acting β_2 agonist (SABA) is recommended for asthma and COPD, as is the case for ACO. Suppose the patient has been treated with budesonide/formoterol in the stable phase. In that case, this drug can also be used to treat attacks, and if SABA inhalation or additional budesonide/formoterol inhalation fails to improve, i.e., moderate or severe exacerbations, systemic administration of steroids is indicated. In COPD, the importance of viral and bacterial infections as a cause of exacerbations has been pointed out, and if sputum becomes purulent, antimicrobials are recommended, given the possibility of bacterial infection. However, there is still no evidence for ACO in these responses.

6 Referral to a Specialist

Referral to a specialist is necessary in the following cases. Symptoms persist or worsen despite treatment; the diagnosis is not confirmed (e.g., suspicion of pulmonary hypertension, cardiovascular disease, or other causes of respiratory symptoms); asthma or COPD is suspected, but features of the condition are atypical, or there are additional symptoms or signs (e.g., hemoptysis, body weight loss, night sweats, fever, findings of bronchiectasis), other pulmonary conditions are suspected, complications or management of dependence is difficult. And bronchiectasis), when other pulmonary diseases are suspected or difficulties or support are difficult to manage.

References

1. Ishiura Y, Fujimura M, Shiba Y, Ohkura N, Hara J, Kasahara K. A comparison of the efficacy of once-daily fluticasone furoate/vilanterole with twice-daily fluticasone propionate/salmeterol in Asthma-COPD overlap syndrome. Pulm Pharmacol Ther. 2015;35:28–33. https://doi.org/10.1016/j.pupt.2015.10.005. Epub 2015 Oct 22.
2. Ishiura Y, Fujimura M, Ohkura N, et al. Effect of triple therapy in patients with asthma-COPD overlap. Int J Clin Pharmacol Ther. 2019;57(8):384–92. https://doi.org/10.5414/CP203382.
3. Ishiura Y, Fujimura M, Ohkura N, et al. Therapy with budesonide/glycopyrrolate/formoterol fumarate improves inspiratory capacity in patients with asthma-chronic obstructive pulmonary disease overlap. Int J Chron Obstruct Pulmon Dis. 2020;15:269–77. https://doi.org/10.2147/COPD.S231004. eCollection 2020.
4. Ishiura Y, Fujimura M, Ohkura N, Hara J, Nakahama K, Sawai Y, Tamaki T, Murai R, Shimizu T, Miyashita N, Nomura S. Tiotropium add-on and treatable traits in asthma-COPD overlap: a real-world pilot study. J Asthma Allergy. 2022;15:703–12. https://doi.org/10.2147/JAA.S360260. eCollection 2022.
5. Menezes AMB, de Oca MM, Pérez-Padilla R, et al. Increased risk of exacerbation and hospitalization in subjects with an overlap phenotype: COPD-asthma. Chest. 2014;145(2):297–304. https://doi.org/10.1378/chest.13-0622.
6. Bateman ED, Reddel HK, van Zyl-Smit RN, Agusti A. The asthma-COPD overlap syndrome: towards a revised taxonomy of chronic airways diseases? Lancet Respir Med. 2015;3(9):719–28. https://doi.org/10.1016/S2213-2600(15)00254-4. Epub 2015 Aug 5.
7. Nielsen M, Bårnes CB, Ulrik CS. Clinical characteristics of the asthma-COPD overlap syndrome—a systematic review. Int J Chron Obstruct Pulmon Dis. 2015;10:1443–54. https://doi.org/10.2147/COPD.S85363. eCollection 2015.
8. Shaya FT, Dongyi D, Akazawa MO, et al. Burden of concomitant asthma and COPD in a Medicaid population. Chest. 2008;134(1):14–9. https://doi.org/10.1378/chest.07-2317. Epub 2008 Mar 13.
9. Kauppi P, Kupiainen H, Lindqvist A, et al. Overlap syndrome of asthma and COPD predicts low quality of life. J Asthma. 2011;48(3):279–85. https://doi.org/10.3109/02770903.2011.555576. Epub 2011 Feb 17.
10. McDonald VM, Simpson JL, Higgins I, et al. Multidimensional assessment of older people with asthma and COPD: clinical management and health status. Age Ageing. 2011;40(1):42–9. https://doi.org/10.1093/ageing/afq134. Epub 2010 Nov 17.
11. Salpeter SR, Buckley NS, Ormiston TM, Salpeter EE. Meta-analysis: effect of long-acting beta-agonists on severe asthma exacerbations and asthma-related deaths. Ann Intern Med. 2006;144(12):904–12. https://doi.org/10.7326/0003-4819-144-12-200606200-00126. Epub 2006 Jun 5.
12. Vogelmeier C, Hederer B, Glaab T, et al. Tiotropium versus salmeterol for the prevention of exacerbations of COPD. N Engl J Med. 2011;364(12):1093–103. https://doi.org/10.1056/NEJMoa1008378.
13. Chalmers GW, Macleod KJ, Little SA, et al. Influence of cigarette smoking on inhaled corticosteroid treatment in mild asthma. Thorax. 2002;57(3):226–30. https://doi.org/10.1136/thorax.57.3.226.

14. Reiter J, Demirel N, Mendy A, et al. Macrolides for the long-term management of asthma—a meta-analysis of randomized clinical trials. Allergy. 2013;68(8):1040–9. https://doi.org/10.1111/all.12199. Epub 2013 Jul 30.
15. Brusselle GG, Vanderstichele C, Jordens P, et al. Azithromycin for prevention of exacerbations in severe asthma (AZISAST): a multicentre randomised double-blind placebo-controlled trial. Thorax. 2013;68(4):322–9. https://doi.org/10.1136/thoraxjnl-2012-202698. Epub 2013 Jan 3.
16. Postma DS, Rabe KF. The asthma-COPD overlap syndrome. N Engl J Med. 2015;373(13):1241–9. https://doi.org/10.1056/NEJMra1411863.

Chapter 18
Potential Treatment Options for ACO, Including Biologics: Are There Any Roles of Biologics?

Nobuhisa Ishikawa

Abstract Anti-immunoglobulin E (IgE) antibody (omalizumab), anti-interleukin (IL)-5 antibodies (mepolizumab and reslizumab), anti-IL-5R antibody (benralizumab), and anti-IL-4Rα antibody (dupilumab, an IL-4 and IL-13 blocker) have been approved to treat severe asthma, targeting individuals with an allergic background or eosinophilic asthma. These biologics have been demonstrated to be selectively effective in patients with type 2 (T2)-high severe asthma; however, studies on their use in patients with chronic pulmonary obstructive disease (COPD) have reported inconsistent results. Therefore, it is important to differentiate severe asthma, especially late-onset asthma, from COPD. However, experience with the use of biologics in patients with asthma and COPD overlap (ACO) is limited. Some patients with ACO predominantly have T2-high inflammation and may respond to these biologics. In patients with severe ACO who exhibit uncontrolled symptoms despite currently available standard treatment, including inhaled triple therapy, advanced treatment with biologics may be considered. Thus, the evaluation of T2-high biomarkers, such as blood eosinophils, fractional exhaled nitric oxide, and IgE, may help select appropriate biologics for ACO. The selection of the most suitable biologics for each patient should be multifaceted, considering the eligibility criteria, clinical characteristics (phenotypes), molecular mechanisms (endotypes), comorbidities, route of administration, and dosing frequency.

Keywords Asthma and chronic obstructive pulmonary disease overlap · Eosinophil · Biologics

N. Ishikawa (✉)
Department of Respiratory Medicine, Hiroshima Prefectural Hospital, Hiroshima, Japan
e-mail: n-ishikawa@hph.pref.hiroshima.jp

H. Nagase et al. (eds.), *Asthma-COPD Overlap*, Respiratory Disease Series: Diagnostic Tools and Disease Managements,
https://doi.org/10.1007/978-981-96-0217-9_18

1 Introduction

Asthma is characterized by eosinophilic inflammation of the airways and respiratory symptoms, such as wheezing, shortness of breath, chest tightness, and cough, which vary over time and in their occurrence, frequency, and intensity. These symptoms are associated with variable expiratory airflow obstruction, airway wall thickening, and increased mucus production. Chronic obstructive pulmonary disease (COPD) is a common, preventable, and treatable disease characterized by persistent respiratory symptoms and airflow limitation due to airway and/or alveolar abnormalities, usually caused by significant exposure to noxious particles or gases. In 2015, 358 million and 174 million individuals were estimated to be affected by asthma and COPD, respectively, worldwide [1]. Deaths from COPD were eight times more common than deaths from asthma. Asthma and COPD are the most common chronic airway diseases but have different etiologies, prognoses, and treatment guidelines. However, asthma and COPD frequently overlap, particularly in smokers and older patients, and distinguishing late-onset asthma from asthma and COPD overlap (ACO) is challenging. Atopy is less frequent, and spirometry values are lower in late-onset asthma than in early-onset asthma. ACO may affect 10–40% of patients with COPD and 15–35% of patients with asthma [2]. In the near future, the incidence of ACO in older patients is expected to increase because of the aging population and the disproportionate increase in the number of individuals aged >65 years. Owing to the increase in the proportion of ACO with age, its significance is currently in focus. Furthermore, patients with ACO exhibit more frequent and severe exacerbations, rapid decline in lung function, high mortality, lower health-related quality of life (HRQOL), and a higher economic burden than those with asthma or COPD alone [3]. Therefore, early screening and diagnosis are crucial in the successful management of ACO. Strategies are needed to reduce the severity or frequency of exacerbations, prevent hospitalization, and improve the HRQOL of patients with ACO.

However, the efficacy and safety of pharmacological therapy for ACO are not well established, as patients with ACO are excluded from clinical trials for asthma or COPD. Most clinical trials for asthma have excluded patients with a significant smoking history, whereas clinical trials for COPD have typically not included patients with a history of asthma. There are several definitions for ACO, and almost all definitions include the following criterion: individuals with smoking-related COPD with a background of T2 inflammation and/or significant airway reversibility. Therefore, most of the available treatment strategies for ACO are currently extrapolated from trials on asthma and COPD. Recently, anti-immunoglobulin E (IgE) antibody (omalizumab), anti-interleukin (IL)-5 antibodies (mepolizumab and reslizumab), anti-IL-5R antibody (benralizumab), and anti-IL-4Rα antibody (dupilumab, an IL-4 and IL-13 blocker) have been approved for the treatment of severe asthma. Although these biologics have been demonstrated to be effective in patients with type 2 (T2)-high severe asthma, there is little evidence regarding the use of biologics in ACO. In this chapter, we propose a therapeutic approach, especially for biologics, for patients with severe uncontrolled ACO.

2 Assessment of T2-High Inflammation for ACO

The lack of a strict definition for ACO results in the need for biomarkers that could help in its identification. However, there is no single biomarker that can be used to identify ACO accurately. T2-high inflammatory biomarkers, such as peripheral blood eosinophil counts, fractional exhaled nitric oxide (FeNO), and serum levels of IgE, could be used to support the diagnosis of ACO [4]. Because each of these biomarkers has low sensitivity and specificity, some guidelines recommend a combination of the biomarkers for improved diagnostic accuracy of ACO [5].

2.1 Eosinophils

Eosinophils are proinflammatory granulocytes that play a major role in the T2-high inflammatory phenotype, including severe eosinophilic asthma and COPD. The pathogenetic role of eosinophils is more apparent in COPD than in asthma. However, it has been shown that increased eosinophil counts in sputum or blood predict clinical response to inhaled corticosteroids (ICS) and oral corticosteroids (OCS). Eosinophilic airway inflammation is one of the most influential treatable traits in chronic airway diseases, including asthma and COPD.

Although the sputum eosinophil count is known to directly reflect the severity of airway inflammation, it is difficult for clinicians to evaluate the inflammatory status of the airways via sputum examination due to its complicated processing. Instead, the blood eosinophil count can be more easily and conveniently measured as a surrogate marker of eosinophilic airway inflammation, and it has been shown to be significantly correlated with sputum eosinophil count. Elevated eosinophil counts in sputum have been defined as ≥2% of the total cell count and are known to be correlated with peripheral blood eosinophil counts. In contrast, elevated blood eosinophil counts in COPD have been classified as either >150 or ≥300 cells/μL in several studies on severe asthma to identify T2-high predominant inflammation, with no clear consensus. However, most studies have suggested an elevated blood eosinophil count of ≥300 cells/μL [6].

2.2 FeNO

Exhaled nitric oxide (NO), derived from the inducible type of NO synthase (iNOS) in airway epithelial cells, reflects the degree of airway eosinophilic inflammation [4]. FeNO is another useful biomarker produced by NO synthase activity that identifies the T2-high phenotype. FeNO quantification offers several advantages over other methods, including being generally easy to perform, inexpensive, reproducible, and less invasive. The FeNO levels in patients with stable COPD range between the levels found in healthy subjects and those observed in patients with asthma. If an elevated FeNO level is observed in a patient with COPD, the possible coexistence of asthma should be considered. The American Thoracic Society/European Respiratory Society has published recommendations in which eosinophilic airway inflammation based on FeNO levels is categorized as low (<25 ppb), intermediate (between 25 and 50 ppb), or high (>50 ppb) [7].

2.3 IgE

IgE levels and skin test results are biomarkers of atopy and allergic asthma. Moreover, they are useful for identifying T2-high phenotypes and are the standard biomarkers in diagnosing allergic diseases. Total and specific IgE levels are often elevated in patients with allergic asthma, whereas skin testing is another useful tool to determine whether atopy exists, with a positive result indicating sensitization to environmental allergens. If patients with ACO have a documented history of allergic disease (early-onset asthma or atopic dermatitis) and elevated levels of serum IgE (total or allergen-specific), the presence of asthma like-features is suggested.

2.4 T2-Inflammation Pattern in Patients with ACO

Asthma is predominantly mediated by eosinophilic inflammation and T2-high inflammation, whereas COPD is predominantly mediated by neutrophilic and T2-low inflammation. Recent progress in clinical characteristics (phenotypes) and molecular mechanisms (endotypes) regarding response to biologics has improved our understanding of the phenotypes/endotypes in patients with severe asthma. When ACO in patients was classified according to the inflammation pattern as "T2-high" or "T2-low" endotype, the complex heterogeneity and different overlapping endotypes pose a challenge for clinicians. After allocating severe ACO to the T2-high endotype, it is necessary to further assess whether the T2-high allergic endotype or the T2-high eosinophilic endotype is predominant. The T2-high allergic endotype most frequently starts in childhood and is defined as at least one positive allergen-specific test result [8]. In contrast, the T2-high eosinophilic endotype (classified as >300 blood eosinophils/μL) is a late-onset disease with no atopy and normal serum IgE. It is more likely to affect males, have greater FeNO values and worse lung function, and affect individuals with a history of chronic rhinosinusitis and nasal polyposis [9]. A clinical cohort study on severe asthma in Japanese adults demonstrated that a substantial proportion of these cases overlap between two or more endotypes, namely, eosinophilic, periostin-high, and allergic [10]. Some patients with ACO exhibit T2-high inflammation and might respond to high doses of ICS and biologics targeting T2-high inflammation.

3 Advanced Treatment for Severe Uncontrolled ACO

3.1 Biologics

In patients with severe asthma, biologics targeting T2-high inflammation such as omalizumab, mepolizumab, reslizumab, benralizumab, dupilumab, and tezepelumab have been successfully developed and have changed treatment paradigms. Treatment with biologics for severe asthma was well-tolerated and resulted in a significant reduction in exacerbations and OCS intake and an improvement in lung function and HRQOL (Table 18.1). However, these biologics have yielded inconsistent results in COPD studies (Table 18.2). There is little experience with the use of biologics in ACO. Thus, it is important to differentiate asthma from COPD, particularly late-onset severe asthma. A recent retrospective study suggested that patients with ACO treated with biologics have worse outcomes than those with asthma alone in terms of exacerbations, asthma control, and OCS use. Taken together with these results, some patients with ACO predominantly have T2-high inflammation and might respond to biologics targeted for T2-high inflammation. Further investigation is necessary to clarify the role of biologics in patients with ACO.

3.1.1 Omalizumab

Omalizumab, a humanized monoclonal anti-IgE antibody of murine origin, is the first biologically approved antibody for clinical use in the management of severe asthma. Omalizumab is approved for patients with evidence of T2-high inflammation with a total serum IgE level between 30 and 1500 IU/mL, positive results on the skin-prick test, allergen-specific IgE to perennial aeroallergens, and symptoms not controlled by ICS. Omalizumab, at a dose between 150 and 375 mg, based on the patient's weight (40–120 kg) and total serum IgE concentration (30–1500 IU/mL), was administered subcutaneously every 2 or 4 weeks. A Cochrane review assessing 25 clinical trials revealed that omalizumab reduced exacerbation, hospitalization, and the required ICS dose [11]. Some studies have shown small improvements in lung function, although a significant effect on lung function has not been observed

Table 18.1 Efficacy of biologics in severe asthma with T2-high phenotype

Efficacy	Omalizumab	Mepolizumab	Reslizumab	Benralizumab	Dupilumab
Frequency of asthma exacerbation	++	++	++	++	++
OCS-sparing effect	±	++	NE	++	++
Lung function	±	+	+	+	++
QOL and symptom control	+	+	+	+	+

Abbreviations: *OCS* Oral corticosteroid, *QOL* Quality of life, ++ High utility, + Moderate utility, ± No clear evidence, *NE* Not evaluated

Table 18.2 Efficacy of biologics in COPD with T2-high phenotype

Efficacy	Omalizumab	Mepolizumab	Reslizumab	Benralizumab	Dupilumab
Frequency of asthma exacerbation	NE	±	NE	±	NE
OCS-sparing effect	NE	NE	NE	NE	NE
Lung function	NE	±	NE	±	NE
QOL and symptom control	NE	±	NE	±	NE

Abbreviations: *COPD* Chronic pulmonary obstructive disease, *OCS* Oral corticosteroid, *QOL* Quality of life, ++ High utility, + Moderate utility, ± Not clear evidence, *NE* Not evaluated

in other studies. However, the OCS-sparing effect of omalizumab in patients with severe asthma requiring daily OCS is still unclear.

Serum IgE levels do not accurately predict the therapeutic response to omalizumab, although the dose of omalizumab is based on body weight and serum levels of IgE. The PROSPERO (Prospective Observational Study to Evaluate Predictors of Clinical Effectiveness in Response to Omalizumab) trial is an open-label, multicenter, single-arm, prospective real-world 48-week observational study that examined patients with asthma who had comorbid COPD or smoking history [12]. Post hoc analysis of PROSPERO suggested that the reduction in asthma exacerbations was greater in the subgroup of patients with T2-high inflammation biomarkers, including FeNO, blood eosinophil counts, and serum periostin, than in the T2-low inflammation subgroups. In contrast, real-world studies of omalizumab suggested that the biomarker status (T2-high or T2-low) had a minimal influence on omalizumab treatment outcomes. Patients treated with omalizumab should be reassessed 16 weeks after treatment initiation to evaluate their response and treatment and decide whether the treatment should be continued.

Data from the Australian Xolair Registry evaluated the response to omalizumab in patients with ACO compared with those with asthma alone [13]. This study suggests that omalizumab improves asthma control and HRQOL in patients with severe allergic asthma and ACO. Similar improvements were observed in individuals with ACO and those with severe asthma alone. Subgroup analysis of PROSPERO showed that similar improvements were reported in the exacerbation rate and symptom control in individuals with ACO or asthma alone [14].

3.1.2 Mepolizumab

Mepolizumab is a high-affinity humanized monoclonal antibody of the IgG1/κ subtype of murine origin that inhibits the binding of IL-5 to the IL-5 receptor (IL-5Rα) expressed on eosinophils, thereby considerably reducing eosinophil production and survival. Mepolizumab 100 mg is administered subcutaneously every 4 weeks to patients with severe asthma who have an eosinophilic phenotype (>150 blood eosinophils/μL at baseline or 300 cells/μL at some point during the previous year).

In several randomized, placebo-controlled, double-blind phase III trials involving patients with severe eosinophilic asthma, mepolizumab treatment significantly reduced the eosinophil count, exacerbations, and OCS intake, and improved QOL and lung function irrespective of the presence or absence of allergy. A secondary analysis of the DREAM (Dose Ranging Efficacy And safety with Mepolizumab) and MENSA (Mepolizumab as Adjunctive Therapy in Patients with Severe Asthma) trials demonstrated a close relationship between the baseline blood eosinophil count and the clinical efficacy of mepolizumab in patients with severe eosinophilic asthma and a history of exacerbations [15]. Thus, higher blood eosinophil counts can predict an enhanced response to mepolizumab. However, an elevated FeNO level does not predict response to mepolizumab, and FeNO is not reliably reduced with mepolizumab.

In contrast, two previous randomized, placebo-controlled, phase III trials METREX (Mepolizumab Versus Placebo as Add-On Treatment for Frequently Exacerbating COPD Patients) and METREO (Mepolizumab Versus Placebo as Add-On Treatment for Frequently Exacerbating COPD Patients Characterised by Eosinophil Level) compared mepolizumab with placebo in patients with COPD who had a history of moderate or severe exacerbations despite triple therapy demonstrated conflicting results [16]. At randomization in METREX, patients were stratified based on blood eosinophil counts as having either an eosinophilic phenotype (≥150 blood eosinophils/μL at screening or ≥300 blood eosinophils/μL at any point in the previous year) or a non-eosinophilic phenotype (<150 blood eosinophils/μL at screening and no evidence of ≥300 blood eosinophils/μL in the previous year). Only one trial (METREX) reached the primary endpoint of a significant reduction in exacerbations in patients with an eosinophilic phenotype. There were no improvements in lung function and the St. George's Respiratory Questionnaire or COPD Assessment Test scores in either trial. Many of these patients with eosinophilic phenotype may be classified as having ACO, depending on the definition used. A phase III trial, MATINEE (Mepolizumab as Add-on Treatment IN Participants With COPD Characterized by Frequent Exacerbations and Eosinophil Level) designed to confirm the benefits of mepolizumab treatment on moderate or severe exacerbations in COPD with T2-high inflammation is ongoing (Clinical Trials.gov Identifier: NCT04133909).

In a single-center retrospective observational study, the efficacy of mepolizumab in older patients with severe asthma alone and in those with ACO was evaluated. Importantly, mepolizumab showed favorable efficacy in reducing blood eosinophil levels, OCS intake, and exacerbation rate in older patients with asthma and ACO [17].

3.1.3 Reslizumab

Reslizumab, an IgG4κ humanized, monoclonal antibody of rat origin, is administered as an intravenous infusion at a recommended weight-based dose of 3 mg/kg once every 4 weeks. Weight-based dosing of intravenous reslizumab significantly reduced the rate of exacerbations and improved lung function and HRQOL in patients with inadequately controlled asthma with blood eosinophil counts of ≥400 cells/μL and a history of asthma exacerbations [18]. Higher blood eosinophil counts (≥400 cells/μL) predicted responses such as improved lung function and asthma control in patients treated with reslizumab. Other studies have also shown that patients with exacerbation-prone late-onset asthma with elevated blood eosinophil levels (≥400 cells/μL) and inadequately controlled symptoms responded particularly well to reslizumab. No study has evaluated the OCS-sparing effects of reslizumab. Furthermore, there are no ongoing studies on the use of reslizumab in COPD and ACO.

3.1.4 Benralizumab

Benralizumab is a humanized, fucosylated monoclonal antibody of murine origin that targets the IL-5 receptor. Unlike other monoclonal antibodies such as mepolizumab and reslizumab, benralizumab binds directly to eosinophils and induces rapid apoptosis in vitro in the presence of natural killer cells via enhanced antibody-dependent cell-mediated cytotoxicity. Thus, benralizumab results in the direct, rapid, and near-complete depletion of blood eosinophils in patients with severe eosinophilic asthma after the first administration. Furthermore, benralizumab also significantly reduces eosinophil counts in airway mucosa/submucosa and sputum. Benralizumab 30 mg is injected subcutaneously every 4 weeks for the first three doses, followed by 30 mg every 8 weeks thereafter in patients with severe asthma who have an eosinophilic phenotype (>300 or >150 blood eosinophils/μL in those receiving treatment with OCS). In several randomized, placebo-controlled, phase III trials, benralizumab significantly decreased the exacerbation rate and OCS intake and improved lung function and HRQOL in patients with severe eosinophilic asthma. Higher baseline blood eosinophil counts and a history of exacerbation can predict an enhanced response to benralizumab. The analysis using pooled data from the SIROCCO (Efficacy and Safety of Benralizumab for Patients with Severe Asthma Uncontrolled with High-Dosage Inhaled Corticosteroids and Long-Acting β(2)-Agonists) and CALIMA (Benralizumab, an Anti-interleukin-5 Receptor α Monoclonal Antibody, as an Add-On Treatment for Patients with Severe, Uncontrolled, Eosinophilic Asthma) for severe asthma demonstrated that baseline OCS use, history of nasal polyps, low lung function, history of frequent exacerbations, and late onset of disease were associated with enhanced response to benralizumab, regardless of baseline blood eosinophil count [19].

In contrast, benralizumab did not improve the rates of exacerbations in two phase III trials, GALATHEA (Benralizumab Efficacy in Moderate-to-Very Severe Chronic Obstructive Pulmonary Disease with Exacerbation History) and TERRANOVA (Efficacy and Safety of Benralizumab in Moderate-to-Very Severe Chronic Obstructive Pulmonary Disease with Exacerbation History), that included patients with moderate-to-severe COPD with eosinophilic phenotypes and a history of exacerbations [20]. Post hoc analysis using data from the original study and pooled results from the GALATHEA and TERRANOVA trials suggested that patients with elevated baseline blood eosinophil counts (≥220 blood eosinophils/μL) with three or more exacerbations in the previous year and who were receiving triple therapy were identified as likely to benefit from benralizumab compared to placebo [21]. A significant reduction in the exacerbation ratio of 0.70 (95% confidence interval, 0.56–0.88) compared to placebo was observed. A phase III RESOLUTE (Efficacy and Safety of Benralizumab in Moderate to Very Severe Chronic Obstructive Pulmonary Disease [COPD] With a History of Frequent Exacerbations) study designed to assess the efficacy and safety of benralizumab in patients with moderate to severe COPD with high exacerbations and a history of frequent exacerbations and elevated blood eosinophil count (≥300/μL) is currently ongoing (Clinical Trials.gov Identifier: NCT04053634).

In a retrospective observational study, the efficacy of switching from mepolizumab to benralizumab in older patients with severe asthma and ACO was evaluated. Although this study was based on a small sample of participants, switching mepolizumab to benralizumab have resulted in clinically relevant asthma control benefits in older patients with severe asthma and ACO [22].

3.1.5 Dupilumab

Dupilumab, a fully human monoclonal IgG4 antibody directed against the α subunit of the IL-4 receptor (IL-4Rα), which acts as a dual inhibitor of both IL-4- and IL-13-mediated signaling pathways, was approved for the treatment of T2 asthma. Dupilumab 600 mg is injected subcutaneously, followed by 300 mg administered subcutaneously every 2 weeks thereafter. Several randomized, placebo-controlled, phase III trials have also demonstrated improvements in asthma exacerbation rates, forced expiratory volume in 1 second, OCS intake, and HRQOL in patients with uncontrolled severe asthma. Furthermore, a reduction in the frequency of exacerbations and improvement in lung function was observed in patients with evidence of T2-high biomarkers at baseline (>150 blood eosinophils/μL at baseline or FeNO >25 ppb). Unlike biologics targeting IL-5, baseline FeNO was a predictor of clinical response to dupilumab. A post hoc analysis of the LIBERTY ASTHMA QUEST (Evaluation of Dupilumab in Patients with Persistent Asthma) study demonstrated that the beneficial effects of dupilumab can be detected in both allergic and non-allergic asthma [23].

A phase III randomized, placebo-controlled study BOREAS (Pivotal Study to Assess the Efficacy, Safety, and Tolerability of Dupilumab in Patients with Moderate-to-Severe COPD with Type 2 Inflammation) to assess the efficacy, safety, and tolerability of dupilumab in patients with moderate-to-severe COPD with T2-high inflammation is ongoing (Clinical Trials.gov Identifier: NCT03930732). There are no ongoing studies on the use of dupilumab in ACO.

3.1.6 Tezepelumab

Alarmins are cytokines that play an important role in the propagation of T2-high and T2-low airway inflammation. Tezepelumab is an anti-thymic stromal lymphopoietin (TSLP) fully human IgG2λ monoclonal antibody that prevents TSLP from binding to its receptor complex. Tezepelumab has been developed to treat asthma, COPD, chronic rhinosinusitis with nasal polyps (CRSwNP), chronic spontaneous urticaria, and eosinophilic esophagitis. A phase IIb trial demonstrated that tezepelumab decreased the annual rates of asthma exacerbation and improved lung function independent of the blood eosinophil count [24]. Tezepelumab lowered T2-high biomarkers such as peripheral blood eosinophil counts, FeNO, and serum IgE. In this study, the annual rate of exacerbations was decreased in patients with low FeNO and blood eosinophil counts, suggesting the involvement of T2-low mediated airway inflammation. A phase III, randomized, placebo-controlled trial demonstrated that tezepelumab significantly reduced exacerbations compared to placebo in patients with severe uncontrolled asthma by 56%, including in those with low blood eosinophil counts (<300 cells/μL at baseline) by 41%, and improved lung function, asthma control, and HRQOL [25].

3.2 *Macrolides*

Various trials to determine whether macrolides can reduce the annual rate of exacerbation have been conducted in patients with severe asthma, reporting varying results. The AMAZES study is a randomized, double-blind, placebo-controlled trial that evaluated the effect of azithromycin on asthma exacerbations and HRQOL in patients with persistent uncontrolled asthma despite the use of ICS/long-acting beta-agonists (LABA) [26]. Compared to placebo, azithromycin 500 mg (both administered three times weekly for 48 weeks) reduced asthma exacerbations and improved HRQOL. Furthermore, azithromycin demonstrated similar improvements in both eosinophilic and non-eosinophilic asthma. In another randomized, placebo-controlled phase III trial in patients with severe asthma, add-on treatment with low-dose azithromycin for 26 weeks did not decrease the frequency of severe exacerbations of asthma or lower respiratory tract infections requiring antibiotics [27]. However, subgroup analysis of patients with non-eosinophilic severe asthma (blood eosinophils ≤200/μL) revealed that azithromycin reduced the frequency of exacerbations.

In contrast, compared with usual treatment only, the addition of low-dose chronic azithromycin therapy has been shown to reduce exacerbations in patients with COPD who are prone to exacerbations and are not actively smoking [28, 29]. Macrolides reduce the risk of acute exacerbations in patients with COPD owing to their antiviral action and ability to suppress the activation of neutrophils. Azithromycin use has been associated with an increased incidence of bacterial resistance, prolonged QT intervals on electrocardiograms, and hearing impairment. No study has prospectively evaluated the effect of macrolides in patients with ACO, and little data exists on the use of macrolides in ACO. These results suggest that macrolides may be effective for treating ACO, which continues to exacerbate in patients with T2-low inflammation despite triple therapy.

3.3 Bronchial Thermoplasty

Bronchial thermoplasty (BT) is a non-pharmacological, bronchoscopic, catheter-based treatment approved for patients with severe asthma at specialized facilities. During BT, radiofrequency energy is applied to heat the airway walls in a controlled manner, leading to a reduction in airway smooth muscle mass and bronchial nerve endings. Previous randomized clinical trials have demonstrated that BT reduces severe exacerbations and improves HRQOL, with the effects lasting for 5 years [30]. Furthermore, a recent international multicenter follow-up study suggested that the efficacy of BT is sustained for 10 years or more with an acceptable safety profile [31]. BT may be effective in patients with severe asthma with marked airway smooth muscle hypertrophy that contributes to the fixed narrowing of the airways; however, it is difficult to identify such patients in real-world clinical settings. BT was found to be effective and safe for treating patients with severe asthma and smoking history [32]. Thus, highly selected patients with severe ACO may benefit from BT. However, the use of biologics and macrolide antibiotics is prioritized, as there are currently no known biomarkers for BT effectiveness.

4 Management of Patients with ACO

4.1 Treatment Algorism for Patients with Severe Uncontrolled ACO

In practice, ACO should be treated more intensively because it tends to be more severe than asthma or COPD alone. The current recommendation for treating patients with ACO refers to asthma and COPD guidelines according to patients' characteristics because most clinical studies on asthma and COPD have excluded patients with ACO. Patients with ACO should initially start ICS therapy with LABA and/or long-acting muscarinic agents (LAMA). The most important aspect of ACO management is avoiding LABA as monotherapy without ICS. Once or twice-daily single triple inhaler therapy (ICS/LABA/LAMA) has been effective in improving lung function in patients with asthma [33]. Furthermore, triple therapy has been shown to reduce exacerbation rates and improve lung function and HRQOL compared with dual therapy in patients with COPD [33]. These results suggest that if a patient with ACO remains symptomatic or has controllable but frequent exacerbations, triple therapy should be considered as an additional therapy.

If ACO remains uncontrolled despite currently available standard treatment, including triple therapy, advanced therapies may be considered (Fig. 18.1). Management of severe ACO in older patients is difficult because they often have multiple comorbid conditions (such as chronic rhinosinusitis with nasal polyps (CRSwNP), atopic dermatitis, osteoporosis, cardiovascular disease, gastroesophageal reflux disease, and depression), poor adherence to therapy, and decreased responsiveness to medications. The inhalation technique, drug adherence, comorbidities, and aggravating factors should be evaluated before treatment with biologics.

As indications for biologics can be identified based on T2-high phenotypes, patients with severe, uncontrolled ACO should be biologically divided into T2-high or T2-low endotypes using biomarkers. This approach is similar to emerging disease management strategies such as treatable traits, precision medicine, and personalized medicine. ACO in patients with predominant T2-high inflammation may have applications for biologics targeted at T2-high inflammation.

With no approved targeted therapy for T2-low endotypes, there is presently an unmet need to treat severe asthma, COPD, and ACO. Low-dose chronic macrolide therapy may be considered for patients with ACO and T2-low endotypes, particularly for those who continue to experience frequent exacerbations despite triple therapy. Moreover, it is important to identify patients who are potential responders

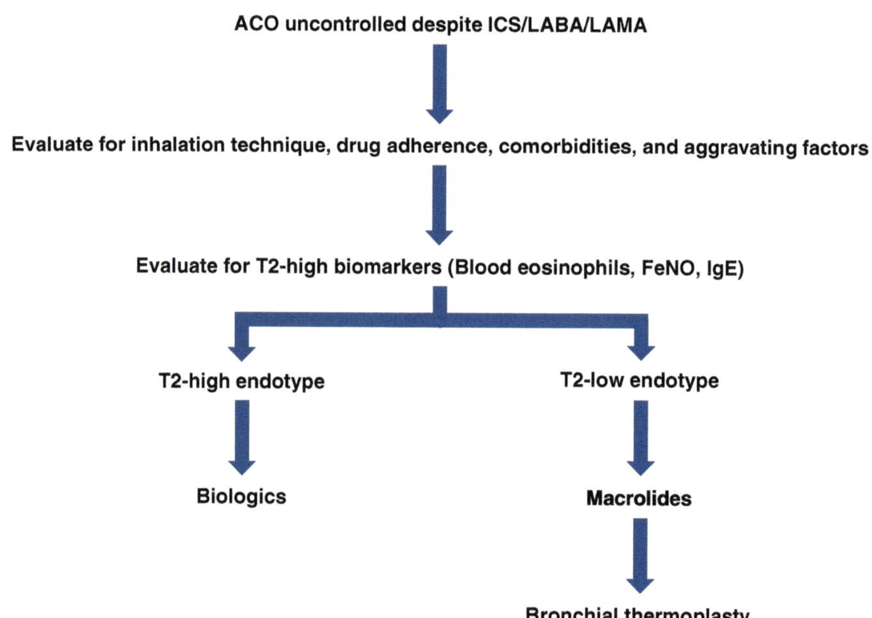

Fig. 18.1 Treatment algorithm for patients with ACO. *ACO* Asthma and chronic pulmonary obstructive disease overlap, *ICS* Inhaled corticosteroids, *LABA* Long-acting beta-agonists, *LAMA* Long-acting muscarinic agents, *FeNO* Fractional exhaled nitric oxide, *IgE* Immunoglobulin E

to BT. As tezepelumab was shown to reduce exacerbation in patients with severe uncontrolled asthma, irrespective of blood eosinophil counts at baseline, tezepelumab might provide additional treatment options for T2-low endotypes in the future.

4.2 Selection of Biologics in Patients with ACO

Severe, uncontrolled ACO with T2-high endotype is a heterogeneous and complex syndrome encompassing several clinical phenotypes/endotypes. Unfortunately, there are no data from head-to-head randomized control trials comparing the efficacy and safety of biologics. The selection of the most suitable biologics for each patient should be multifaceted, considering clinical characteristics (phenotypes) and molecular mechanisms (endotypes). Before biological therapy is initiated, phenotypes, such as the frequency of exacerbations, OCS intake, lung function, asthma control, and HRQOL, should be recorded. Eligibility criteria, route of administration, duration of therapy, approval of self-administration, endotype, T2-high biomarkers, comorbidities, insurance coverage, cost, and patient choice should be integrated with clinical phenotyping to select the appropriate initial biological treatment.

4.2.1 Eligibility Criteria

Biomarkers for T2-high populations, such as blood eosinophils, FeNO, and serum IgE, can be used to identify patients who may benefit from biologics. Table 18.3 shows the commonly used criteria for the use of biologics for severe asthma. The use of omalizumab is limited to patients with an allergy to a perennial allergen whose weight and serum IgE levels are within the manufacturer's recommended limits. As shown in Table 18.3, predictive biomarkers could also help clinicians determine the biological treatment leading to the most beneficial response. At present, omalizumab has no useful biomarker for predicting or monitoring responses. In the cases of mepolizumab and benralizumab, blood eosinophil counts greater than 150 cells/μL at baseline or 300 cells/μL at some point during the previous year appeared to identify patients most likely to respond. In clinical studies, reslizumab has been evaluated in patients with blood eosinophil counts >300 cells/μL. Baseline FeNO is a predictor of clinical response to dupilumab as IL-4 or IL-13 induces iNOS through a STAT-6 mediated pathway [4]; hence, dupilumab should be considered for patients with FeNO levels ≥25 ppb and blood eosinophil counts ≥150 cells/μL [34]. Thus, blood eosinophil counts and FeNO levels are complementary biomarkers for predicting therapeutic responses to biologics.

Table 18.3 Summary of biologics approved for severe asthma with T2-high phenotype

Biologics	Omalizumab	Mepolizumab	Reslizumab	Benralizumab	Dupilumab
Target	IgE	IL-5	IL-5	IL-5 receptor α	IL-4 receptor α
Commonly used criteria	30 ≤ IgE ≤ 1500 IU/mL, positive results on allergen test	Blood eosinophil counts ≥300 cells/μL	Blood eosinophil counts ≥400 cells/μL	Blood eosinophil counts ≥300 cells/μL	Blood eosinophil counts ≥300 cells/mL FeNO ≥25 ppb
Predictive biomarkers for response to biologics					
Blood eosinophil counts	++	++	++	++	++
FeNO	±	–	–	–	++
IgE	±	–	–	–	±
Endotype	Allergic	Eosinophilic	Eosinophilic	Eosinophilic	Allergic, eosinophilic
Indication of comorbidities	Chronic idiopathic urticaria	Eosinophilic granulomatosis with polyangiitis			Atopic dermatitis, Chronic rhinosinusitis with nasal polyps
Route of administration, duration of therapy	150–375 mg (based on patient weight and total serum IgE) SC, every 2 or 4 weeks	100 mg SC, every 4 weeks	weight-based dose of 3 mg/kg IV, every 4 weeks	30 mg SC every 4 weeks for three doses followed by 30 mg SC every 8 weeks thereafter.	600 mg SC starting dose followed by 300 mg SC every 2 weeks thereafter.
Self-administration	Approved	Approved	Not approved	Not approved	Approved

Abbreviations: *IL* Interleukin, *IgE* Immunoglobulin E, *FeNO* Fractional exhaled nitric oxide, *IV* Intravenous, *SC* Subcutaneous, ++ High utility, + Moderate utility, ± No clear evidence, – No utility

4.2.2 Clinical Characteristics (Phenotypes)

Exacerbation-Prone

A recent Cochrane review of 13 studies on 6000 participants indicated that three anti-IL-5 (rα)-targeted biologics, namely mepolizumab, benralizumab, and reslizumab, reduced the rates of clinically significant asthma exacerbations by approximately 50% in patients with severe eosinophilic asthma [35]. Additionally, dupilumab and omalizumab reduced asthma exacerbations by approximately 50% and 25%, respectively [11].

OCS-Sparing Effect

Mepolizumab, benralizumab, and dupilumab have been studied specifically in patients who are OCS-dependent and have been found to reduce the burden of OCS usage. When choosing a biologic for patients who are attempting to wean off chronic OCSs and have evidence of eosinophilia (≥150–300 cells/μL), mepolizumab, benralizumab, or dupilumab would be appropriate [36].

Fixed Airway Obstruction

Many, but not all, studies on biologics have shown significant improvement in lung function in patients with reversible airflow obstruction. The effect of dupilumab on lung function and symptoms may be greater than that of anti-IL-5 or IgE alone, although there is less convincing evidence regarding the effect of omalizumab on lung function.

4.2.3 Molecular Mechanisms (Endotypes)

After allocating severe ACO to the T2-high endotype, it is necessary to further assess whether the T2-high allergic endotype or the T2-high eosinophilic endotype is predominant. In allergic endotypes, omalizumab and dupilumab are the treatments of choice, although biologics targeting IL-5 might be effective in some of these patients. In eosinophilic endotypes, anti-IL-5 treatment and dupilumab are reasonable therapeutic approaches.

4.2.4 Comorbidities

Clinicians should consider comorbidities when selecting optimal biologics. CRSwNP and atopic dermatitis are chronic diseases characterized by T2-high inflammation and frequently co-exist with asthma. CRSwNP is frequently associated with the T2-high allergic endotype, whereas atopic dermatitis is primarily associated with the T2-high allergic endotype. As dupilumab has been approved to treat CRSwNP and atopic dermatitis, it is effective in treating these relevant asthma comorbidities. The T2-high allergic endotype of severe, uncontrolled asthma with concomitant refractory chronic idiopathic urticaria should be treated with omalizumab because omalizumab is approved for use in patients with chronic idiopathic urticaria. Mepolizumab is approved to treat eosinophilic granulomatosis with polyangiitis and uncontrolled asthma at a higher dose (300 mg subcutaneously every 4 weeks). If blood eosinophil counts are elevated above 1000/μL, along with other pertinent clinical features, clinicians should consider the diagnosis of eosinophilic granulomatosis with polyangiitis.

4.2.5 Route of Administration, Duration of Therapy, and Self-Administration

The route of administration and duration of therapy should be considered when selecting biologics. Mepolizumab should be administered subcutaneously every 4 weeks; reslizumab, intravenously at a weight-adjusted dose every 4 weeks; and benralizumab, subcutaneously every 4 weeks for the first three doses, followed by every 8 weeks thereafter. These differences might be important when selecting biologics that target IL-5 for individual patients. Furthermore, omalizumab, mepolizumab, and dupilumab are biologics that can be self-administered by patients at home after proper training. Patients with a busy life might prefer the convenience of receiving maintenance therapy with benralizumab every 8 weeks or self-administration of omalizumab, mepolizumab, and dupilumab at home every 2–4 weeks.

5 Conclusion

Although biologics have been demonstrated to be effective in T2-high severe patients with asthma, there is little evidence regarding their use in ACO. Newly developed biologics targeted at T2-high inflammation might be effective, probably in a highly selected group of people who predominantly have asthma components with T2-high inflammation.

This approach is similar to emerging disease management strategies, such as treatable traits, precision medicine, and personalized medicine. Further investigations are needed to elucidate the role of biologics in the near future, such as anti-TSLP, to manage ACO for both T2-high and T2-low endotypes in clinical practice. In particular, it is unclear whether there is a threshold blood eosinophil level and FeNO values above which these drugs may be effective.

References

1. GBD 2015 Chronic Respiratory Disease Collaborators. Global, regional, and national deaths, prevalence, disability-adjusted life years, and years lived with disability for chronic obstructive pulmonary disease and asthma, 1990–2015: a systematic analysis for the Global Burden of Disease Study 2015. Lancet Respir Med. 2017;5(9):691–706.
2. Mekov E, Nuñez A, Sin DD, Ichinose M, Rhee CK, Maselli DJ, et al. Update on asthma-COPD overlap (ACO): a narrative review. Int J Chron Obstruct Pulmon Dis. 2021;16:1783–99.
3. Bateman ED, Reddel HK, van Zyl-Smit RN, Agusti A. The asthma-COPD overlap syndrome: towards a revised taxonomy of chronic airways diseases? Lancet Respir Med. 2015;3:719–28.
4. Yanagisawa S, Ichinose M. Definition and diagnosis of asthma-COPD overlap (ACO). Allergol Int. 2018;67:172–8.
5. Kondo M, Tamaoki J. Therapeutic approaches of asthma and COPD overlap. Allergol Int. 2018;67:187–90.
6. Toledo-Pons N, van Boven JFM, Román-Rodríguez M, Pérez N, Valera Felices JL, Soriano JB, et al. ACO: time to move from the description of different phenotypes to the treatable traits. PLoS One. 2019;14:e0210915.
7. American Thoracic Society; European Respiratory Society. ATS/ERS recommendations for standardized procedures for the online and offline measurement of exhaled lower respiratory nitric oxide and nasal nitric oxide, 2005. Am J Respir Crit Care Med. 2005;171:912–30.
8. Brusselle GG, Koppelman GH. Biologic therapies for severe asthma. N Engl J Med. 2022;386:157–71.
9. Zervas E, Samitas K, Papaioannou AI, Bakakos P, Loukides S, Gaga M. An algorithmic approach to treat severe uncontrolled asthma. ERJ Open Res. 2018;4:00125–2017.
10. Matsusaka M, Fukunaga K, Kabata H, Izuhara K, Asano K, Betsuyaku T. Subphenotypes of type 2 severe asthma in adults. J Allergy Clin Immunol Pract. 2018;6:274–6.e2.
11. Normansell R, Walker S, Milan SJ, Walters EH, Nair P. Omalizumab for asthma in adults and children. Cochrane Database Syst Rev. 2014:CD003559. https://doi.org/10.1002/14651858.CD003559.pub4.
12. Casale TB, Luskin AT, Busse W, Zeiger RS, Trzaskoma B, Yang M, et al. Omalizumab effectiveness by biomarker status in patients with asthma: evidence from PROSPERO, a prospective real-world study. J Allergy Clin Immunol Pract. 2019;7:156–64.e1.
13. Maltby S, Gibson PG, Powell H, McDonald VM. Omalizumab treatment response in a population with severe allergic asthma and overlapping COPD. Chest. 2017;151:78–89.
14. Hanania NA, Chipps BE, Griffin NM, Yoo B, Iqbal A, Casale TB. Omalizumab effectiveness in asthma-COPD overlap: Post hoc analysis of PROSPERO. J Allergy Clin Immunol. 2019;143:1629–33.e2.
15. Ortega HG, Yancey SW, Mayer B, Gunsoy NB, Keene ON, Bleecker ER, et al. Severe eosinophilic asthma treated with mepolizumab stratified by baseline eosinophil thresholds: a secondary analysis of the DREAM and MENSA studies. Lancet Respir Med. 2016;4:549–56.
16. Pavord ID, Chanez P, Criner GJ, Kerstjens HAM, Korn S, Lugogo N, et al. Mepolizumab for eosinophilic chronic obstructive pulmonary disease. N Engl J Med. 2017;377:1613–29.
17. Isoyama S, Ishikawa N, Hamai K, Matsumura M, Kobayashi H, Nomura A, et al. Efficacy of mepolizumab in elderly patients with severe asthma and overlapping COPD in real-world settings: a retrospective observational study. Respir Investig. 2021;59:478–86.
18. Castro M, Zangrilli J, Wechsler ME, Bateman ED, Brusselle GG, Bardin P, et al. Reslizumab for inadequately controlled asthma with elevated blood eosinophil counts: results from two multicentre, parallel, double-blind, randomised, placebo-controlled, phase 3 trials. Lancet Respir Med. 2015;3:355–66.
19. Bleecker ER, Wechsler ME, FitzGerald JM, Menzies-Gow A, Wu Y, Hirsch I, et al. Baseline patient factors impact on the clinical efficacy of benralizumab for severe asthma. Eur Respir J. 2018;52:1800936.

20. Criner GJ, Celli BR, Brightling CE, Agusti A, Papi A, Singh D, et al. Benralizumab for the prevention of COPD exacerbations. N Engl J Med. 2019;381:1023–34.
21. Criner GJ, Celli BR, Singh D, Agusti A, Papi A, Jison M, et al. Predicting response to benralizumab in chronic obstructive pulmonary disease: analyses of GALATHEA and TERRANOVA studies. Lancet Respir Med. 2020;8:158–70.
22. Isoyama S, Ishikawa N, Hamai K, Matsumura M, Kobayashi H, Nomura A, et al. Switching treatment from mepolizumab to benralizumab for elderly patients with severe eosinophilic asthma: a retrospective observational study. Intern Med. 2022;61:1663–71.
23. Corren J, Castro M, O'Riordan T, Hanania NA, Pavord ID, Quirce S, et al. Dupilumab efficacy in patients with uncontrolled, moderate-to-severe allergic asthma. J Allergy Clin Immunol Pract. 2020;8:516–26.
24. Corren J, Parnes JR, Wang L, Mo M, Roseti SL, Griffiths JM, et al. Tezepelumab in adults with uncontrolled asthma. N Engl J Med. 2017;377:936–46.
25. Menzies-Gow A, Corren J, Bourdin A, Chupp G, Israel E, Wechsler ME, et al. Tezepelumab in adults and adolescents with severe, uncontrolled asthma. N Engl J Med. 2021;384:1800–9.
26. Gibson PG, Yang IA, Upham JW, Reynolds PN, Hodge S, James AL, et al. Effect of azithromycin on asthma exacerbations and quality of life in adults with persistent uncontrolled asthma (AMAZES): a randomised, double-blind, placebo-controlled trial. Lancet. 2017;390:659–68.
27. Brusselle GG, Vanderstichele C, Jordens P, Deman R, Slabbynck H, Ringoet V, et al. Azithromycin for prevention of exacerbations in severe asthma (AZISAST): a multicentre randomised double-blind placebo-controlled trial. Thorax. 2013;68:322–9.
28. Uzun S, Djamin RS, Kluytmans JA, Mulder PGH, van't Veer NE, Ermens AA, et al. Azithromycin maintenance treatment in patients with frequent exacerbations of chronic obstructive pulmonary disease (COLUMBUS): a randomised, double-blind, placebo-controlled trial. Lancet Respir Med. 2014;2:361–8.
29. Albert RK, Connett J, Bailey WC, Casaburi R, Cooper JAD Jr, Criner GJ, et al. Azithromycin for prevention of exacerbations of COPD. N Engl J Med. 2011;365:689–98.
30. Castro M, Rubin AS, Laviolette M, Fiterman J, De Andrade LM, Shah PL, et al. Effectiveness and safety of bronchial thermoplasty in the treatment of severe asthma: a multicenter, randomized, double-blind, sham-controlled clinical trial. Am J Respir Crit Care Med. 2010;181:116–24.
31. Chaudhuri R, Rubin A, Sumino K, Lapa E, Silva JR, Niven R, Siddiqui S, et al. Safety and effectiveness of bronchial thermoplasty after 10 years in patients with persistent asthma (BT10+): a follow-up of three randomised controlled trials. Lancet Respir Med. 2021;9:457–66.
32. Otoshi R, Baba T, Aiko N, Tabata E, Sadoyama S, Nakagawa H, et al. Effectiveness and safety of bronchial thermoplasty in the treatment of severe asthma with smoking history: a single-center experience. Int Arch Allergy Immunol. 2020;181:522–8.
33. Rogliani P, Ritondo BL, Calzetta L. Triple therapy in uncontrolled asthma: a network meta-analysis of phase III studies. Eur Respir J. 2021;58:2004233.
34. Chan R, RuiWen Kuo C, Lipworth B. Pragmatic clinical perspective on biologics for severe refractory type 2 asthma. J Allergy Clin Immunol Pract. 2020;8:3363–70.
35. Farne HA, Wilson A, Powell C, Bax L, Milan SJ. Anti-IL5 therapies for asthma. Cochrane Database Syst Rev. 2017;9:CD010834.
36. Krings JG, McGregor MC, Bacharier LB, Castro M. Biologics for severe asthma: treatment-specific effects are important in choosing a specific agent. J Allergy Clin Immunol Pract. 2019;7:1379–92.

GPSR Compliance

The European Union's (EU) General Product Safety Regulation (GPSR) is a set of rules that requires consumer products to be safe and our obligations to ensure this.

If you have any concerns about our products, you can contact us on ProductSafety@springernature.com

In case Publisher is established outside the EU, the EU authorized representative is:

Springer Nature Customer Service Center GmbH
Europaplatz 3
69115 Heidelberg, Germany

Batch number: 10370708

Printed by Printforce, the Netherlands